THE ARSENIC CENTURY

THE
Arsenic century

*How Victorian Britain was
Poisoned at Home, Work, and Play*

JAMES C. WHORTON

OXFORD
UNIVERSITY PRESS

OXFORD
UNIVERSITY PRESS

Great Clarendon Street, Oxford ox2 6DP

Oxford University Press is a department of the University of Oxford.
It furthers the University's objective of excellence in research, scholarship,
and education by publishing worldwide in

Oxford New York

Auckland Cape Town Dar es Salaam Hong Kong Karachi
Kuala Lumpur Madrid Melbourne Mexico City Nairobi
New Delhi Shanghai Taipei Toronto

With offices in

Argentina Austria Brazil Chile Czech Republic France Greece
Guatemala Hungary Italy Japan Poland Portugal Singapore
South Korea Switzerland Thailand Turkey Ukraine Vietnam

Oxford is a registered trade mark of Oxford University Press
in the UK and in certain other countries

Published in the United States
by Oxford University Press Inc., New York

British Library Cataloguing in Publication Data

Data available

Library of Congress Control Number: 2009939961

Typeset by SPI Publisher Services, Pondicherry, India
Printed in Great Britain
on acid-free paper by
Clays Ltd, St Ives plc

ISBN 978-0-19-957470-4

1 3 5 7 9 10 8 6 4 2

For Charlotte and Johnny

PREFACE

The bizarre and the grotesque have ever been the daily bread of journalists, and the reporters of Victorian Britain were no exceptions: 'Wife Driven Insane by Husband Tickling Her Feet' (1869), 'Death From Swallowing a Mouse' (1876). But even when judged by such a standard as 'Child Stolen by a Monkey' (1870), the story that greeted readers on page eight of *The Times* (of London) for 13 December 1848 was extraordinary, a tale so macabre as scarcely to be believed. 'For some months past,' it was revealed, hunters in certain rural districts had been coming upon entire coveys of partridges nestled together, sitting on the ground 'with their heads erect and their eyes open, presenting all the semblances of life.' Yet when approached the birds refused to take wing and provide sport, for, appearances notwithstanding, they were as stone dead as statues.[1]

A curious Hampshire outdoorsman who discovered a group of ten such birds sent two of them up to London to a physician he hoped might determine what was going on. Dr Fuller found the animals 'plump and in good condition' externally. But within, each one's oesophagus was severely inflamed and its intestines abnormally clean, as if they had been vigorously rinsed with water—or cleared by diarrhoea. Suspecting poison, he cut some meat from the breast and legs of one of the birds and offered it, along with the liver, to his cat, which ate it 'with avidity'. Within half an hour, the deceived creature was overcome by vomiting 'and vomited almost incessantly for nearly 12 hours, during the whole of which time she

evidently suffered excessive pain'. Happily, Puss recovered, and all
the wiser for her ordeal: even after an enforced fast of a full twenty-
four hours she remained resolute in her refusal to eat even 'an atom
more of the bird'.[2]

The cat's symptoms were suggestive of arsenic poisoning, so
the flesh of the second partridge was subjected to chemical testing,
along with grains of wheat taken from the crops of all ten of the
birds: considerable quantities of arsenic were found in every sample. As it turned out, all the dead partridges, and many dead pheasants as well, had been found in areas where farmers had recently
adopted the practice of soaking their wheat seed in an arsenic solution to protect against parasitic infestations. Clearly the animals
were being killed by eating the seeds scattered in planting; why they
expired so eerily, sitting up with eyes open instead of keeling over
as proper birds did, has yet to be explained.

The case of the poisoned partridges is but one illustration of
a social problem of no little significance in nineteenth-century
Britain: arsenic was everywhere. The poison was not confined to
country fields, its depredations were by no means limited to wildfowl. Arsenic lurked at every turn in the Victorian world, and chief
among its victims were human beings.

First, it reigned throughout the century as the poison of choice
for committing homicide, and for suicide was second only to
opium. Through much of the 1800s, upwards of a third of all
cases of criminal poisoning in Britain were due to arsenic, giving
the poison so lurid a reputation as an agent of mayhem as to set
it apart from all other methods of ending life. By 1849, a London
physician could complain that the odious crime of arsenical murder had become 'a *national disgrace*' (all italicized words appearing
in quotations throughout this book were given that emphasis in the
original), an offence that had increased so dramatically in recent

years as to make it 'the greatest blot upon the civilization of the nineteenth century'. The *greatest* blot overstates the case certainly, but a serious enough blot it was, and would remain so down to the end of the century. Despite the enactment of a law to make purchase of the deadly substance more difficult, and despite the development of more reliable tests for detecting it in the bodies of the slain, rendering arsenical murder a notably chancier proposition, victims continued to fall. As late as 1889, the editor of the nation's leading medical journal, reporting on a recent incident in which a man had killed his father-in-law with arsenic, worried that the 'very sordid' crime was of a type 'which has been unhappily too frequent of late'; the entire past year, he regretted, 'will be ever memorable for its many [arsenic] poisoning cases'.[3]

Yet arsenic also claimed countless subjects who were not the targets of acts of malice or self-loathing, people who succumbed, rather, to accident and even well-intentioned consumption of the poison. Seemingly every week, one paper or another published an account of a wife or servant mistaking the arsenic purchased to poison rats for baking powder or sugar and sickening if not killing the entire family with dumplings or pudding. At the opposite pole from rat poison, arsenic was also a component of an array of medicines, being frequently prescribed by physicians and almost as liberally purveyed by quacks. It was, moreover, a substance that could be adapted to a great variety of industrial applications. An inexpensive byproduct of the mining industry, arsenic was being produced in astonishing quantities by the mid-nineteenth century. When government inspectors visited a smelter in Cornwall in the 1870s, they were shocked into 'startling reflection' on being shown the contents of the warehouse, where ready for shipment was 'a quantity of white arsenic probably sufficient to destroy every living animal upon the face of the earth'. It was one month's output for this single factory. How so much of the material could be sent out into the world on a monthly basis without in fact exterminating humankind and the rest of creation was a question that perplexed even the experts: where, asked J.T. Arlidge, a medical authority of the 1890s, 'does all this most poisonous substance go?'[4]

Most arsenic went ultimately into the oceans, but where did all the rest go? A great deal of it was introduced purposely into many of the components of everyday life, with the result that people took it in with fruits and vegetables, swallowed it with wine, inhaled it from cigarettes, absorbed it from cosmetics, and imbibed it even from the pint glass. Arsenic was released from fireworks and exploded from dynamite (arsenical nitroglycerine! A double-barrelled weapon if ever one existed). The substance was present in a broad assortment of household items from candies and candles to cookware, concert tickets, and preserved partridge heads used to ornament ladies' headdresses (of this last, there was a ready supply from wheat-growing regions). Christmas tree ornaments and children's stuffed animals, no less, were often arsenical, and the money used to purchase all these products was itself sometimes contaminated. Not even professors of medicine were secure from the poison, the cadavers they and their pupils dissected in anatomical studies being oft-times preserved from decomposition with arsenic.

Further, unlike infectious disease, which concentrated its ravages on the poor, those whose lives played out in crowded squalour, arsenic was an equal-opportunity threat. With the poison present as commonly in the most fashionable home furnishings and apparel as in products made for the masses, barristers were no safer than barrow boys. Small wonder, then, that Victorians came to fear that their homes, venerated as tranquil havens from the hurly-burly of the outside world, had, through arsenic, been transformed from 'the abode of health and happiness [into] a sepulcher instead'.[5]

Arsenic compounds were regularly encountered in the workplace as well, not just by employees in smelters and chemical manufactories but by other labourers as diverse as shepherds and dressmakers (arsenic *in* old lace was the true danger). Thus whether at home amidst arsenical curtains and wallpapers, at work manufacturing arsenical curtains and papers, or at play swirling about the papered, curtained ballroom in arsenical gowns and gloves, no one was beyond the poison's reach. The very air people breathed carried arsenic, since it was released from the coal that heated homes and powered industry: house and factory chimneys 'unceasingly vomited forth arsenic by the ton', *The Times* reported, with the consequence that 'every shower of rain washes arsenic out of the air and distributes it over the land.... Traces of arsenic are all-pervading.' All-pervading was a refrain that resounded through the century. As late as the end of the 1870s, physicians were still complaining that 'scarcely a week passes without some fresh and startling revelation of the presence of that poison in the most unlikely substances'. Arsenic in odd places: such was the insidious threat against which the British public had to stay perpetually on guard throughout the Victorian age. As the scene was painted by one of London's most respected medical practitioners, 'grim death is made to surround the domestic hearth, and hover over the easy chair'.[6]

Today, as we squirm uneasily in our own chairs reading accounts of lead-painted toys and glycol-tainted toothpaste, of foetuses injured by mercury-contaminated seafood, babies killed by melamine-infused milk formula—and children sickened by contact with playground equipment built from arsenic-treated wood—the Victorian experience should resonate powerfully. The infiltration of arsenic into nineteenth-century domestic life was the template for pollution in the modern industrial world, the pilot episode, if you will, for a series of dramas of environmental poisoning that has no end in sight. When the administrator of America's Environmental Protection Agency warned in 1983 that 'life now takes place in a minefield of risks from hundreds, perhaps thousands, of substances', he might have added 'and the first mine to be laid was arsenic.'[7]

Nevertheless, the damage done by arsenic must not be overstated. While it was everywhere, it generally was present in amounts well below the lethal dose; indeed it commonly occurred in such small concentrations as to be innocuous to many people. 'It is perfectly true,' a critic of the inclusion of arsenic in textile products conceded, 'that the majority of mankind can bear exposure to arsenical fabrics without apparent injury.' But, he hastened to add, 'they also bear exposure to...all kinds of infectious diseases with impunity'. Individual susceptibilities to microbes, and to small doses of poison, vary widely: 'were this not the case,' our critic reminded, 'the world would soon be depopulated'. Nineteenth-century Britain was not depopulated by arsenic any more than it was by cholera or smallpox. Even so, while most people survived smallpox epidemics, enough died to make vaccination a desirable public health policy. Likewise, the fact that—as an American physician put it—'a portion of mankind is...arsenic-proof' did not obviate the necessity of keeping the poison away from those who were not so blessed.[8]

It is also true that most of those who were injured by environmental arsenic did not meet the wretched end of the murderer's prey or the suicide. Their discomforts came not in the form of torment that appeared suddenly and killed in a matter of hours. They suffered instead an infirmity that grew slowly, over weeks and months as a rule, but it was illness whose insults, while less intense than those of acute intoxication, were still incapacitating—and on occasion, mortal. If less violent than acute arsenic poisoning, chronic arsenicism was fearful enough, and it was an ailment experienced by thousands in nineteenth-century Britain. There was, one expert informed the public in the 1870s, 'a very large amount of sickness and mortality amongst all classes... attributable to chronic arsenical poisoning, and,' he continued ominously, 'it may eventually prove to be the true cause of many of the mysterious diseases of the present day, which so continually baffle medical skill'.[9]

There are, then, two tightly interwoven plot lines in the story of arsenic poisoning in the nineteenth century. One is the convoluted account of how arsenic became a nearly inescapable element of daily life, the toll it exacted as environmental hazard, and the ways by which the threat came to be recognized and either removed or regulated. The other is the grisly tale of its repeated employment as a tool of murder and self-annihilation, and attempts at suppression on that front. Together they present a tangled web of human imperfection, commercial avarice, medical uncertainty, and legislative dithering that conspired to allow arsenic to spread suffering through every level of nineteenth-century British society.

I have chosen to concentrate on *nineteenth-century* Britain because in the broad sweep of arsenic's history, the 1800s witnessed the most widespread occurrence of arsenic poisoning, both intentional and otherwise. The substance had been employed purposely for centuries before, primarily in connection with European aristocracy accelerating inheritances or eliminating political competition. During the nineteenth century, in ways to be discussed, the criminal employment of arsenic was democratized, so much so that the prevailing view of arsenical murder became that expressed by the University of London's professor of forensic medicine, who assured his students in the 1830s that the crime was largely the work of 'the lower orders of society'.[10] At that same time, the lower orders—

indeed, all orders—also became exposed to arsenic in ways that
assured accidental poisoning, ways that have become less common
since 1900. The 1800s, in sum, were the arsenic century. And even
though Victoria did not ascend to the throne until 1837, more than
a third of the way into the century, it is fair to call this a study of the
poisoning of Victorian Britain because it was not until the decade
of her coronation that the magnitude of the arsenic threat began
to be clearly perceived.

I have chosen to focus on nineteenth-century *Britain* because
the problems associated with arsenic were both more pronounced
there and more complex. The same arsenical hazards existed
on the Continent, but there strong traditions of state control
ensured that arsenic would be more tightly regulated and thus
less damaging. The prohibitory approach favoured in Europe
did not play well in *laissez-faire* Britain, where business was pretty
much given free rein, to the unending chagrin of advocates of
public health. 'How long,' a physician wailed in the 1850s, 'will
money-hunters be allowed, in the pursuit of their game, to viti-
ate the necessaries of life with the deadliest poisons?'[11] The same
lamentations could be heard in America, where could be found
all the same arsenic problems that afflicted the mother country
and where regulation was, if anything, more lax. But the British,
who overall were the pioneers of modern public health, recognized and addressed the arsenic threat a good bit earlier than
Americans, and largely shaped the American response. Thus if
it is permissible to speak of a golden age of arsenic, a time when
poisoning flourished as in no other, that age was the 1800s and
Great Britain was at its centre, the nation providing the most
compelling narrative of the impact of the poison on society. The
decision to concentrate on the British experience with arsenic
was also influenced, in no small degree I have to confess, by

the fact that for an aficionado of traditional ale, there are no more congenial locations in the world for conducting historical research than London and Edinburgh.

Even at its peak of popularity, arsenic was still just one of a number of poisons that claimed the lives and health of Britons. Murderers and suicides were nothing if not resourceful, and they pursued their ends with a host of noxious materials. They could choose from corrosive sublimate (a mercury compound as destructive as its name implies), antimony, prussic acid (cyanide), strychnine, opium, the reputed aphrodisiac Spanish fly (a caustic preparation of powdered beetles), and carbolic acid, to cite just a few. Nevertheless, no single substance seriously challenged arsenic in frequency of use, its reputation for unfailing deadliness making it the people's choice.[12]

Similarly, chronic intoxication could result from a plethora of environmental poisons besides arsenic. Lead, for example, was taken in from paints, glazed pottery, enamelled cooking utensils, wine and cider, and still other items. Mercury affected miners, felt hat makers, and dentists; phosphorous poisoned workers in match factories; zinc injured labourers in brass foundries; carcinogens in soot induced skin cancer in chimney sweeps and shale oil caused skin cancer in cotton spinners; several compounds produced bladder cancer in dye workers. The list could run on, but it would yield no substance other than lead that could even begin to rival the extent and variety of arsenic-laden threats in the environment. As both murder weapon and environmental toxin, arsenic was the poisoner par excellence of Victorian Britain and, for those who struggled to control it, a matter of national embarrassment. Britons should arise in 'universal indignation', an author railed in 1871, that 'such wholesale murder, for it amounts to nothing less, should have gone on...unchecked during the greater part of this century', and flourished in a country 'which considers herself foremost in the ranks of civilised nations'.[13] The chapters that follow will attempt to show how the most self-consciously civilized society in modern times found itself countenancing wholesale murder and wide-scale poisoning.

*

As with previous books, I owe an immeasurable debt of gratitude to Colleen Weum, acquisitions and collection management librarian for the University of Washington Health Sciences Library. Colleen was exceedingly generous with time and effort in helping me locate obscure publications, calling my attention to (and explaining how to use) research databases on the Internet, and granting access to the otherwise off-limits chamber in the entrails of the Library where pre-twentieth-century medical texts and journals are kept. Thanks yet again, Colleen.

Other University of Washington librarians also provided much-appreciated assistance, particularly Kathy Sisak and Cheyenne Roduin. Margaret Mitchell and Sarah Edwards, of the Department of Bioethics and Humanities, offered invaluable, and patient, technical guidance in the preparation of the manuscript and illustrations.

I was greatly aided as well by staff at the Wellcome Library, the British Library, and Senate House Library, in London; Edinburgh University Library, the Royal College of Physicians Library, and the National Library of Scotland, in Edinburgh; the National Library of Medicine in Washington, DC; the New York Academy of Medicine Library in New York City; the Francis Countway Library of Medicine of Harvard University in Boston; and the Bernard Becker Medical Library of Washington University in Saint Louis. Helpful suggestions were also received from Ian Burney, of the University of Manchester, England, Mary Jo Nye and Robert

Nye of Oregon State University, Corvallis, and Connie Staudohar, of Montana State University, Bozeman. My son Adrian cleared up more than one medical uncertainty for me.

Sincere thanks go to the editors at Oxford University Press. Sylvie Jaffrey, my copy editor, was a pleasure to work with. She not only expertly discharged the usual duties of detecting errors and proposing stylistic improvements, but also gave meticulous attention to translating my American English into the mother tongue. Matthew Cotton coordinated a variety of tasks involved with transforming the manuscript into a book. Also contributing at various stages of the process were Luciana O'Flaherty, Natasha Knight, and Kate Hind.

Finally, I am deeply grateful to my wife Jackie both for vetting my translations of French works and for uncomplainingly tolerating years of books and papers stacked about the home office-space we share. Completion of this project will be as great a relief to her as to me, not least because she will now be spared my dinnertime stories of people dying in torment.

J.W.
Tacoma, Washington
September 2009

CONTENTS

LIST OF ILLUSTRATIONS

Of all the varieties of death by poison, none is so important to the medical jurist as poisoning with Arsenic. On account of the facility with which it may be procured in this country, even by the lowest of the vulgar, and the ease with which it may be secretly administered, it is the poison most frequently chosen for the purpose of committing murder.

Robert Christison, physician and toxicologist,
Edinburgh, 1829

The preparations of arsenic are, of all the poisonous substances in the mineral kingdom, the most fatal; and are those, the properties of which the physician ought to be best acquainted with. Being of considerable use in the arts, disposed of in commerce for the purpose of destroying noxious animals, administered and applied every day under various forms, for the cure of several species of diseases, frequently the instrument of crime and suicide, it is not to be wondered at, that they should furnish, more frequently than any others, the opportunity of exercising the talents of professional men.

Mathieu Orfila, physician and toxicologist, Paris, 1817

1

'Such an Instrument of Death and Agony'

'Of all kinds of murders that by poison is the most dreadful, as it takes a man unguarded, and gives him no opportunity to defend himself.' So spoke a Counsel for the Crown in the 1752 trial of an accused murderess. In making that observation, he had in mind a particular man unguarded, Mr Francis Blandy, prominent citizen of Henley-on-Thames, prosperous attorney, and parent *extraordinaire*, 'the most fond, the most tender, the most indulgent that ever lived'. Too indulgent, it would seem, much too indulgent for his own good, for despite seeing that she was 'educated with the utmost tenderness,' and taking 'every possible care . . . to impress her mind with sentiments of virtue and religion', Francis Blandy reared a daughter so lacking in judgement as to be seduced by a scheming bounder into carrying out the murder of her own doting father.[1]

Like so many women of the eighteenth century, Mary Blandy had been disfigured in childhood by an attack of smallpox ('That dire disease, whose ruthless power, Withers the beauty's transient flower': Goldsmith). Yet if her face was pocked, her figure was comely enough, she possessed wit and charm to match, and when those gifts were coupled with a reputed dowry of £10,000 she was assured of no shortage of suitors. Not one of her wooers, however, met with her father's approval; not one, that is, until Captain William Henry Cranstoun turned up in the summer of 1746. On the surface, the 32-year-old soldier was hardly a likely candidate for Mary's hand. He too had been pitted by the pox, 'so marked...that his face was in seams, and he squinted very much'. His seamed face was also dotted so thickly with freckles as to excite comment, his legs were 'clumsy', his stature was well below the average, and all in all he impressed others as nothing more than 'a mean-looking little ugly fellow'. As to his intellect, it was 'by no means striking...his mental powers [having] been chiefly exerted in attacks upon women and artifices at play'. A cad and a gambler and physically off-putting to boot was Captain Cranstoun. Yet even a freckle-faced, squinty-eyed wastrel can make himself dashing when inspired by a vision of £10,000, and soon the 26-year-old Mary was yielding to the soldier's advances. For Mr Blandy, the man's appeal was that he was the scion of Scottish aristocracy, so an opportunity for significant social advancement for both daughter and self. When, a year after their meeting, Cranstoun asked for Mary's hand, the father was only too pleased to assent.[2]

Before long, however, it came out that Captain Cranstoun was already wed, to a woman back in Scotland who had borne him a daughter two years before. And though Mary fell for his lie that he had been nothing more than the woman's lover, never her legal husband, Mr Blandy's opinion of the aspiring son-in-law turned sour and wedding plans were set aside. Feeling the dowry slipping through his fingers, Cranstoun turned to beguiling Mary with stories of a special powder known to certain cunning women in Scotland that made all who swallowed it forgive their enemies, and would surely soften her father's heart towards him.

Conveniently having himself called to Scotland to tend his ailing mother, Cranstoun posted the powder of forgiveness to Mary with instructions that if she put it in her father's tea he would be won over. This, at least, was Mary's version of things when brought to trial. Yet even if it were true that she did not initially know the real nature of the powder, events quickly demonstrated it to be toxic. As Counsel for the Crown later recounted, 'The effects of the poison were soon perceived.... The poor man frequently complained of pains in his bowels; had frequent reachings [retchings] and sickness.' But he proved most reluctant to die, forcing Cranstoun to urge Mary to double the dose. Mr Blandy now grew worse, suffering with 'a fireball in his stomach', while his child continued 'adding fuel to the fire, till it had consumed her father's entrails'. His mouth was consumed as well, 'one of the effects [being] the teeth dropping out of his head, whole from their sockets. Yet what do you think, gentlemen [of the jury], the daughter did when she perceived it? She damned him for a toothless old rogue, and wished him at hell.'[3]

It is far from clear that these were Mary Blandy's true feelings. That she expressed a wish that her father go to hell was the testimony of a servant, as was the assertion that more than once she had complained of her father's strong constitution and bemoaned what 'a monstrous thing' it was 'that old fellows should keep girls out of their fortunes so long'. Mary denied under oath making either statement, and would continue to protest her innocence of any malice towards her parent or any knowledge of the nature of the powder to the very hour of her death. Further to her credit are the facts that her father's first complaints, of stomach pain and heartburn, were symptoms she knew him to have experienced in the past before passing kidney stones, and so did not alarm her; and that when it became evident her father was more seriously ill, she sent at once for medical assistance.[4]

As Mr Blandy's condition worsened, two of his servants chanced to notice a strange-looking white powder at the bottom of a bowl of gruel, the only food their toothless master could any longer eat. Suspicious, they handed it over to a physician, who determined it to be arsenic. In the interim, the father's pains had worsened. Yet when the servants informed him he was likely being poisoned by his daughter, the ill-used man could feel nothing but pity. 'Poor love-sick girl!' he despaired. 'What will not a woman do for the man she loves!'⁵

That Mary was aware of what she was doing is suggested by an act that would be the most damning piece of evidence at her trial. She was observed by one of the now omnipresent servants throwing a bundle of her lover's letters into the fire—along with a paper packet that was retrieved by the servant before it took flame and found to contain a white powder like that in the gruel. Had Mary attempted to destroy the poison to preserve herself from detection? Or was she throwing it away in horror at the discovery she had been duped? Whatever her motivation, she by now realized she had poisoned her father, and rushed to his bedside to beg him not to condemn her. Yet despite her mistreatment, he refused to curse his only child, blessing her instead and vowing he would 'pray to God to bless you, and to amend your life'. A few days later, on 14 August 1751, Francis Blandy passed away in the sixty-second year of his age, the tragedy heightened by the fact he was in part the author of his own undoing. When his estate was settled, it became apparent he had considerably exaggerated his worth in order to attract potential husbands for his daughter. One wonders would Cranstoun have been quite so ready to resort to a capital offence had he known the old man's total wealth amounted to not much more than a third of the £10,000 he had advertised as a dowry.⁶

With her father's passing, Mary unwisely left the house, only to be accosted by a mob that had heard of the death and of the suspicion she was responsible. With 'half the town at my heels', she took refuge in The Angel, a pub that stands still at the foot of Henley's bridge, until being persuaded to return home under protection and to surrender herself to the authorities. That she had apparently taken flight would weigh heavily against her in court, where jurors found it hard to credit her story that she had left home only because her father was to be autopsied and she could not bear to stay in the house during the procedure. Nor were they persuaded by her additional observations that she had left on foot instead of horseback, and had not dressed heavily enough for the long outing of an escape attempt.[7]

Mary Blandy was imprisoned at Oxford, and eventually brought to trial (brought there, so the prosecutor declaimed, by the very power to which her father had appealed to amend her life: 'For what but the hand of Providence could have preserved the paper thrown by her into the fire, and have snatched it unburnt from the devouring flame? Good God! How wonderful are all Thy ways!'). Her trial stirred up tremendous excitement throughout the nation. Newspapers were dominated by the story of her shameful acts, and it was not because there was nothing else to write about. Among other things, the movement to replace the Julian with the Gregorian calendar was underway; Parliament had decreed that next 2 September would be followed by 14 September, and many had interpreted this to mean that the government had just cut short everyone's life by eleven days. Mary Blandy got more attention. In addition, pamphlets dramatizing the cruel deeds of Mary and her lover rolled from the presses, books were written on the crime, and even a theatrical drama was penned. *The Fair Parricide. A Tragedy in Three Acts. Founded on a late Melancholy Event* sided with the

accused, presenting heroine Maria Blandford as one whose 'Hands
are guilty' but 'Heart is clear', a lesson to other young women to
'henceforth shun the enticing Wiles of Love's pernicious Lure'.[8]

Small wonder, then, that a 'vast concourse of people' gathered
for the trial, including many students from the university (whom
one prosecutor could not resist lecturing: 'See here the dreadful consequences of disobedience to a parent'). The proceedings
lasted but a single day, albeit a long one, running from eight in
the morning till nine at night. Conducting herself 'with more than
masculine firmness', Mary continued to insist she was the victim
of a cruel deception ('What woman can stand the arguments and
persuasions men will make of us?'), but the jury would have none
of it. Devoting only five minutes to deliberation, not even retiring
from the courtroom, they pronounced the defendant guilty.[9]

The prisoner was hanged five weeks later, on 6 April 1752, still
avowing her innocence: 'May I not meet with eternal salvation,'
she declared from the scaffold, 'nor be acquitted by almighty God,
in whose awful presence I am instantly to appear' if guilty. Then,
'without shedding one tear', Mary Blandy pulled her handkerchief
over her face and was dropped into eternity. The throng of some
5,000 onlookers was not so stoic, many being themselves moved
to tears, 'particularly several gentlemen of the university'. Even
more must have taken in the moral lesson of the event, the exhor-
tation that accompanied an etching of the execution: 'With horror . . . behold, The parricide in murder bold. . . . Warned by her fate
ye children be, And dread her sad catastrophe.'[10]

Yet if the parricide could not escape the executioner, she did
baffle the surgeons. Mary Blandy was laid to rest in Henley only
weeks ahead of the enactment of a Parliamentary statute 'for better preventing the Horrid Crime of Murder', a law that provided
for the bodies of executed criminals to be immediately turned

over to the Surgeons' Company of London for the purposes of anatomical dissection (there was at the time a shortage of legally supplied cadavers for the practical study of anatomy, so the act promoted medical education and research at the same time as it futilely attempted to deter murder). Cranstoun, that 'base and barbarous man', that 'abandoned, insidious and execrable wretch', that 'unspeakable Scot' (feeling against Mary's 'cruel Spoiler' ran high), got off scot-free, fleeing to France at the news of Mary's arrest. He could not, however, escape the long arm of poetic justice. Nine months later, now in Belgium, he was stricken by an ailment marked by 'such Torments' and such 'great agonies' as to make him 'wish for Death for some days before he died'. His was much the same sort of end, in short, as he had arranged for Francis Blandy.[11]

*

The Blandy case, interesting though it is, predates the Victorian era by the greater part of a century and would seem to lie outside our focus on arsenic in the 1800s. Appreciating the uses and abuses of the poison in the nineteenth century, however, requires some understanding of its earlier history, as well as of its chemical properties and effects on the living frame. And for those purposes, the melancholy tale of the Blandy family is admirably adapted to serve as the centrepiece for a chapter outlining the pre-Victorian experience with arsenic.

To the chemist, arsenic (As) is element number 33 in the periodic table. A shiny steel-gray substance, it is the twentieth most common element in the earth's crust, and occurs as well in spring and sea water, in volcanic emissions, and even in space: meteorites are composed of as much as a tenth of a percent of arsenic (the illness that affected residents of a village in Peru after a meteorite crashed to earth in 2007 was blamed on vaporized arsenic compounds).

But the most striking thing about elemental arsenic—at least to the layman accustomed to equate the word with certain death—is that it is perfectly safe to swallow.[12]

Arsenic becomes toxic only when it combines with other elements to form compounds, and it is in the form of compounds with sulphur (S) and iron (Fe) that it exists in soil and water. Arsenopyrite (FeAsS), realgar (AsS), and orpiment (As_2S_3) are particularly common in mineral ores and coal. Yellow-hued orpiment, in fact, was the original 'arsenic', being dubbed *arsenikon* by the ancient Greeks, who probably derived the name from a Persian word for yellow.[13]

Orpiment and realgar are both poisonous (the fourteenth-century artist Cennino advised fellow painters to avoid using the deep-red realgar as a pigment: 'There is no keeping company with it.... Look out for yourself.'). Yet what the average person has in mind when using the word 'arsenic' is a combination of the element with oxygen, the compound arsenic trioxide (As_2O_3). Known to nineteenth-century chemists as arsenious acid (the name is now antiquated, but will be maintained here for purposes of historical accuracy), the compound is generated in the smelting of ores, primarily those of copper, lead, zinc, tin, and gold. As the ore is heated, elemental arsenic is driven off in gaseous form and combines with oxygen in the atmosphere. Popularly referred to as 'white arsenic', it is a substance that the *Merck Index of Chemicals and Drugs*, a generally sober reference work, singles out as '*intensely poisonous*!'; other medical writers have dubbed it simply 'the poison of poisons'.[14] It is arsenious acid—white arsenic—that historically has been the favourite of the poisoner, and that, understandably, has come to be referred to as arsenic in popular usage. Unless otherwise specified, that common meaning will be followed throughout the book.

Arsenic is toxic to all animals with a central nervous system, and to most plants. Although it usually enters the body through the alimentary tract, it can also be taken in by inhalation and by absorption through the skin or through mucous membranes such as those of the urethra or rectum. Thus when an eighteenth-century French servant failed to eliminate his lady employer with arsenical soup, he turned to putting the substance into her enema liquid—and succeeded. It was equally effective to introduce arsenic into the vagina, as was occasionally done to induce abortion or as a means of suicide. There are also several cases recorded of vaginal administration for purposes of murder, such as that of the sixteenth-century German farmer who poisoned three wives in succession by inserting an arsenic-covered finger into their sexual organs after a farewell act of coition (an eighteenth-century Finn rid himself of two wives similarly). Rumour had it that the trick could be used against men as well. In what must rank as one of the most ingenious homicides in history (in the unlikely event it actually occurred), the sudden death of King Ladislas of Naples in 1414 was caused by an enemy concealing arsenic in the vagina of the ruler's mistress (she is supposed to have died also; but through what machinations did the perpetrator have to go in order to plant the poison?). Further, since arsenic is excreted from the body through milk, it can be delivered even to the nursing babe. In a shocking incident in France in the 1880s, a man was convicted of killing his year-old child while trying to poison his wife.[15]

The great attraction of arsenious acid to those contemplating murder is that it has no distinctive taste or smell and, since it resembles flour and sugar, can be added to foods and beverages without arousing suspicion. On the other hand, white arsenic is only sparingly soluble in cold water, and thus often precipitates as a food or drink cools, imparting to it a distinct granular texture. On more than one occasion, Mr Blandy told his physician that he 'perceived an extraordinary grittiness in his mouth' when eating his gruel. Other victims compared the experience to having sand in the mouth, and at least one woman escaped possible death by rejecting an apple on which her husband had sprinkled arsenic after the first bite produced a sensation of sand between her teeth.[16]

Another attraction of arsenious acid is that it can do the desired job in small, hardly noticeable amounts. As little as 300 milligrams (mg), a mere hundredth of an ounce, can be counted on to kill. In the nineteenth century, however, physicians and apothecaries generally measured doses in units of grains rather than the modern milligrams (a grain represented the weight of an average grain of wheat). One grain is equivalent to 64.8 mg, meaning four to five grains would be adequate to dispatch most victims, and as little as two grains has been known to kill. Hence even the tiniest pinch of the poison can exert profound effects. An eighteenth-century lady who mistakenly ingested 'only so small a Quantity of *White Arsenic* as adhered to the Tip of her Finger, found herself within two Hours in great Disorder, grew faint, fell in a Swoon, and lost her Senses before she could be laid in Bed'.[17]

She should have considered herself fortunate, not merely for surviving, but for so quickly losing her senses. Most victims of arsenic poisoning passed through a far unhappier experience than simply finding themselves in great disorder of a sudden, then fainting into oblivion. Arsenic, after all, is the chief example of what early toxicologists called irritant poisons, substances that 'irritate, inflame, and corrode the texture' of internal organs. The irritant poisons classification was a large one, including compounds of mercury, antimony, copper and other metals, lye, ammonia, and Spanish fly. But few even in that category could challenge arsenic in violence, as a multitude of case histories to be gleaned from the pages of nineteenth-century medical and legal literature vividly demonstrate: arsenical poisoning was 'the most deplorable state that the imagination can possibly conceive'; arsenical death involved 'agonies that would soften the heart of a savage'.[18]

The agonies do not usually begin at once, for arsenic does not irritate, inflame, and corrode as soon as it makes contact with interior tissues. Rather, the poison must first be absorbed into the circulation. Thus, in most instances, nothing much at all happens for the first quarter of an hour or more after arsenic is ingested. This should be borne in mind when attending Joseph Kesselring's 1942 stage classic *Arsenic and Old Lace*: when the elderly men poisoned by the spinster aunts are said to have dropped on the spot ('One of our gentlemen found time to say "How delicious." '), it is not from the arsenic dissolved in the elderberry wine, or even the strychnine, but from the cyanide the determined old ladies have added. There are, to be sure, significant variations from one person to another, variations of both kind and degree. There are cases on record of individuals becoming ill almost immediately, and of others experiencing no untoward sensations for several hours, as many as ten: among a group of hotel guests poisoned in 1867 by biscuits prepared with arsenic that had been mistaken for flour, one fell ill shortly after the first bite while the onset of others' symptoms spread over the course of several hours, even though all had partaken of the poison at the same time. As a rule, the first indications of poisoning appear after a period of fifteen to thirty minutes, when sensations of warmth and tightness are experienced in the esophagus, creating difficulty in swallowing. In the trial of Mary Blandy, there was testimony that her father had much trouble swallowing, and experienced 'a very painful burning and pricking' in his tongue and throat, 'which prickings he compared to an infinite number of needles darting into him all at once'. In the arsenic poisoning trial of another Mary, a Mrs Hunter, in 1842, it was stated that her husband complained he felt 'as if he had swallowed cayenne pepper'.[19]

As the arsenic is taken into the bloodstream, it causes inflammation of the capillaries, a process that is particularly severe in the alimentary tract. The inflammation of the stomach causes 'enormous anguish', the anguish that for Mr Blandy was 'almost intolerable burnings and pains in his stomach and bowels', the fireball that consumed his entrails. A century after Blandy's death, a Yorkshire woman would cry out on her deathbed that the arsenic she had been given (probably by her husband) 'fair burnt her inside out'; other sufferers likened its effects to 'a furnace' or 'a ball of red hot iron'. Lucky the French woman (had she survived) who, intent on suicide, swallowed a Herculean dose of arsenic, then set about her day's work. From mid-morning until eight in the evening, she felt no discomfort at all, and even when abdominal pain did begin it was not enough to keep her from going to bed, and to sleep, at eleven. At three, she awoke, sat up, complained of nausea, then expired—'without the least appearance of suffering'.[20] Such are the vagaries of arsenic's action.

Nausea generally appears at the same time as the stomach pain and is shortly followed by vomiting (the 'reachings' that wracked Mr Blandy). Typically described by attending physicians as 'violent' and 'incessant', projectile vomiting continues for hours; the quantities evacuated can be such that an Essex man who lived below the bedroom of two children poisoned with arsenic in the 1840s had to leave his quarters when their vomit began to drip through the ceiling and onto his dining table. The first regurgitations contain any food that was in the stomach (and also remove much of any unabsorbed arsenic). But subsequently the vomit may be any combination of mucus and blood, as well as bile pulled from the intestines by the violence of the retching. In the instance of a young woman who attempted suicide in 1851, the ejection was 'dark and glutinous, mixed with clots of coagulated blood; and after each effort of vomiting, about a tablespoon of bright, florid, fluid blood was brought up'. In another case, 'on examining the contents of the utensils in which he had vomited, a fluid was perceived of a yellowish and greenish colour, and in two of them stercoraceous [faecal] matter'; and in yet another, 'the appearance of the matter vomited was...peculiar, in the colour especially, which was of a reddish yellow' (the colour variations are due to the mixing of bile with stomach contents). There was generally the added misery that 'each effort of vomiting...was preceded and followed by...painful gripings and spasmodic contractions of the abdominal muscles', and sometimes persistent and painful hiccupping occurred as well.[21]

While stomach fluids are being evacuated by vomiting, water from the body is draining into the gut, and as the bowel fills, purging of a violent and incessant nature begins: 'such purging and vomiting I never before has seen', a Scottish woman commented of a friend she witnessed die from arsenic. Similarly, soon after Mr Blandy's charwoman inadvisedly sampled some of his leftover gruel, her bowels became agitated and she was compelled to dash 'to the necessary, and was not able to return in less than two hours'.[22]

The purging occurs at first in the form of profuse watery diarrhoea. These rice-water stools (so named for having the milky appearance of water used to rinse rice) may eventually give way to bloody evacuations as capillaries rupture, or to other appalling discharges. Mr Blandy 'had a great many stools, and some bloody ones' during nights after he ate poisoned gruel. 'He passed dark bloody stools of a very offensive character,' one doctor noted of a patient in the 1850s; in the case of a suicidal French woman, the intestinal discharges were 'blackish, and of a horrible foetor'; a London practitioner characterized the odour of arsenical stools as 'cadaverous'; 'on examining the alvine [bowel] secretions', a practitioner recorded in another case, 'the singularity of their appearance excited great surprise; they were all of a bright homogeneous green colour, like paint'. An eighteenth-century lady who accidentally swallowed white arsenic 'voided by Stool several globules of greenish Coagulum, of the Bigness, Colour, and nearly the Consistency of Pickled Olives'.[23]

If the victim lives long enough, the purging may well end, but only to be replaced by tenesmus, a painful spasm of the anal sphincter that creates a feeling of urgency to defecate unaccompanied by the ability to do so: in the 1880s, a Liverpool man was racked for hours by 'persistent and constant, but fruitless, endeavours to go to stool'. The violent evacuations and the fruitless straining play havoc with a victim's rectum and anus, of course. Blandy's bowel opening was 'almost surrounded with gleety [pus-streaked] excoriations and ulcers', while 'an ulcerous matter generally issued from his fundament'.[24]

The expulsion of fluid upwards and downwards, coupled with the burning pain throughout the alimentary tract, creates extreme thirst: 'The thirst of each patient was so urgent, that they would readily have drank [sic] quarts, had they been permitted.' They were usually not permitted, however, because intake of fluid would simply trigger renewed retching; the most that was normally allowed was rinsing of the mouth with water. The action of the kidneys is also inhibited by inflammation, and urination becomes difficult and painful (and often bloody), or is suspended altogether. Sharp pains in the muscles and bones commonly occur, a man who attempted suicide comparing them 'to the gnawing of rats, or the boring of a gimblet [gimlet] into the bones'. At last, degeneration of heart muscle brings on circulatory collapse and hard-earned death.[25]

Arsenic worked its evil in a multitude of ways. It presented 'the greatest possible variety in the character, combination, and severity of the symptoms' (modern research has confirmed that opinion, demonstrating that genetic variations and other personal characteristics make for a broad range of susceptibility to arsenic among individuals). The action of the poison, further, was marked by 'exceptions and anomalies of the most perplexing kind': in at least one case, death occurred not following the usual coma, but 'after a horrible fit of convulsive laughter'. By a jurisprudence professor's analogy, it was 'the very Proteus of poisons', capable of assuming almost any form.[26]

The whole agonizing experience of acute arsenic poisoning may last as little as two hours, or extend to forty-eight hours or even three or four days (for some victims the misery is drawn out to a fortnight; Francis Blandy's final sufferings stretched to a week and a half, during which time he received several doses of the poison). A calculation performed in the 1880s determined that the average time from ingestion of the poison to death was eleven hours and five minutes, but most experts have placed the average at upwards of twenty-four hours. Even those who recover may continue to suffer gastric and intestinal disturbances for months, as well as neurological damage producing tingling sensations one survivor likened to 'being in a bagful of fleas'. There is almost no end to the aftereffects of arsenic poisoning. An eighteenth-century English surgeon who attended the favourite wife of the ruler of Morocco after she was given arsenic by rivals reported that 'her beauty, the fatal cause of her misfortune, was completely destroyed', so that while her enemies failed in their goal of killing her, they 'yet enjoyed the malignant triumph of seeing those charms which had excited their jealousy, reduced below the standard of other women'. Fortunately, happier endings do sometimes occur, as in the case of the mental patient who tried to kill himself with arsenic, suffered horribly, but survived and found his reason had been so fully restored that he could return to his former life as a businessman. His case was the exception. The rule was that arsenic fully deserved the description given it by a mid-nineteenth-century newspaper editor: 'such an instrument of death and agony'.[27]

*

The foregoing catalogue of agonies applies to acute arsenic intoxication, the result of a single large dose that produces marked symptoms within a matter of hours (as with MrBlandy, the large doses may be given several times before death results). Smaller but repeated doses of arsenic lead to sub-acute poisoning, a state in which symptoms appear more gradually and in less violent form. Over the space of days to weeks, the victim experiences loss of appetite, fatigue and weakness, vomiting, and diarrhoea. As injuries accumulate, intoxication takes the form of depressed urination, skin eruptions, muscular pain, numbness and tingling in the extremities, and finally paralysis, convulsions, coma, and death. Victorian physicians held that slow, sub-acute poisoning was the method preferred by 'ingenious criminals', and that it was employed frequently but often went undetected because its gradual development made it appear to be simply a general decline in vitality. Still smaller doses could produce an even more subtle and drawn-out level of poisoning, the chronic arsenicism that will feature in many of the later chapters. Finally, to complete the picture, it should be noted that arsenic is also an escharotic, a substance that exerts a caustic effect on the skin, producing sores, scabs, and sloughing of the damaged tissue, and sometimes being absorbed through the abraded surface in amounts sufficient to kill. A man who for some reason washed his entire body with a solution of arsenic at once felt severe burning pain all over, as if 'laid on a fire', saw his skin soon 'raised in blisters', and ultimately died in anguish.[28]

Acute poisoning naturally got the greatest share of attention, and so fearsome was arsenic's reputation in that regard one could forgive physicians if they had just thrown up their hands when presented with a case ('No animal, great or small, is capable of resisting its fatal energy,' a professor of medical jurisprudence exclaimed; another authority declared, 'I defy the imagination to conceive of a poison more irresistible in its operation'). Antidotes aplenty were suggested: milk, vinegar, castor oil, bloodletting, the application of leeches to the abdomen, even the ashes of burned leather. It was nevertheless generally agreed that the only thing that had a chance of working was induction of vomiting either with large quantities of warm water or oil, or a finger down the patient's throat. And one had better be quick about it. 'No remedy can ever alleviate these melancholy preludes of death,' an American doctor maintained with a touch of excess, 'unless it operate with the velocity of light.' That helps explain why the mortality rate from arsenic poisoning was close to, if not beyond, 50 per cent.[29]

In antiquity and for some centuries after, poisoning with arsenic was restricted to the use of its sulphides, the yellow orpiment and the red realgar (because of their intense colours, these substances were also much in demand as pigments and cosmetics; a container of orpiment was even placed in King Tutankhamen's tomb for use in the next world). At this remove, it is next to impossible to determine just how frequently orpiment and realgar were employed by assassins, but stories abound. The best is the tale that Nero rid himself of his potential rival Britannicus by putting an arsenic compound in his soup. Initially, it is told, untainted soup was presented to Britannicus's taster, who determined it to be wholesome but objected that the liquid was too hot for his master. Accordingly, water—laced with one of the arsenic sulphides, of course—was added to the soup to cool it down. That produced the desired result. It was an ingenious trick, to be sure, but it is highly unlikely any compound of arsenic was involved, not if Suetonius is correct in reporting that 'Britannicus dropped dead at the very first taste'. Death at first taste is not one of arsenic's effects.[30]

Indeed, the bright colours that made orpiment and realgar so desirable for ornamental purposes militated against their use as poisons; they had to be cleverly disguised, and even then their strong taste would probably give the game away. Consequently, arsenic poisoning did not begin to flourish until the discovery of arsenious acid during the Middle Ages. That momentous event is thought to have occurred in the laboratory of the eighth-century Arabic alchemist Jabir ibn Hayyan (for the chemically literate, it can be explained that Jabir sublimated elemental arsenic by heating realgar, then collected the arsenious acid that formed when the sublimate combined with atmospheric oxygen). Having neither colour, taste, nor smell, and producing symptoms easily mistaken for those of natural disease, white arsenic was virtually designed for murder. To the criminally inclined, it was a godsend.[31]

None welcomed it with such delight as the Italians. The name of de Medici, the ruling family of Florence during the fifteenth century, is synonymous with poison as a tool of statecraft (their tradition was carried into the sixteenth century in the hands of Catherine de Medici, queen of France until 1589). Even more notorious were the Borgias, also of the fifteenth century. Pope Alexander VI (nee Rodrigo Borgia), his son Cesare (the model for Machiavelli's *Prince*), and daughter Lucrezia have become infamous over the centuries for using poison in the pursuit of politics and profit: in Max Beerbohm's witticism, Renaissance Romans liked to brag they would be dining with the wealthy Borgias tonight, but none was ever heard to say he had dined with the Borgias *last* night. In fact, reports of the deaths they caused have been greatly exaggerated. Most who accepted invitations from a Borgia did live to tell about it. The trick to survival was to avoid dining *chez Cesare*; the prince was the one ready to poison anybody who stood in the way of what he wanted. The case against the Pope is much less certain, and Lucrezia, whose name has been most thickly tarred of all, was probably altogether innocent. Nevertheless, the rumours were such that a new term entered English during the sixteenth century: to be removed by poison was to be 'Italianated'.[32]

The Italianator supreme was a Sicilian woman of the later 1600s named Toffana (sometimes Toffania or Tophana or Tophania— contemporaries disagreed on just how her name should be spelled). Residing first in Palermo, then Naples, she dispensed the arsenic-impregnated 'Acqua Toffana' under the guise of a cosmetic lotion. As will be discussed in Chapter 10, arsenic does have certain cosmetic properties when taken in the right doses, but Toffana's clients were more intent on removing husbands than dermal blemishes. And they succeeded, because the Acqua operated very slowly, and so failed to arouse suspicion. It produced, an eighteenth-century physician stated, 'a gradual sinking of the powers of life, without any violent symptoms; a nameless feeling of illness, failure of strength, slight feverishness, want of sleep, an aversion to food, drink, and the other enjoyments of life', until finally life itself came to an end. Properly administered, it was believed, the Acqua Toffana could actually bring about death on any predetermined day. (Slow sub-acute poisoning was an ideal of long standing; nearly a century before Toffana's reputation was established, Camillo, in *The Winter's*

Tale, boasted of having the skill to prepare a poison that was 'no rash potion, but... a lingering dram'.)[33]

Through strict secrecy and frequent changes of address and disguise, Toffana managed to elude detection for decades. By the time she was at last found out, in 1709, an estimated 600 people had been felled by her Acqua, including, rumour had it, two popes. So it was not *just* husbands who had to fear Toffana. As always, people in power were vulnerable: the governor of Naples reported that the Acqua 'was the dread of every noble family in the city'.[34]

When the poisonings were finally traced to Toffana, the now 70-year-old woman took sanctuary in a convent, whence, supposedly, she continued to market her product until exasperated authorities repudiated the privilege of church asylum, dragged her out against clerical protests, strapped her to the rack, and extracted a confession (a confession was almost essential for a poisoning charge, as chemistry at that time was incapable of identifying any poison in the body of the deceased; about the only test was to give the suspected substance to a dog and see what happened). Toffana was then strangled and her body dumped in the courtyard of the convent. A similar fate befell her most notable imitator, the Roman woman Hieronyma Spara, who from 1659 onwards supplied an arsenic preparation to ladies of the city for use against their husbands or other family members. 'La Spara' too escaped discovery for years, and even when she was at last arrested, 'the hardened old hag', as one chronicler described her, refused to confess her crimes even under the ordeal of the rack. She was hanged anyway, along with a dozen other women implicated in her crimes.[35]

Fear of the Acqua Toffana lingered long after its originator's death, down to the opening of the nineteenth century. For one, Mozart was sure he was a victim of the notorious poison. After finishing *Die Zauberflöte*, in 1791, the composer returned from Prague to Vienna, weak and pale and convinced he was dying; he even intimated to his wife that the Requiem on which he had begun work was to be for himself. He indeed did die before the year was out, from chronic kidney disease in the opinion of modern physicians. His wife, however, reported that Mozart had told her he was certain he had somehow been dosed with Aqua Toffana, an account that fuelled the rumour that has survived to the present, that the composer was poisoned by envious rival Antonio Salieri; in the award-winning drama *Amadeus*, Peter Shaffer has Mozart die slowly from poison administered by Salieri, a lingering dram that produced the stomach pain and cramping to be expected from arsenic. Two decades later, in 1815, an Irish nobleman incurred 'most distressing complaints for the remainder of his life ... through the jealousy of an Italian lady', a devotee of Toffana, while about the same time an Englishman travelling in Calabria learned that '*several hundred* persons are poisoned there *annually*' by the Acqua.[36]

Tales of Toffana moulded a public perception of arsenic poisoning as a highly mysterious, almost magical process, and one, moreover, that exerted a preternatural appeal to feminine nature (arsenic's attraction for the fairer sex was buttressed further by two seventeenth-century French poisoners, the Marquise de Brinvilliers and Catherine Monvoisin, who relied on *la poudre de succession* to hasten inheritances). The perception, which would hold on to the end of the Victorian era, was presented with particular clarity in an 1846 novel by Edward Bulwer Lytton (he in whose name an annual award for bad writing is given today). The unsubtly named title character of *Lucretia or The Children of Night* is set upon her evil course by reading a book recounting 'that singular epoch of terror in Italy' when arsenic poisoning was rampant, when hundreds of husbands perished, 'but not one wife!' Lucretia is particularly struck by the book's revelations of 'the astonishing craft brought daily to bear on the victim, the wondrous perfidy of the subtle means, the variation of the certain murder—here swift as epilepsy, there slow and wasting as long decline'. Thus inspired, she goes on to poison her own husband, and then her niece, with what Bulwer Lytton eventually identifies as 'the celebrated acqua di Tufania'.[37]

Even if not wielded by a woman, arsenic had so nefarious a history that it sparked in the popular imagination a credulous belief in far greater potency than it possessed, in essentially supernatural qualities. Cesare Borgia was supposed to have relied on a preparation he called 'La Cantarella', prepared by removing the abdominal organs of a sow poisoned with arsenic, salting the organs with more arsenic, then letting them slowly putrefy. The fluids that dripped from the rotting viscera were then evaporated to dryness and collected as a white powder resembling sugar: Voila! La Cantarella! In some tellings, the sow was replaced by a bear, in others by a toad, but the finished product was the same. Shirts secretly washed with arsenical soap, it was averred, could slowly destroy the wearer, as could poisoned gloves and shoes, or handkerchiefs or towels or rings. A priest was said to have contemplated killing Elizabeth I by rubbing arsenic on her saddle. It was common knowledge that killing a toad with arsenic, then crushing the animal in a goblet would infuse the glass with such venom that any drinking from it would be doomed; that when mice were exterminated by arsenic, 'the very smell of the dead will destroy the living of that species'; that Pope Clement VII had been killed by a poisoned torch borne ahead of him in a ceremonial procession ... and so on (it is, however, conceivable that a torch could be prepared in such a way as to give off vapours of the deadly arsenic-based gas arsine). Part of arsenical mythology was that wolves, alone among animals, were immune to the poison.[38]

Possibly the most extreme bit of arsenic folly was 'Sympathetic Ink', an amazing preparation for which respectable authors were still giving out instructions as late as the mid-1700s. Make a water solution of sugar of lead (lead acetate), readers were told, and use it to write a message on a sheet of paper: 'When it is dry nothing will be seen at all.' This might seem just the tired old invisible ink trick—but it came with a twist. The directions next required the sheet of invisible writing to be placed between the first pages of a large book, and that there be inserted at the back of the volume a similar sheet of paper that had been brushed with a solution of orpiment: 'Shut the Book nimbly, and with your Hand strike on it two or three smart Blows ... or sit upon it for a few Minutes; after which, on opening the book, you'll find the invisible Writing, black and legible, by the subtile Penetration of the Steams of the Orpiment through all the Leaves.' The experiment, this writer added in a cautionary note, 'should be made in the open Air ... the Fumes of the Orpiment stinking most abominably, and being productive of great Mischief if taken into the Lungs'.[39]

Arsenic's potency hardly needed such mystical amplification. Its true action was productive of Mischief enough—just ask Francis Blandy. Even so, the total amount of mischief done by arsenic was about to increase markedly.

2

'A New Race of Poisoners'

The British public, a journalist announced in the 1850s, had lately become more anxious about arsenic poisoning 'than ever men were in the worst age of Italian profligacy. We dread it of nights.... We inquire actively as to its presence in our bread, and in our wine, and in our sauce.' Things had come to such a pass, he reported, that 'to take heed against poison' was now 'one of the waking thoughts common to all'.[1]

Were people really *that* possessed by the fear of being poisoned, that they opened their eyes each morning calculating the odds of making it through the day? They may well have been if they took seriously the alarms that resounded through newspapers and periodicals of the time, that 'the poison fiend is abroad' through the land, that poisoning had become a 'horrid taint in the national mind', that the employment of arsenic now constituted 'a tendency to crime more wild, more brutal, more abominable, than the darkest ages of the world ever heard of', that the threat was so out-of-hand that 'the only way [the *only* way] of grappling with it now will be by... instruction of our population in the doctrines of Christianity'.[2]

This picture of poison-wielders running amok has coloured perceptions of the Victorian era down to the present. It is, however, a somewhat distorted one. For the entire decade of the 1840s, the peak period in the use of arsenic, there were only ninety-eight trials for criminal poisoning in England and Wales, fewer than one a month for a population of nearly twenty million. Granted, some of the trials involved more than one victim, and there were assuredly instances of poisoning that passed unrecognized. Still, a degree of hysteria is evident in the contention of *The Times* that poisoning cases uncovered by the police were merely isolated samples 'of countless undetected crimes'. While the possibility of being poisoned was not so remote that it could be put entirely out of mind, cases were hardly countless. Warnings that 'the fell spirit of the Borgias is stalking through English society' were just a bit exaggerated.[3]

Why was the danger so overstated? First, while poisoning was certainly not so commonplace that everyone had to analyse his bread and wine daily, the crime had indeed grown significantly over the first half of the century, the number of trials for murder by poison during the 1830s was triple the number of trials for the 1810s, then rose by more than 50 per cent the following decade. Further, the most frequently used material, by far, was arsenic (some 70 per cent of poisoning trials in the 1840s involved that agent), the substance damned by history as the poison of poisons, the tool of the Borgias, the instrument of Italian profligacy. Arsenic's dreadful reputation all but guaranteed an overreaction as poisoning crimes increased. So pervasive was arsenic-phobia that the substance was automatically presumed guilty in any situation in which it was found. When a house fire in Bloomsbury in 1858 killed fifteen people, a physician proposed to an inquest jury the fanciful explanation that the deaths had actually been caused by arsenic. As he interpreted it, arsenic present in samples kept by a mineralogist in a room adjacent to where the blaze started was vaporized by the heat, the fumes were inhaled by the building's residents, and since with arsenic vapours 'prostration immediately succeeds', all collapsed on the spot and were then finished off by smoke and fire.[4]

The flames of overreaction were fanned still higher by the popular press, which had grown dramatically since the early 1800s, when improvements in printing technology allowed production of newspapers at significantly lower cost than before. Then, in 1836, Parliament reduced the tax imposed on newspapers by 75 per cent (and abolished it altogether in 1855), reducing costs still further. The price of an issue of *The Times*, for example, fell from 7 *d.* in 1830 to 3 *d.* in 1870. Meanwhile, both state and church were expanding schooling for the lower classes, promoting a rise in the basic literacy rate from 50 per cent in 1830 to 95 per cent by the end of the century. Newspaper publishers recognized opportunity when they saw it and began aggressively marketing their product to the newly literate, bringing about an extraordinary increase of circulation among working-class readers. *Lloyd's Weekly Newspaper*, to choose one example, began in 1843 with a circulation of 21,000; by 1863, the number of readers had swelled to 350,000. As much then as now, people were drawn to stories of sex and violence. But while sexual themes had to be muted to meet standards of propriety, murder most foul could be trumpeted to the heavens, and lurid accounts of arsenical homicide made particularly compelling copy. The press of the early Victorian era thus sharply elevated public awareness of poisoning, and created the illusion the crime was more common than in truth it was.[5]

Yet if death by arsenic was not an everyday occurrence, it still was happening more frequently than in the past. Why? The answer is partly that the poison was more available and affordable than it had previously been. Industrial production of white arsenic began in the 1400s as a by-product of iron smelting in Austria. The poison was not produced in significant quantity, though, until an expansion of metal refining in the later 1600s. As a waste product, arsenic was cheap, and as supplies became plentiful, it was eagerly adopted as a measure superior to traps or cats for combating the hordes of rats that infested city and countryside alike: arsenic soon became ratsbane to the English, *mort-aux-rats* to the French. It has even been proposed that the disappearance of bubonic plague from Europe after 1720 was due to the adoption of arsenic to eliminate rodents (if so, it was an unwitting attack on plague, as the role of the rat as the chief reservoir of the infection was not understood until the end of the nineteenth century).[6]

Working hand-in-hand with the ready availability of arsenic was an intensification of the temptation to use it for murder. Temptation had always existed, of course: an anticipated inheritance, a tiresome spouse, any number of considerations might move the impatient to act. Among the poor, a frequent motivator was too many mouths to feed. Mortality among children was naturally high anyway, especially from intestinal infections that mimicked the action of arsenic, so a few more deaths here and there from poison would scarcely be noticed. Such murders might even be carried out as mercy killings. In 1849, a Wiltshire woman, Rebecca Smith, was executed for destroying eight of her babies shortly after birth because she was bound to a ne'er-do-well alcoholic husband and feared the children 'might come to want' and die the crueller death of starvation. From both good intentions and bad, infanticide had long been commonplace among the poverty-ridden (and would continue so: on into the 1880s, it is estimated that some 60 per cent of all victims of homicide were less than a year old).[7]

But in the middle third of the century, the temptation to poison underwent a growth spurt, stimulated by the rise of the insurance industry. The first life insurance company organized along modern lines was founded in London in 1762, and though only seven more companies went into business in Britain before 1800, by 1825 seventeen new ones had been launched, and over the next decade another fourteen were added to the list. By then it had become apparent that a life insurance policy cut two ways, providing families peace of mind, but also opening a door to quick wealth: 'by insuring a life and destroying it', one poison authority noted, 'thousands of pounds can, as it were, be called into existence'. Lucretia, the villainess of the Bulwer Lytton novel cited in Chapter 1, put the principle into action, taking out a £15,000 policy on her niece before poisoning her.[8]

Policies paying out thousands of pounds were, of course, an option for only the more highly placed. Yet the limited means of the lower classes did not keep them from poisoning for profit too; it merely restricted them to lower gains. Throughout the nineteenth century, tradesmen of all stripes—bakers and blacksmiths, carpenters and coopers, weavers and wool-combers—joined together to form 'friendly societies' whose purpose was only partly to support the convivial social interactions their name implied. The more important object of the societies was to provide members some degree of protection against life's more trying contingencies: unemployment, sickness, death. Workers paid in weekly contributions in return for the promise of subsistence financial support if they became incapacitated through illness or accident, and funeral expenses if they died. For a higher contribution, some friendly societies also provided basic medical care.[9]

Friendly societies appeared in the later 1600s, began to enlarge in numbers towards the end of the 1700s in response to the quickening pace of industrialization, then grew even more rapidly from the 1830s as workers acquired somewhat more discretionary income. Reliable estimates put the membership in friendly

societies in 1815 at just under a million. By 1870, roughly four million tradesmen were enrolled in more than 30,000 societies, some
groups operating at the local level (the Cannon Street Adult Male
Provident Institution of Birmingham, for example), others being
national in scope (most notably the Ancient Order of Foresters and
the various congregations of Oddfellows).[10]

Friendly society membership had the same built-in enticement to do away with family members as the life insurance policies purchased by the more well-to-do, and in certain societies that
enticement was placed front and centre. There were entities called
'burial clubs' that had as their sole purpose the dispensation of
funeral expenses for departed members, catering to the desire to
avoid the humiliation of a pauper's burial. However squalid the
realities of their earthly existence, the poor wanted their leaving
of it at least to be respectable, and being dumped into a pit with
a dozen or more other corpses, as occurred with funerals 'on the
parish', was a shameful end not to be incurred if possible. Further,
after passage of the 1832 Warburton Anatomy Act, bodies turned
over for parish disposal were liable to be given to anatomists for
dissection. Burial societies thus flourished with their promise to pay
for a decent funeral.[11]

Yet there were, inevitably, some subscribers who were not at
all averse to a child or spouse receiving a pauper's send-off, and if
sufficient economies were adopted in their disposal, there would
be enough money left over to make murder worthwhile. By the
mid-1800s, it was widely held that young children were frequently
destroyed for the burial money their deaths would bring. If done
right, profits were not inconsiderable. First of all, club dues were
affordable for virtually anyone. The Liverpool Victoria Legal Burial Society, which was representative, levied a half-penny to a penny
per week, depending on the age of the child. Second, benefits were

relatively generous. Manchester clubs, for example, paid out £3 as a rule, but some paid £4, or even £5; a basic funeral for a child could be financed for only £1 or £2. There was a saying among women in the Manchester tenements, 'Aye, aye, that child will not live, it is in the burial club!' Not without reason were club membership rolls referred to as 'catalogues of the doomed'.[12]

Profits were multiplied, further, when children were enrolled in several clubs at once. A clergyman's wife who visited a family shortly after a child's death was shocked to hear a neighbour comment on what 'a fine thing' it was for the mother, as 'the child's in two clubs!' Some children were enrolled in quite a few more, the probable record being the nineteen to which a Manchester child belonged. It was not unheard of for parents to reap £20 from a death, a mighty enticement for people such as the father in a poem titled 'The Burial Club':

> I was once, I confess, chicken-hearted:
> His moans made me tremble and shrink:
> But I thought of the club and the money,
> Grew bolder, and gave him the drink.

'The drink' was arsenic ('How curled up he is! I wonder | How the blue came into his face'), and such crimes, it was charged by mid-century, were undergoing 'frightful progress'. Women were producing babies 'with no more heart than a woman would plant a row of cabbages or let a hen hatch a nestfull of eggs'. To mothers of this strain, a child was 'simply a crop to be planted, watered, and then gathered in... a useful animal to be bred, and converted into money in due time... a speculation to be wound up at the earliest opportunity'. In response to this the-earlier-the-better philosophy, Parliament in 1850 enacted a statute prohibiting the insuring of children under the age of 10 for more than £3.[13]

The law did nothing, however, to protect adult members of burial clubs. Such a one was the Devon man whose wife killed him with arsenic in 1819 after having 'put him into two clubs with a view to obtain twenty pounds to spend at his death'. As membership in burial clubs grew in subsequent decades, reports of poisoning for funeral benefits increased proportionately. The 'DEATH CLUB' came to be widely regarded as the 'prolific mother' of arsenical murder, the institution from which 'a new race of poisoners has sprung'.[14]

That new race had sprung forth because in order to call into existence those thousands of pounds from an insurance company or simply the five or ten pounds provided by a burial club, one had to destroy the insured life without being detected, and for that purpose poison was ideal. Unlike the bullet to the head or knife to the gut, poison produced a death that could be passed off as natural. Arsenic was particularly well suited for the purpose, imitating, as it did, some of the most common symptoms of disease. When its deadliness, ready availability, and cheapness (it cost notably less than any comparably lethal poison) were figured in as well, it was clearly the best choice for cashing in on insurance.

Any number of villains capitalized on that fact, but none so fruitfully as Mary Ann Cotton. A 'comely-looking' woman of the coal-mining regions of County Durham, Cotton was the undisputed champion of the game of murder for insurance money, if one awards the title on the basis of number of insured victims (if the title is determined according to total income, however, she was an also-ran, typically collecting only a few pounds per death). She was, in fact, the most prodigious serial killer in English history, at least until Cheshire physician Harold Shipman's multiple murders came to light in the 1990s. From the early 1860s until her arrest in 1872, Cotton, a one-time Sunday-school teacher, employed arsenic to murder her mother, three husbands,

a lodger who became—briefly—her fiancé, and most of her fifteen children and stepchildren. In every case, death was diagnosed as some form of gastric complaint, and in nearly every case
Cotton was the beneficiary of an insurance policy (one of the
uninsured was the fiancé, but he paid off in his own way, having
been charmed into writing a will that left her all his possessions,
meagre though they were; there was also a fourth husband, but
he escaped the others' fate when Cotton left him after he declined
to be insured).[15]

Through all this, no one seems to have suspected a thing, neither the Prudential, the insurance company which paid out benefits
for a number of her victims, nor her neighbours, who might have
thought it an improbably nasty run of luck for six of her children
to die suddenly within a single year (1867). Not until weeks after
the death of a stepson in 1872 did suspicions surface at last, trig-
gering an inquest that led to a trial and conviction. Yet to the very
end, Cotton appears to have believed her uncanny luck would hold.
Even though the jury returned an unequivocal verdict, she 'seemed
to be stunned' when the judge 'assumed the black cap [and] passed
upon her the awful sentence', so taken aback, in fact, that she had to
be 'removed in a fainting condition'. Up to the day of her execution
she still, it was reported, believed clemency would be granted by the
throne. Victoria, predictably, was not amused, and a pardon did not
come. Five days before her death, Cotton gave up for adoption her
one remaining child, an infant born while she was in prison, charg-
ing the new parents to bring the little one up in the fear of God.[16]

Cotton's execution, it is worth noting, was presided over by the
most famous hangman of the century, William Calcraft. This was
a man so dedicated to his craft that once when a prisoner who had
been dropped through the scaffold managed to get his feet up to
the platform again so as to support himself, Calcraft pushed him

back into the drop, then jumped down into the opening himself and held the man's legs until he was dead. Calcraft gave his subjects (approximately 500 in number) a short rope, being put off by the decapitation that sometimes resulted when the victim gained too much momentum before being snapped to a halt. Consequently, prisoners did not die quickly, but struggled for a period; Cotton fought against death for a full three minutes. Such struggles were the inspiration for Calcraft's autobiography, *The Groans of the Gallows*.[17]

*

Mary Ann Cotton was representative of the new race of poisoner in at least two other ways. First, she was of humble social standing. In the burst of poisoning trials that roiled the 1840s, three-quarters of the defendants came from the lower classes, to no one's surprise. It made sense that the poor would choose poison, arsenic particularly. It was inexpensive and easily available. One no longer need be an aristocratic Borgia, or even a middle-class scoundrel like William Cranstoun, to take advantage of the opportunity. Poisoning had been made available to the masses, a fact that further stimulated arsenic paranoia. 'Buried in sensuality and hardened by want; dark and moody, aimless and miserable', the poor, it was agreed, were largely untouched by Christian teaching. Society's dregs, 'longing for... indulgences beyond [their] means, and... having no pure and kindly influences to correct the horrid craving', they were far more likely to turn to arsenic than were decent folk. 'Who does this horrid deed,' a *Times* editorial inquired, 'but the occupant of some cellar or garret under the smoke of tall chimneys.' Poisoners were wretches such as Betty Eccles, killer of three daughters and a stepson for burial money, 'an abandoned woman... given to drinking', wife of an unskilled labourer whose address in the factory town of Bolton bore the designation Bugbear-hole. She was hanged in the spring of 1843, along with a man who had slit his wife's throat.[18]

Cotton exemplified the new poisoners also by virtue of being female. Poisoning had long been associated with the sex, from Locusta, who was employed by Nero to concoct potions to use against his rivals, to Catherine de Medici and Toffana in more recent times. But during the 1840s there took hold a suspicion that women in general, not just individual females of vicious disposition, were inclined to turn to poison to gain their ends. There was, admittedly, a shred of truth to the suspicion, for when women did kill they were much more likely to do so through means not requiring physical force. Consider the crime of spousal homicide. More than 90 per cent of the murders of a spouse in nineteenth-century England were committed by men against their wives, usually by beating or stabbing; only 5 per cent of the men convicted of killing their wives used poison. Among women convicted of murdering their husbands, the percentage relying on poison was 55, and was even higher in the 1840s and 1850s, when almost as many cases of husband-poisoning were tried as had been done in the entire century preceding or the half-century to follow. Over the course of the Victorian era, twice as many women as men were tried on charges of killing their mates with poison. Other types of murder followed a similar pattern. Men committed the crime much more often than women, but female killers were much more likely to use poison.[19]

Public perceptions were that even more women, many more, were doling out poison to their husbands, their children, and anyone else who got in the way. At a time when the newly organized feminist movement was agitating for greater social and professional roles for women, challenging traditional male authority, threatening to unleash sexual anarchy, it was all too easy to suppose that the female poisoners who now made such regular appearances in newspaper headlines were a much more numerous species than, in fact, they were. When Anne Merritt was sentenced for poisoning her husband in 1850, the judge professed himself aghast over the 'frequency of the crime with which you are charged'.[20]

He also declared that hers was a particularly 'strange and horrible' crime. 'Horrible,' of course, applied not just to the supposed frequency of husband-poisoning, but even more aptly to the nature of the woman who would do such a thing. When a man beat his wife, it might be regrettable, but it was, after all, an expression of masculine nature—men were physical creatures, governed by violent temperament. Women were cut from finer cloth, so when they turned to murder it was a shocking, indeed monstrous perversion of their essential nobility of spirit. At the same time, their preference for poisoning, a secretive, skulking act, confirmed male suspicions that at bottom women truly were sinister, deceitful beings. With respect to poisoning, a newspaper correspondent asserted, 'it is the softer sex who are everywhere addicted to this amiable propensity', possessed, as was said of Betty Eccles, by an 'extraordinary and unaccountable predilection for poisoning'. Woman was easily pictured, in the imagery of one historian, as 'Circe in crinoline', a demure seductress who behind her skirts carried a chalice filled with poison.[21]

In the summer of 1846, there came to light in the county of Essex a situation so shocking as to be deemed without parallel 'in the truths or fictions of even French life', and that would elevate the fear of female poisoners to absurd heights. At the centre of the storm was one Sarah Chesham, aka 'Sally Arsenic', responsible, it appeared, for a whole string of poisonings: 'deeds which the imagination connects with the Medicis', *The Times* blared, 'are seen at this moment naturalized in an uneducated English county'. Chesham, 'a masculine-looking woman', resided in the village of Clavering (when, only months later, Bulwer Lytton published his novel of poisoning, he gave the title-character Lucretia the last name of Clavering so as to send extra chills through readers). There and in neighbouring settlements, she was 'well known' to be a poisoner, so well known that 'mothers used to keep their infants within doors when she was seen to be prowling about the village, and snatch their children out of her path, as they would from that of any noxious animal'. She had a habit, according to gossip, of carrying about poisoned lozenges which she offered to children as treats; one woman swore that she had just barely managed to snatch her own infant from the jaws of death 'by plucking the deadly morsel from its lips'.[22]

Yet nothing had been done to interfere with her murderous career until that summer of 1846, when her actions led to her arrest on suspicion of poisoning an acquaintance's illegitimate baby. Two of her sons had died suddenly several months previously, presumably of intestinal illness, and, it now came out, the entire village suspected she had poisoned them yet had said 'little more about it than if she had killed her pigs'. Now that she was in custody, every tongue began wagging. The two children, who had been buried in a single coffin, were exhumed, and found to have large amounts of arsenic in their stomachs. An inquest quickly led to Chesham being indicted for murder, and she was brought to trial in the spring of 1847. The evidence against her seemed conclusive: her sons had arsenic in their bodies, police had found 'an assortment of poisons' in her house, and during the trial there were clear attempts to coerce witnesses not to testify against her. Sarah Chesham was nevertheless acquitted of all charges. The verdict struck most observers as outrageous, but even if it was correct, something very disturbing was going on. The woman's neighbours had believed her to be spreading poison for years, yet had uttered not a word to the authorities. 'What is to be said', a newspaper asked, 'of a district where cold-blooded murder meets with all the popular favour which is shown to smuggling in Sussex?'[23]

The bad news was only beginning. One of the rumours about Chesham was that she was 'zealous in making proselytes', teaching other women the secrets of poisoning 'as a good useful trick of management' for husbands and children (when one woman complained to Chesham of her husband's treatment of her, she was told she should 'make him up a pie of sheep's liver, lights [lungs], etc., and if she brought it down to her [Chesham] she would season it for her').[24]

One of her recruits was Mary May, convicted in 1848 of poisoning her brother with arsenic for his burial club pay-out. Police had reason to believe May had also poisoned her husband and some of her fourteen children ('most of whom died suddenly'). But what was most upsetting was that shortly before her execution, the poisoner confessed that she had been schooled in her deadly art by Sarah Chesham—and, it soon appeared, had in turn passed her knowledge on to another woman, Hannah Ham (readers will have noticed in journalists' reports on Cotton and Chesham a propensity to describe female murderers' physical appearance; Ham, we are told, was 'rather good-looking', while May was 'a repulsive-looking woman'). Ham's husband died suddenly in the spring of 1847, apparently of natural causes. But the trials of Chesham and May had aroused anxiety that a rash of poisonings had broken out, and it was common knowledge among the Hams' neighbours that their marriage had been somewhat less than happy. Thus shortly after May's execution the body of Thomas Ham was exhumed—and found to be rich in arsenic. His wife had been known to be having an affair with a farmer named John Southgate, once having run off with him for a fortnight, taunting her husband on her return with the news she had been to see 'my Johnny'. Then, less than four months after her husband's burial, she had married her Johnny. Hannah Southgate was arrested on suspicion of murder in August, 1848 and tried the following spring.[25]

The case against her was strong. Testimony revealed she had had arsenic in her possession; that her six children had also 'dropped off short'; that not long before her husband's death, she had entertained Mary May at lunch and May had suggested getting rid of the husband; and that she had more than once voiced the wish her husband would die, had referred to him as 'a nasty little blackguard', had been caught beating him with a whip, and had told a friend that she 'liked John's little finger better than the deceased's whole carcase'. The jury deliberated only a few minutes before declaring her—not guilty.[26]

That a jury could return such a verdict confirmed the public's worst fears: Essex had become a hotbed of female poisoners, villages being now so overrun with the vipers that no one dared offend them. Hysteria was set into full gallop. The women of Essex, the papers reported, were given to 'wholesale indiscriminate and almost gratuitous assassination', killing for both love (a new husband, such as John Southgate) and money. The latter they got from the burial clubs in which nearly all, it was supposed, enrolled their offspring. When passing through an Essex village, an over-agitated journalist wrote, and 'you...see the children playing in the sunshine', you must realize that many 'are predoomed to a painful and lingering destruction; that the blooming cheek *must* soon grow pale, the rounded form be worn down by an emaciating fire from within, and the changing expression of childhood give way to the monotonous aspect of death'. And if you would know just how many of them 'are destined to so premature a fate, ascertain how many have been entered by their parents in the BURIAL CLUBS, and you may then guess with tolerable accuracy the number marked for death'.[27]

Arsenical murder had become so everyday an occurrence that women in the area talked openly of 'white powdering' their mates and offspring (or they might 'season a pie' for them, as Chesham had advised, or 'give him a dose'; such terms held on for some time, it being the practice after Jack the Ripper terrorized Whitechapel in 1888 for husbands upset with their wives to threaten to 'whitechapel' them, and the wives to retort with a promise to 'white powder' them first). White-powderers were so commonplace they could practice their art 'without incurring thereby any greater disrepute than if they had been poachers or smugglers'. Everyone knew what they were doing, but no one felt it a duty to notify the authorities for, through repetition, 'murder itself no longer wore any hideous or repulsive aspect in the eyes' of these provincials.[28]

Stories circulated of mass exhumations of children and husbands to test for arsenic, and of women taking on new mates, men with whom they had been intimate before their husbands had died. Nor did the women limit themselves to family members, for poisoning 'seems to acquire a zest of its own [and] becomes a frightful kind of gratification', cascading into 'a moral epidemic far more formidable than any plague'. Reputedly, there were actually clubs scattered through Essex that placed poison and knowledge of its use in women's hands so they could do away with any bothersome person. Only execution could stop them, and indeed these deadly women were cited more than once as the best refutation of the fledgling campaign to abolish the death penalty. The movement to end capital punishment had no chance of success in any event, not in the mid-1800s. But when confronted with the threat of the Essex 'dabblers in death', it was as doomed as any convicted murderer.[29]

Execution was, however, the fate of only one other of the supposed legion of Essex poisoners besides Mary May. Sarah Chesham was acquitted of killing her children in 1847. Two years later, her husband died after weeks of painful illness. Given her past, and all the excitement stirred up over Essex women in general, it was inevitable she would be suspected of murder. A neighbour related she had said of her husband that 'it would be no more harm to kill such a man...than it would be to kill a mouse'. When arsenic was found in the man's body, and the rice she had used for some of his meals was determined to be 'all over arsenic' (the pound of rice remaining contained sixteen grains of the poison), there could be no escape. She was promptly tried and executed. With her death, the Essex poisoning epidemic at last subsided, though it would be a topic of conversation for years to come: nearly a decade after Chesham's hanging, *The Times* was still wondering 'how long had the Essex poisonings flourished before the system was discovered?'[30]

*

The arsenic panic of the 1840s was not all that different from the anthrax anxiety that gripped America in the months after the September 11 terrorist attacks, when a mysterious white powder seemed to be turning up everywhere and more than one person was wrongly suspected of scattering spores among the public. A Victorian man likewise was accused of killing his wife with poison because a servant girl with whom he was suspected of being intimate was found carrying a packet of white powder. When the wife's body was disinterred and tested for arsenic, none was found—and the suspicious packet was determined to contain sugar. Amidst all this patent overreaction, alarmists nevertheless hit upon certain vital elements of truth. However serious this moral epidemic might be, it could not be brought under control until physicians became more alert to signs of suspicious death, regulations were imposed on the sale of arsenic, and 'beyond all other measures', adequate funding was provided for arresting and trying poisoners. Here was a

second economic factor tempting people into the crime of poisoning: financial constraints on judicial institutions resulted in many
crimes going uninvestigated, and this being a widely known secret,
it encouraged potential killers to calculate that their act might well
be ignored if it were subtle enough in nature.[31]

Funds allotted by government for the work of police and judiciary had always fallen short of need, no doubt, but during the
1830s, a ratepayer revolt against rising taxes forced legal institutions to tighten their belts still further. More than ever, enforcement
of the law had to be rationed. 'Punishment of every crime that is
committed is clearly unattainable,' a barrister observed; 'the only
attainable object is example.' In particular, authorities had to select
the suspicious deaths they would investigate, and hope that the
example made of the unfortunates they chose would deter at least
some others from committing similar acts. It has been argued, in
fact, that capital punishment for murder was maintained primarily
because the most extreme deterrent was needed as a counterweight
to the laxness with which the crime was prosecuted.[32]

'Many a suspicious case of death is slurred over without notice
in order to save the fees incurred by the inquest.'[33] With that comment, a journalist pinpointed the critical stage in the workings of
justice that was disrupted by pecuniary constraints. The inquest
was the preliminary hearing and evaluation of evidence related to
a suspicious death. It determined whether a suspect was committed to trial or cleared of the charge. An inquest cost money. If it
was not held, money was saved.

When it was held, the inquest was directed by the coroner of the
jurisdiction in which the death occurred. The office of the coroner
(derived from *corona*, or crown) had existed since medieval times
as the agency representing the Crown's interests in investigating
all violent or unexplained deaths. By the nineteenth century, there

were over 300 coroners in England and Wales, the majority being lawyers by training (in Scotland a slightly different system and terminology prevailed). Each served for life, or at least for as long as he did 'well behave himself in his office'.[34]

The chief duty of the coroner was to convene inquests when there was reason to believe a death was unnatural, an event that during the 1800s applied to 5–7 per cent of all deaths annually. As soon as possible after receiving notice of such a death, the coroner was supposed to issue a warrant summoning from twelve to twenty-four 'good and lawful men' to appear before him at a specified time and place to be sworn in as jurors. After viewing the body, the jury sat to hear testimony from anyone having knowledge of the circumstances of the death, most questions being directed to witnesses by the coroner, the rest coming from individual jurors. At the end of the hearing, the jury rendered a verdict that either ordered the suspect be jailed and held for trial or dismissed the allegations as unsubstantiated.[35]

Like other of society's institutions, the inquest worked far better in theory than in practice. To begin with, not every coroner was a model of astuteness whose steel-trap mind instantly snapped shut on any inconsistency in testimony or uncertainty in evidence. Rather, it is clear that many were poorly equipped by intellect and/or temperament to direct investigations skilfully and were prone to errors of both omission and commission.[36]

Second, inquests, by long tradition, were held in the community's social centre, the pub ('the Coroner', Dickens quipped in *Bleak House*, 'frequents more public-houses than any man alive'). Whether it was the Horse and Groom or the White Hart, a public house did not provide an environment conducive to sober judicial inquiry. The *Bleak House* inquest at the Sol's Arms, in which the coroner struggles to make himself heard over the ale-swilling rowdies playing at skittles, was the norm. An inquest, sometimes with the body of the deceased available for public viewing, was welcome entertainment for the diversion-hungry masses, an occasion for tippling and merriment at the moment and a fount of sordid conversation for weeks to come. Not just spectators, but witnesses too might partake of the publican's offerings, and even the jurors were not disallowed from having a dram to sustain them through the proceedings. 'The majesty of death', it was said of the atmosphere of the pub inquest, 'evaporated with the fumes from the gin of the jury.'[37]

An inquiry into the deaths of three children near Ely in 1847 (they were determined to have been killed by arsenic) was most notable for 'the ignorance and brutality of the wretched inhabitants' who attended, people 'totally devoid of any moral feeling or restraint', a rabble that 'laugh at the proceedings of the coroner, and devote the day of the inquest to revelry and drunkenness'. While the jury deliberated in an upstairs room, 'the scene below beggared description', what with the fathers of the dead children 'in a state of intoxication' and the mothers holding forth in 'the most obscene language'. One of the fathers did stir from his stupor long enough to opine that the suspected murderess had done the right thing in getting rid of the children: 'There was a deal too many of 'em, and nine out of every ten ought to be put out of the way.' Not until the closing years of the century would inquests be moved from pubs to more solemn surroundings such as court rooms or quarters in other municipal institutions, though in some rural areas the public house continued to serve the purpose until the 1920s.[38]

Inquiries undertaken in such a mood of frivolity were, unavoidably, sometimes less serious and searching than they ought to have been. A commentator on the inquest into a series of arsenic poisonings in Somerset in 1844 voiced an oft-heard complaint, that such investigations were 'too frequently mockeries', 'loose and careless' affairs in which juries returned verdicts 'totally at variance with the evidence adduced'. But at least those inquests took place. In all too many instances, questionable deaths were left unquestioned. First off, coroners could not initiate inquests on their own. They were empowered to act only after a complaint had been registered that a death might be due to a criminal act. Complaints often came from the doctors who attended the deceased and, once the institution of police forces began to spread to communities beyond London during the 1830s, from policemen investigating a report of death. But when there was no clear evidence of violence (as was so commonly the case with arsenic), it was up to lay citizens who might suspect murder to act. As was shown in Essex, citizens did not always take their suspicions to the authorities. 'The coroner is not often enough called upon to hold his inquest in cases of suspected death by foul means,' a medical editor in the 1850s stated as a widely recognized fact. Relatives and acquaintances of poisoning victims 'commonly talked about their having been put out of the way' without doing anything about it, or else they got around to acting only after the passing of considerable time. 'Are not the ghastly remains of parent, child, or friend', he asked rhetorically, 'being continually disinterred, years after their burial, in consequence of suspicions having incidentally come to the ears of justice, long after they were the public talk of the village?'[39]

Often, though, it was not indolent citizens who were at fault, but the authorities themselves. Coroners had to be paid for their time (for most of the century on a straight fee-per-inquest basis), and physicians called to examine the body also had to be compensated. The purse strings for allocations for inquests, however, were held by justices of the peace, in the nineteenth century the chief officers for local law enforcement. Almost to a man, it seems, justices were reluctant to dispense their limited financial resources unless there was overwhelming reason to suspect a death had been unnatural. In Devon by mid-century, justices were applying such pressure to conserve funds that even highly suspicious cases were commonly passed over with the classification 'died by the visitation of God' rather than subjected to an inquest. In 1857, Yorkshire justices actually denied payment for the coroner's expenses in ten inquests because they had been held 'needlessly', that is, no foul play had been uncovered, though the fact they were 'needless' could be determined only by holding the inquest.[40]

Such penuriousness is difficult to justify given the national outrage stirred up in the mid-1840s by a series of murders in a village on the Norfolk coast. Within a span of three years, three grandchildren and the wife of one Jonathan Balls died suddenly with the classic symptoms of arsenic intoxication. The village rumour mill cranked out suspicions of poisoning, but no one took the step of contacting the coroner. The local justice of the peace, moreover, along with others throughout the county, had been directed to proceed conservatively in calling for inquiries, 'there having been a deal of complaint at the magistrates' meetings as to the heavy expense of coroners' inquests'. After old man Balls himself died with vomiting and purging, the coroner was at last notified of a problem, but he too stalled until being forced into action by a deluge of complaints from villagers. When the inquest was finally held, the bodies of all five of the deceased were disinterred and analysed for arsenic. The poison was detected in four (Balls's stomach 'contained arsenic enough to poison the whole parish'); the remains of the fifth, a 9-week-old girl, were 'so much decomposed that its various parts could not be distinguished'. The jury decided that at least four of the deaths were due to arsenic, and that Jonathan Balls was likely responsible, though he was now, they regretted, 'beyond the reach of the law'.[41]

'The Norfolk poisonings' were detected only three months before the Essex scandal, and no doubt served to make the response to Chesham and Southgate even more extreme than it would otherwise have been. Balls was, in fact, excoriated in the press much the way the female poisoners would be. He was 'the arch-murderer,' possessed by a 'master-propensity' to poisoning that was 'irresistible', driven 'solely by the lust for murder'. He had killed, it was reckoned, not just his wife and three grandchildren, but five other grandchildren, one of his own children, and his parents. The near-octogenarian's fellow villagers now recalled that 'strangers with whom this wretch had no imaginable connexion have died suddenly, after calling at his home or being in his company'; these included 'a casual wayfarer' destroyed by a cup of ale offered by Balls. Evidently, the man had carried on 'a system of wholesale murder' for years, a series of crimes 'so incredibly stupendous as not yet to have been dramatized in a French novel'. When Balls finally began to fear his deeds would be uncovered, he took arsenic himself, controlled by his master-propensity to the end.[42]

The Balls case was particularly upsetting because it was a demonstration of the tragic consequences of the law being 'negatived by the criminal parsimony of county officers'. In the name of frugality, people were being allowed not only to get away with murder, but emboldened to get away with it more than once. Had an inquest been held at the death of the first victim, Balls could have been stopped before passing beyond reach of the law and prevented from killing at least three other people and finally himself. The affair so shocked the public that the Home Secretary was compelled to intervene personally, sending 'a chemist of eminence' from London to Norfolk to examine the remains of other suspected victims (poison was found in several, including a child who had been buried ten years). The whole mishandled affair was a disturbing proof that undertaking inquests with such evident reluctance was bound to persuade poisoners that their form of murder was 'a deed as safe as they had found it to be easy'. The lesson was not taken to heart, unfortunately, and ten years later the *British Medical Journal* could still ask 'how many persons now sleep under the turf with arsenic in their intestines who would have been alive at this moment' if their killers had known that an inquest was certain to follow the deaths. The forgoing of inquests was 'nothing less than offering a premium upon poisoning'.[43]

Sometimes financial considerations resulted in an incomplete inquest. In 1845, Sarah Freeman was executed for having poisoned her child, mother, husband, and brother. On the death of her first victim, the 7-year-old son, an inquest was held, but when the surgeon who had cared for the child suggested performing an autopsy, which would have doubled his remuneration, he was informed that 'the magistrates were particular as regarded the expenses'. Discouraged from doing the post-mortem, he assigned the death to natural causes and the jury agreed. Sarah Freeman was left to go her murderous way for another fifteen months, until, with the death of her brother under circumstances too suspicious to be ignored, she was subjected to another inquest. At that point, the child was exhumed and the autopsy finally carried out. Lethal amounts of arsenic were found in his remains.[44]

Such stories could be duplicated at length. They might also be summarized by disturbing statistics. During a four-month period in Manchester in 1846, for example, 279 deaths of children were recorded. Fewer than half of those children were attended by physicians, so the cause of many of the deaths was anybody's guess. It was by then no

secret that parents frequently poisoned children for the burial benefits
or to save money, yet for that same four-month period, only eighty-
seven inquests were held in Manchester on people of all ages. The
odds, clearly, were against getting caught, and it was not without reason that some argued that justices of the peace, by neglecting to fund
inquests, encouraged the killing of children. Such concerns led at last
to an 1860 Coroners Act that provided for coroners to be salaried;
they would henceforth not have to worry that a justice of the peace
would deny their application for expenses incurred for inquests. The
frequency of inquests began to rise at once.[45]

*

Through all of these events and the growing public fear of poisoners, the crime of poisoning itself took on a special mystique. Ian
Burney has described how during the 1800s the administration of
arsenic, and other poisons, came to be regarded as the type of
crime characteristic of civilized societies. In less advanced cultures,
murder was most often committed as a spontaneous, unpremedi-
tated act of passion using weapons of a direct, physical nature—
bludgeons, swords, guns. In more mature, sophisticated societies,
subtlety was the ideal. Now, a nineteenth-century English coroner
observed, 'villainy is so refined' that killers planned and schemed
before acting, employed means that were not perceptible and created no wounds, and that caught victims unawares and unable to
defend themselves. The bold and violent assassin of yore was being
replaced by 'a smoothfaced, plausible person, without any external
symptoms of depravity'.[46]

But labelling poisoning a crime of refinement was not intended
to compliment the poisoner. By acting secretly and in cold blood,
usually against trusting family or friends, those who killed with poison were 'murderers of the blackest dye', their crimes 'so foul and
hideous as to haunt the guilty to death by its mere image'. Such
people deserved the full measure of retribution prescribed by law.

During the reign of Henry VIII, poisoners were held to be so despicable the punishment prescribed for them was to be boiled alive, lowered ever so slowly feet first into the steaming water. The statute was repealed after Henry's death, yet public feeling against poisoning still ran hot in Victorian times: 'Incensed at the most cowardly of crimes', the upright citizen 'regards with horror the execrable assassin; and loudly demands the punishment of a monster'.[47]

Consequently, while hangings drew a crowd no matter what the crime involved (at least until public executions were ended in 1868), the punishments meted out to poisoners were special events. Thousands turned out for Mary Blandy's hanging, we have seen, but that was nothing exceptional. For another example, there was the 1849 execution of Rebecca Smith for poisoning her children to save them from want:

It is impossible to give anything like a correct calculation of the numbers of persons present to witness the awful scene—they were countless. From 9 until 11 o'clock people poured into the town [Devizes] in shoals, on foot, in waggons, in boats; and by the latter hour, the prison yard, the banks of the canal, every tree, hedge, and field that could command a view of the drop appeared crammed. Still the roads were lined with persons thronging to the spot. People were there from every part of the county—old, young, and infants; but they were chiefly of the labouring classes, and there were thousands more of women than of men.[48]

The fact that most attendees were women did not mean that the crowd's comportment was polite or respectful. Several gentlemen of the University may have been moved to tears at Mary Blandy's execution, but she was a sympathetic figure believed by many to have been manipulated by the true killer. Most poisoners and other murderers were seen as receiving their just desserts when they swung, and onlookers were moved to jeers and cheers, not tears. The atmosphere that reigned at public hangings has often been portrayed in literature and film, but a brief reminder would do no harm. The estimated 7,000 people who attended Sarah Chesham's hanging began gathering before dawn, taut with impatience, 'thinking the minutes hours until the condemned made [her] appearance'. As usual, their ranks included 'a disgusting number of women', some of whom 'had gay flowers in their bonnets', while 'others were mothers, giving suck to infants'. Elderly matrons, veterans of these festivities, were seen 'pointing out to their young daughters how they could best see the execution', while the calls of fruit vendors rang out in the background.[49]

The circus atmosphere only added to the horror for the prisoner facing imminent extinction, and it is difficult not to feel at least some small measure of sympathy for the poisoner brought to the scaffold, no matter how black her or his dye. Sarah Chesham was a model of composure at her trial: 'the prisoner did not betray the least emotion' when the death sentence was pronounced, and once the judge concluded, 'she walked with a firm step from the dock'. But when it came time to walk to the rope, her legs turned to jelly. The second participant in an 1851 double hanging, she watched her predecessor (who had strangled a lady friend he had impregnated) jerk and writhe for nearly five minutes after the trap was sprung. After that, 'the terrors of a violent and disgraceful death were too strong for her [and] she required the assistance of two persons as she moved forward'. On reaching the steps to the platform she fought off being carried up for several minutes, making the crowd restive at this delay of their gratification. But at last she was—'with difficulty'—conveyed to the noose, still held upright by two attendants. 'And then while with "bated breath," the thousands of spectators below looked on, the bolt was drawn; a faint murmur of horror spread among the crowd as they saw the sentence of the law carried into effect, which was prolonged as the convulsive struggles of the dying…woman were painfully visible.'

She took even longer than the man to expire: 'they were both light figures, and they "died hard"'.[50]

In the case of Mary Gallop, executed in 1844 for poisoning her father with arsenic, the fear was so paralysing she had to be carried to the scaffold in a chair. She soon must have wished she had found the fortitude to stand, for by sitting she did not fall so far, and 'the mortal struggle...was of frightful duration'. Eventually, 'the convulsion of the countenance and the quivering of the limb announced that suffering was at an end', and the crowd began to disperse, besieged no doubt, as they were after Chesham's death, by 'hawkers of ballads and "true and correct accounts" of the execution, and all kinds of edibles [who] appeared among them', so that 'the assemblage was a sort of moving fair on its way back to town'. One can empathize fully with Mary Milner, sentenced in 1847 to hang for using arsenic to kill her mother-in-law, sister-in-law, and niece for burial club money (she poisoned her father-in-law as well, though he survived, 'reduced to imbecility'). Unwilling to be made a spectacle before the brutish mob, she hanged herself in her cell the night before her appointment with Calcraft.[51]

One might feel a touch of sympathy for this new race of poisoners for a second reason: by the 1840s, arsenic-wielding predators were themselves being stalked by a new breed of detective, the forensic toxicologist.

3

A New Breed of Detectives

It might seem that Sarah Chesham has suffered enough abuse, what with vilification as 'Sally Arsenic' and 'noxious animal' topped off by slow strangulation. There was, however, still another line of attack against the woman: characterization of her as a monster not just for poisoning her husband, but even for the *way* she poisoned him. When she killed her sons in 1846 (everyone presumed she did, despite the decision of the jury), she finished them off quickly, with large doses of arsenic. She was not so considerate of her mate. With him, she administered the poison 'at intervals and in small doses, consuming him by slow tortures', tortures that lasted no less than six months. Sally Arsenic put this victim away through the sub-acute poisoning described in Chapter 1, slow but steady destruction of life by repetition of debilitating but not immediately lethal doses. Throughout his half-year decline, Mr Chesham endured vomiting, chest pain, disordered bowels, and a sensation of 'gnawing' in his stomach, 'as though something was feeding on it'. In between the intermittent doses, he might improve for a bit, but soon relapsed, sicker than before.[1]

Slow poisoning was described as early as ancient Rome, and in later centuries, Toffana was believed to have mastered the art, though her skills, physicians knew by 1800, had been 'exaggerated by vulgar credulity': she could not have been capable of managing doses so as to produce death on any predetermined day. Yet open-ended slow poisoning, with death resulting simply sooner or later, was a reality, and an important element of the arsenic panic of the mid-1800s was the conviction that sub-acute poisoning was occurring ever more commonly. This was highly troubling, because, marked by milder symptoms, slow poisoning was more difficult to recognize; these new murderers operated 'with a skill and a nicety' that defied easy discovery.[2]

Would-be poisoners thus had a choice. They could give large doses, which would kill quickly and more surely but with greater chance of detection. Or they could give small doses, which were less certain and took more time but were not so likely to draw attention (Thomas Smethurst, whose trial will be considered in the next chapter, was representative of the extended, low-risk option: 'he neither spared her nor injured his own chances of impunity by precipitancy'). It was all a matter of tension between the perpetrator's level of patience and tolerance for risk. How much longer could she put up with him? How ready was he to chance precipitancy in getting rid of her?[3]

Although either course of action was reprehensible, the protracted one struck physicians and public alike as the greater abomination. It was not just that suffering was spread out over a much longer span of time. What was more disturbing was the cold-bloodedness of the deed, its calculated scheme of doing just enough injury to day-by-day nudge the victim down the path to dissolution without producing symptoms alarming enough to arouse suspicion. 'Wives destroy their husbands by means of the long agonies of days or weeks,' a censor of this new 'murder mania' fumed, sitting 'like Gouls [*sic*] by their bedside... gloating on the struggles of their despair' while pretending to the last to be loving caregivers:

> The cursed crimes of the secret poisoner
> We must confess are the worst of all,
> You bless the hand that smooths your pillow
> But by that hand you surely fall.
> You put your trust in those about you,
> When you lie sick upon your bed,
> While you are blessing they are wishing
> The very next moment would find you dead.[4]

'Murder mania' had another bothersome aspect, which was that it seemed due in a way to the actions of physicians themselves. Every trial for murder by poison involved testimony by at least one doctor or surgeon on the properties and effects and modes of administration of the poison involved. Court proceedings were, in effect, public seminars on how to kill. Much was made of Sarah Chesham's first trial, where famed toxicologist Alfred Taylor had elaborated on the differences between acute and sub-acute poisoning. The prisoner 'stood quietly at the bar, listened, and learnt'. No sooner was she acquitted than she began to apply Taylor's instruction. Whereas previously 'she had...poisoned her people out-of-hand after a coarse and unscientific fashion of proceeding', she now turned to a plan of 'intervals' and 'small doses' and 'slow tortures'.[5]

That prisoners and court audiences and even jurymen were educated in the ways of murder by poison was bad enough. But when every poisoning trial received detailed coverage in the press, with word-for-word reporting of medical evidence, there seemed good reason to fear the entire populace might be initiated into the mysteries of assassination by poison. 'A murder occurs,' one alarmist imagined; 'the journalist does his work; and the poison he gives forth floats over the country like a pestilence.' Decent people would be repulsed by the information, of course, 'but the vulgar drink in the details with a hideous delight', and soon another murder is done. Bulwer Lytton's *Lucretia* was condemned for the same reason. Coming hard on the heels of the discovery of the Essex poisoning epidemic, the book was an instant hit, being 'devoured' by readers, *The Times* announced, despite—or for many because of—being filled with 'sickening and unpardonable revelations'. It was a 'precious catalogue of sin', a 'crowning work of hideousness' certain to bring about 'incalculable evil': such umbrage, particularly when in actuality the author provided far too little detail to educate anyone to be an accomplished poisoner.[6]

There was nearly as much paranoia over court reporters and novelists as over the sickening deeds they related, paranoia that inflated the possibility of being secretly poisoned beyond all reality. 'If you feel a deadly sensation within,' one newspaper asked, 'and grow gradually weaker, how do you know you are not poisoned? If your hands tingle, do you not fancy that it is arsenic?' Of course people did after reading passages like that. After all, 'how can you be sure that it is not?...Your friends and relations all smile kindly upon you; the meal...looks correct; but how can you possibly tell that there is not arsenic in the curry?' How indeed? When properly done, it was supposed, slow poisoning was so subtle that the usual signs of arsenic intoxication simply didn't appear. The only external evidence of poison in Smethurst's victim, one writer said, was 'a strange look of concentrated terror about the face, which could not be explained on any other hypothesis'. With the public being conditioned to live in mortal fear of being poisoned, a look of concentrated terror must have been the near-universal expression.[7]

Yet if there was exaggerated despair over slow arsenic poisoning sweeping the land by mid-century, there was also a burgeoning optimism that medicine and chemistry were catching up to villainy, and that through science the detection of poisoning both fast and slow was being made far more reliable than in the past. During the early 1800s, a new field of study, medical jurisprudence—medicine in the service of the law—had arisen to place new obstacles in the path of the poisoner.

This is not to say that the physicians of previous centuries had been powerless to assist legal authorities in cases of violent death. Since the Renaissance, at least, their expertise had been regularly tapped to answer such questions as whether a knife wound had been self-inflicted or administered by another, if strangling had been performed manually or by garotte, or if a dead newborn had ever breathed (i.e. had there been a stillbirth or might the mother have killed the baby after delivery). Doctors had been called upon as well to help settle other physical matters of legal import, such as rape, or the determination of virginity or impotence in claims of unconsummated marriage.[8]

Books on these topics began to be published as early as the 1500s, but it was not until the later 1700s that medical jurisprudence truly came of age. During those years, an important transition in medical thought occurred, diseases coming to be characterized less in terms of their outward symptoms and more by the specific pathological lesions to be found internally in individual organs and tissues. To take an example, 'consumption', an ailment marked by emaciation (the body was seemingly being consumed), coughing, and spitting of blood came to be thought of as pulmonary tuberculosis, a disease in which distinctive nodules of a cheese-like consistency—tubercles—developed in the lungs. The discovery of internal lesions required the performance of autopsies, a practice that came into widespread use in the later 1700s. The autopsy provided much more, and more reliable, information about cause of death, and thus markedly expanded the range of medical jurisprudence (this was particularly true in cases of poisoning, where symptoms alone were often insufficient to allow confident determination of the exact agent involved). The field's new sophistication is evident in the stream of textbooks on the subject that flowed forth in the early 1800s and in the establishment of university professorships in the field. By the 1820s, would-be poisoners should have been thinking twice before slipping arsenic into the teapot.[9]

Through texts and lectures, medical students and physicians were now enjoined to be on the lookout for any signs of foul play when called to attend a patient, and to bring any suspicions to the attention of the local coroner: they were the ones with the knowledge to uncover 'the first clue of many a hideous maze of crime'. That expertise could also be decisive at the inquest, where the practitioner testified as to the meaning of the patient's symptoms and, if an autopsy had been performed, his internal lesions. As has been seen, post-mortem examination was often opposed by the authorities on economic grounds (it doubled the doctor's compensation), but the criminals themselves, with much more to lose than money, were even less eager for an autopsy. It would only add to their terrible emotional distress, they protested, while simultaneously insulting the dignity of the departed loved one. Sarah Chesham's two sons were not autopsied at the time of death because their physician was swayed by the mother's tears: 'I could not bear to see them cut about.' Resistance of a parent or spouse to a post-mortem, physicians recognized, might well be one of those clues to a hideous maze of crime.[10]

When poisoners got away with crime, however, the error could not all be laid at the feet of penny-pinching justices of the peace and empathic doctors. An additional reason for the failures of inquests and trials to snare the guilty was that the physicians who were called upon to testify had not all kept abreast of the discoveries of medical jurisprudence. Doctors were repeatedly enjoined by professional leaders to educate themselves to better fulfil their legal obligations, yet despite the exhortations, many doctors appear to have lagged behind in knowledge, not least in their familiarity with the action of poisons. As one critic remonstrated in the 1850s, one of the most startling revelations of recent poisoning trials was the fact that many physicians had not 'noted with sufficient accuracy the effect of arsenic and other poisons upon the human body'. It was unconscionable 'when prisoners at the bar are trembling between life and death' for medical men to 'be found guessing upon matters which may send them to the scaffold'.[11]

Yet the value of even the best-informed physician's testimony was only as strong as the intelligence of the juror who heard it— and that too provoked cynicism. The ideal of the jury of judicious peers was repeatedly undone, doctors complained, by the reality of the 'under-educated, dull-brained Englishmen who compose a normal jury.' How could unlettered tradesmen be expected to comprehend the words of men of lofty scientific attainments? When jurymen sometimes fainted during the presentation of the details of a post-mortem, how could they be counted on for an informed judgement of guilt or innocence?[12]

Trying to impart scientific understanding to commoners was child's play, however, compared to communicating with attorneys. Any physician today who has been delivered to the tender mercies of a trial attorney will readily relate to the indignant reminiscences of Victorian doctors made to undergo that experience. There was no situation in which 'so much personal uneasiness is endured', a practitioner of the 1820s moaned, as being called to the witness box. There, the doctor was nothing more than a 'butt for forensic impertinence', buffeted by 'the brow-beating and bullying behaviour of rude lawyers' from one side while being 'foully aspersed by the counsel for the defence' from the other.

Expected to answer unerringly questions which he could not fully anticipate, a physician had to be possessed of exceptional knowledge and *sang-froid* both to come through the trial with reputation intact—and to avoid mistakes that might let the guilty go free, or the innocent hang.[13]

Those who did possess the requisite knowledge and nerve could be the critical figures in solving murders committed through poison. It has been seen with Cotton, Balls, and others that their crimes came to light only with the discovery of arsenic in the remains of their victims. These discoveries were the work of medical jurisprudence, of course, but most particularly of a new sub-speciality within the field, forensic toxicology, the science of poisons related to crime.

*

Like medical jurisprudence in general, forensic toxicology took form in the early 1800s. That is not to suggest that the properties of poisons had been left unexplored before that time, but not even Toffana could be called a toxicologist, not in the sense of carrying out systematic investigations of the physiological effects of toxic substances, methods of detecting their presence, and means of neutralizing their action. As a genuine scientific discipline, toxicology came into being only at the beginning of the nineteenth century, thanks in greatest measure to the extraordinary labours of the Spaniard Mateu Orfila.

Orfila (1787–1853) studied medicine and chemistry in his native land, then moved to Paris at the age of 20. There he stayed until his death, working first as professor of medicine, then of chemistry, at the University of Paris, and winning renown as the author of *Traité des Poisons (Treatise on Poisons)*, the first true textbook of toxicology. Published in 1814, under his Gallicized name *Mathieu* Orfila, the 1,300-plus pages of the *Traité* surveyed the full catalogue of mineral, vegetable, and animal poisons, describing the physical and chemical properties of each and placing it within a classificatory framework according to its mechanism of toxic action (there were corrosive and irritant poisons, for example, arsenic's category, along with astringents, narcotics, and other types). This last area—the determination of each poison's manner of destroying life—was especially challenging, as it involved administering the different materials to animals, establishing the lethal dose for each, closely observing and recording symptoms and the length of time till death, and then autopsying the dead subjects to characterize the pathological lesions produced. These researches, covering a span of three years, involved the sacrifice of several thousand dogs (as well as lesser numbers of other species), and, it must be remembered, the animals were not anaesthetized. Anesthetics did not come into use until the 1840s, and in any event could not be given to animals on which a poison was being tested without invalidating the experiment. The object of the trial, after all, was to determine the effects of the poison, not the effects of poison mixed with anaesthetic. Orfila's animals suffered terribly in the cause of science (arsenic affects dogs, cats, and horses the same as it does people), and his peers did not fail to take notice. For them, those experiments were the most impressive demonstration of the professor's dedication to the advancement of knowledge: 'he has often been under the necessity of sitting up whole nights, in watching the animals submitted to his trials, and it has required no small degree of courage, to overcome the disgust which accompanies so painful a task'. What was more, the man had drawn 'considerable sums' from his own pocket to purchase all the animals.[14]

One should not, however, be left with an impression of Orfila as cold and unfeeling, even sadistic. Animal experimentation was common throughout the biological sciences, and there were other researchers who inflicted considerably more pain and voiced less remorse (French physiologist François Magendie comes to mind). To people, Orfila could be charming. He was much beloved by students, who found him an entrancing lecturer. Under his 'quick and sparkling delivery', we are told, the subject of chemistry 'seemed to dance'. Apparently no topic was beyond his magic; even on a matter as unpromising as the iodide of potassium, a student enthused, he could 'convulse his hearers' with anecdote-filled discourse. And in his spare time, Orfila was a highly accomplished singer, one, his friends believed, who could have starred on the lyric stage had he chosen that over the attractions of potassium salts. He had a spirited competitive streak, though, and with fellow scientists he could be trying. Unyielding in his opinions and making little allowance for the abilities of those who disagreed with him, he kept himself almost constantly embroiled in controversy. One suspects that when it was learned he had bequeathed his body for dissection by the University's medical students, there was no shortage of peers volunteering to direct the proceedings.[15]

Prior to Orfila, the understanding of poisons had been muddled with myths and hearsay. The skin of a poisoning victim soon turns black, or blue, or spotted, it had been believed, and the body is given to grotesque swelling. In a trial in the 1840s, the wife testified she gave her aged husband only half the dose of arsenic recommended by her youthful lover 'because he'd swell, and it would be found out'. Conventional wisdom also had it that putrefaction advanced more rapidly in poisoned than in normal corpses. A treatise published as recently as the 1770s assured readers that in instances of arsenic poisoning the body 'quickly liquefies into a pulp', though the definitive sign of poisoning was that the victim's heart would not burn when placed in the fire.[16]

Putting an end to such fanciful notions was not, however, the work of Orfila alone. He was the trailblazer of toxicology, without question, but close behind came several others whose researches also added greatly to the developing science. In Britain, the pioneer was Edinburgh's Robert Christison, a physician whose 1829 *Treatise on Poisons* was the first thorough work on the subject in English. Christison made a brief acquaintance with Orfila while studying in Paris in 1820, and greatly admired his work while holding less generous feelings about the man. On the subject of the taste of arsenic, for example, he was amazed that Orfila asserted the poison had an acrid flavour. His own experiments, using very small amounts of arsenic and 'extending the poison along the tongue as far back, as we thought safe' before spitting it out, had demonstrated it to have 'hardly any taste at all'. Orfila's perceptions of bitterness 'must be either imaginary', Christison concluded, or the reaction of a tongue 'peculiarly constituted'. It appears peculiar lingual constitutions were common, for while most nineteenth-century toxicologists agreed with Christison that arsenic had no distinct taste, some sided with Orfila in finding it biting, and still others maintained it had a sweet edge.[17]

Christison naturally shared the professional consensus that forensic toxicology was the most useful area of knowledge within medical jurisprudence. With most violent deaths, the cause of fatality was clear even to the non-medical observer, though whether homicide or suicide might not be immediately apparent. With poisoning, however, toxicology was needed to link the victim's pre-death symptoms and post-mortem appearances with the presence of a specific poison in his blood and tissues, and thus build an airtight case beyond the circumstantial evidence. Such demonstrations were additionally important, Christison stressed, because with poisoning there was no question of murder in the heat of passion or as an act of self-defence. Poisoning was premeditated: hence forensic toxicology could remove ambiguity from a jury's deliberations.[18]

Forensic toxicologists typically began their court testimony with identification of the probable poison based on the symptoms experienced by the victim—with arsenic, the vomiting, purging, and gastric pain. But rarely was the task so straightforward as that sounds. First, any combination of symptoms might be caused by more than one poison: irritant poisons all commonly induced vomiting and purging to some degree. Second, the symptoms produced by any poison, arsenic most of all, could vary considerably from one individual to another, and in rare cases the standard signs of arsenic might be missing altogether. Finally, symptoms of poisoning were often duplicated to a confusing extent by infectious diseases, leading physicians to attribute to nature a death that had been inflicted by man or woman. 'In how many poisoning cases', the *British Medical Journal* wondered, 'have the victims of jealousy and all other evil passions slept their last sleep, whilst the register of death, in place of noting "the deep damnation of their taking off," speaks only of ordinary disease?' Many presumed to have died from dysentery or gastritis, the *Journal* explained, were in truth martyrs to arsenic, and one could not think of them 'without a shudder'.[19]

With arsenic, the disease most commonly confounding the diagnosis was cholera. In today's usage, 'cholera' applies to a specific acute intestinal infection endemic in undeveloped nations and caused by a certain micro-organism that thrives in unprotected water supplies. But in the nineteenth century, cholera was a generic term, applied to just about any ailment characterized by pronounced diarrhoea (cholera was derived from the Greek for bile). There was, for example, *cholera infantum*, or childhood diarrhoea (which remains the primary killer of young children in poor countries today). The chief reason life expectancy in Europe did not exceed 40 until the second half of the 1800s was that a quarter or more of all children died within their first five years, due above all to the ravages of *cholera infantum*. The various food- and water-borne microbes that caused that infection in youngsters, furthermore, produced *cholera morbus*, or morbid diarrhoea, in adults. Grown-ups were better able to survive the dehydrating effects of the infection than were babies, but a significant percentage died nonetheless. And in both those types of cholera, symptoms (diarrhoea, vomiting, abdominal discomfort) imitated those of arsenic.

Far the most serious form of cholera was *cholera Asiatica*, Asiatic cholera, the severe infection intended by use of the word 'cholera' today. C*holera Asiatica*, it is important to stress, was the most feared of all diseases in Europe and America in the nineteenth century, partly because it was a new disease: endemic to India, it did not spread into Western Europe until the summer of 1831. Unfamiliar and exotic, it excited a good deal more dread than long-known ailments such as tuberculosis, even though the latter claimed many more lives year by year. Asiatic cholera was embarrassing, generally announcing itself with a copious and uncontrollable eruption of liquid (cloudy rice-water stools) from the intestines; it was painful, violent muscular cramping resulting as electrolytes were eliminated from the body; and it was deadly, killing fully 50 per cent of those affected. In the panic of a cholera outbreak, the most likely diagnosis for a patient experiencing purging, stomach pain, and cramping of the legs was *cholera Asiatica*. Cholera epidemics thus provided a screen for poisoners to work behind, and it was axiomatic that advantage was often taken of the opportunity. 'When a rapidly fatal pestilence is abroad, is the time when many a fearful deed of blood is perpetrated,' a London physician observed of several arsenic deaths during an 1854 cholera epidemic.[20]

Yet when considered calmly, there were significant differences to be seen between arsenic poisoning and an attack of Asiatic cholera with respect to the order of vomiting and purging and the appearance of stools. Such distinctions were less easily made between cases of arsenic poisoning and *cholera morbus* or, as British doctors also called it, the English cholera. *Cholera morbus* usually took several days to kill, longer than the typical time for arsenic. But it was marked by diarrhoea, vomiting, and violent abdominal pain, and the attack generally came on fairly soon after a meal (in this case, a meal contaminated with malignant germs instead of poison). It was, in short, quite difficult to distinguish between the two conditions on the basis of symptoms alone.

Consequently, physicians repeatedly diagnosed arsenic cases as attacks of *cholera morbus*, or as gastroenteritis, or dysentery, or, as in the case of most of Mary Ann Cotton's victims, gastric fever. Sarah Chesham's two sons were initially assumed to have died from the English cholera. In the 1857 trial of Madeline Smith, a contender for most-publicized arsenic case of the century, the doctor to the deceased testified he 'took his complaint to be a bilious derangement', and admitted he 'never suspected irritant poison'. Nineteenth-century medical journals abounded with such examples, providing lawyers with a when-all-else-fails tactic, the argument that the alleged victim had died not from arsenic but from some intestinal ailment. In a prominent trial in 1843, the accused was acquitted in spite of weighty circumstantial evidence thanks to his attorney's ability to convince the jury that death might have come from gastroenteritis.[21]

Prior to the nineteenth century, symptoms were the chief source of evidence relied on by physicians to reach a diagnosis of poisoning. But as the ease of confusing the symptoms of poisoning for those of intestinal illness became more apparent, forensic toxicologists turned to other sources of evidence. At first, confidence was placed primarily in linking pathological changes found in internal organs after death with the action of particular poisons. Orfila's dissections of the dogs killed in his experiments were a valuable source of information in this area, reinforced by the observations of a number of other scientists doing experiments on animals, introducing arsenic through the mouth, anus, or other orifices, injecting it into veins, or applying it to open wounds.

Typical of such investigations were those conducted by Anthony Thomson, professor of forensic medicine at the University of London, in 1838. Working with dogs, he employed a standard technique in poisoning tests: he opened the animal's neck, made an incision in its oesophagus, injected a water solution of the poison downward into the opening, then quickly tied off the oesophagus so that the arsenic could not be regurgitated back. In a matter of minutes, there began 'most severe and almost unremitting efforts to vomit'. The dog appeared to be experiencing severe abdominal pain, its heartbeat became 'extremely rapid', and it soon fell to the floor, its legs convulsing violently. 'The moanings of the animal indicated increased suffering,' yet it continued to suffer for two and a half hours more until at last dying. The experiment was repeated on two more dogs, 'merely with the intention of confirming the results'. The results were confirmed in every detail, except that these dogs did not expire quite so soon as the first. With a fourth dog, the initial attempts to vomit were so violent as to cause the oesophagus to burst, and the trial was discontinued. The animals were autopsied for examination of pathological alterations: in each, the stomach and intestinal tract were found to have 'a deep red colour', a finding different in no material respect from what had been observed by Orfila and others.[22]

Nor were the pathology findings on dogs appreciably different from what had been observed since the 1700s in numerous autopsies performed on human beings determined to have died from arsenic. Autopsy was a standard procedure in cases of suspicious death in the eighteenth and nineteenth centuries, and even if suspicions did not arise until after burial of the victim, the law provided for exhumation for purposes of dissection: we have already seen a number of people disinterred months, and even years, after burial. Through that means primarily, an extensive picture of arsenic pathology had been filled in by the early 1800s and incorporated into textbooks of medical jurisprudence.

That picture showed, not surprisingly, that the most striking damages were to be seen in the digestive tract. The stomach typically is observed to be highly inflamed, its inner surface 'covered with tenacious mucus, streaked or deeply tinged with blood', with pronounced reddening of tissue. Physicians' descriptions of the inflammatory tint characteristic of arsenic were themselves highly colourful, ranging from 'red velvet' to 'port wine' to 'the sides of a boiled lobster'. Bright yellow tones were not infrequently met with also, the result of hydrogen sulphide gas generated by putrefaction converting some of the poison into arsenic trisulphide: in several bodies autopsied by a London physician, 'the stomach looked as if coated thickly with yellow paint'.[23]

These gastric changes occur whether the arsenic is introduced by the mouth, rectum, or vagina, or through the lungs in the form of vapours such as the gas arsine. But in cases of oral ingestion, gritty particles of arsenious acid are often discovered adhering in patches to the stomach wall, the organ's mucus lining keeping such a hold on the particles as to prevent them from being expelled even during the most violent fits of vomiting (the stomach of one arsenic victim was determined to hold nearly 100 grains of white arsenic even though the poor man had thrown up repeatedly in his last hours). If the stomach lining is exposed to sunlight, it will glisten with 'diamond-like specks' of arsenic crystals. Reddish- to dark-brown clumps of digested blood, generally described as resembling coffee grounds, are also often present in the deceased's stomach, and if death is drawn out for several days, the stomach may become perforated, 'riddled like a sieve' in one account.[24]

Inflammation is not restricted to the stomach, but generally occurs throughout the intestinal tract. When Francis Blandy was opened two days after death, his bowels, coated with 'a slimy bloody froth', were found to be 'prodigiously inflamed and excoriated', as red, his physician recorded, as the bloodshot white of an eye that had been rubbed with some irritating substance. On the other hand, inflammation of the alimentary tract is not an inevitable result of arsenic poisoning, and a normal-looking stomach could not be cited as proof that arsenic had not been used. Notwithstanding, the absence of inflammation was repeatedly seized by nineteenth-century defence lawyers to argue the victim could not have died from the alleged arsenic, the 'if his stomach isn't red, my client didn't make him dead' stratagem.[25]

Telltale pathological changes showed up in other organs, as well. Inflammation was found in the heart, windpipe, and lungs: Christison reported a case in which the lungs were 'so congested as to resemble a lump of clotted blood'. The tongue, too, was often inflamed and thickened, and the urinary bladder greatly contracted, sometimes so much 'as not to exceed the size of a walnut'. In Mr Blandy, not only was the heart 'variegated with purple Spots', but the 'Liver looked as if boiled'.[26]

Physicians regarded such pathological changes as reliable indicators of arsenic poisoning. But, interestingly, they sometimes arrived at that same diagnosis on the basis of absence of change in organs. This is not the paradox it may seem. With arsenic, once a tissue is altered by the irritant influence of the poison, it will often resist any further alteration when the person dies. Ordinarily, death brings on the greatest alteration of all, putrefaction, the rotting and dissolution of all body parts but bones. Arsenic, though, is toxic for the micro-organisms that cause putrefaction, and if enough of the poison impregnates an organ the decomposition process can be greatly retarded. The stomach, for instance, with its deep red discoloration, might remain intact for months, even years, allowing for a drama that was re-enacted a number of times: a man was presumed to have died of cholera; he was buried and forgotten until, some considerable time later, information came to light that raised suspicion; his body was disinterred and autopsied; and the telltale stomach, whole and solid and as prodigiously inflamed as the day he had died, revealed the truth—and perhaps a killer.

It was not uncommon for physicians to diagnose arsenic poisoning on the basis of well-preserved organs. Thus the surgeon who performed a post-mortem on a Welsh man two months after burial concluded arsenic must have been the cause of death 'from the fresh state of the viscera'. An arsenic victim buried five months was found to have an alimentary tract 'in a most perfect state of preservation, looking as fresh as if death had occurred only a few days previously'. And in yet another case, that of a man who had been in the grave more than three years, arsenic was implicated by his abdominal organs being so well preserved they 'might have been used for an anatomical demonstration'. According to Alfred Taylor, arsenic's preservative influence extended even to the food in the person's stomach at the time of death: 'I have thus been able to recognize . . . the nature of the last meal which the deceased had taken after the body had been lying many months in the grave.'

That was the sort of evidence, of course, that could prove highly useful in court, either corroborating or contradicting statements made by witnesses.[27]

Impressive as it was, arsenic's action was hardly confined to the viscera and their contents. It will be recalled that until very near the end of the eighteenth century it had been supposed that a body poisoned by arsenic 'quickly liquefies into a pulp'. By 1810, that perception had shifted to the opposite extreme. In several cases of poisoning in Germany at the beginning of the century, the entire bodies of arsenic victims were found to be unusually well preserved. That observation inspired a Dr Klanck to carry out a series of experiments in which he poisoned dogs with arsenic and buried them in a cellar prone to flooding. When dug up ten months after death, the dogs were found to be essentially unaltered, in stark contrast to dogs he had killed with opium or by clubbing, whose 'carcasses were converted into a greasy mass'. Repeating the experiment but leaving the arsenicated dogs in the open air, Klanck found their bodies still intact after three years (while 'all flies that settled on the carcasses died').[28]

If done right, then, arsenic poisoning could result in extended preservation of the entire body. If the victim took enough poison into his circulation, and if he vomited and purged so freely as to produce extreme dehydration, he could keep as well as the man cited above who was exhumed after five months. When the lid of his casket was raised, onlookers (and there usually were quite a number at these events) found themselves staring into a face whose features were 'sufficiently preserved to enable the witnesses to identify the body'. Victorian medical literature fairly reverberates with such eerie tales of arsenical mummies unearthed after lengthy stays in the grave. Even in the case of the man who had been below ground more than three years, 'the face and body generally were found in a remarkable state of preservation, and were easily identified'. Only 'slight indications' of putrefaction were found.[29]

For some Victorian physicians, arsenical mummification was akin to a science. Thus when in the 1880s the bodies of a man and woman killed by arsenic were exhumed two and a half years after burial, and she was found to be badly decomposed while he was almost perfectly intact, his skin still 'firm and moist', doctors had no trouble accounting for the difference. Medical records showed that she had died in two days, while he had taken five: in his case, there had been time for all the arsenic to diffuse through the body, while for her most was still in the stomach (which was the only part of her body still preserved). Similarly in a series of four poisonings in Liverpool that same decade, uncovered three years after the first victim's death, one of the doctors involved determined that there was a direct correlation between the amount of arsenic found in the viscera of the deceased and their state of preservation. In the woman in whom only a quarter of a grain had been discovered, 'decomposition was advancing', even though she had been dead only ten months. The woman whose organs had yielded a full grain of arsenic 'was much less decomposed', while the man in whom three and a quarter grains had been found 'was in a most remarkably preserved state', more so than any of the others, even though he had been dead the longest.[30]

There were, in fact, several cases in which the remarkable state of preservation of remains played an influential role in the conviction of suspects for arsenical murder when the usual evidence of poisoning was limited. The most interesting was that of Thomas Bacon, who in 1855 killed his mother. Poisoning was not suspected at the time, and the woman was buried. But a year and a half later, Bacon's wife slashed the throats of their two children, was convicted of murder but acquitted on grounds of insanity, and committed to the madhouse. During all these proceedings, however, she voiced the suspicion that her husband had poisoned his mother. Local authorities called for an exhumation and analysis of the woman's tissues, which was performed by Alfred Taylor. Although small amounts of arsenic were found in several organs, the viscera did not show the usual pathological indications of arsenic's action, and Taylor was hesitant about declaring arsenic to have been the cause of death. But there was one other telling piece of evidence. When Mrs Bacon's coffin was opened, after nearly two years underground, her facial features were seen to be 'so far perfect as to elicit exclamations of recognition from those present'. Only large amounts of arsenic, deadly amounts, could have produced such effective preservation, it was concluded. The fact that he had purchased arsenic only a few days before his mother's death also told against Bacon, though one has to wonder if it was not his mentally unstable wife who administered the poison. In any event, it was the husband who was convicted (one might say his number had come up, as he had escaped in two previous trials, one for arson and the other for collusion in the killing of his children. No wonder *The Times* opened its commentary on the verdict with 'Thomas Fuller Bacon has been convicted at last').[31]

Yet there seems to have been as much variation in individual reactions to arsenic in death as in life, many victims of the poison decomposing as rapidly as ordinary folk. Recall the disinterred infant poisoned by Jonathan Balls, its body so thoroughly putrefied as to make individual parts indistinguishable. And remains could be worse. In another incident involving Orfila, the casket of a man believed to have been poisoned by his wife was opened to disclose 'a hideous spectacle', a body 'so much decomposed that instead

of the usual instruments, it was necessary, in order to take from it
what was wanted, to use a spoon'.[32]

*

What was wanted from the hideous spectacle of a body, of course,
was tissue to be used for analysis for arsenic. A number of allusions
have already been made to the discovery of arsenic in the bodies of
poisoning victims. That was the forensic toxicologist's trump card,
the piece of evidence that outweighed all others. Symptoms and
pathology could be inconclusive, but if arsenic could be demonstrated by chemical test to be present in the dead person's organs,
or in ingested food or evacuated fluids, the fate of the accused was
virtually sealed. Mary Ann Cotton, Sarah Freeman, and Sarah
Chesham could all attest to that.

Chemical analysis was a newly acquired tool, having played no
role at all in poisoning trials until the mid-1700s and the case of *The
Crown* v. *Blandy*. Prior to that time, prosecutors had relied for the
most part on what was described as the 'moral evidence', meaning instances of incriminating behaviour: the defendant had been
heard to say he would get even with the victim, or had been seen
to add some mysterious substance to the victim's food or drink, or
was known to have purchased a poisonous substance recently, or
found to be in possession of a poison, or otherwise acted in ways
corroborative of the charges. Toxicology was involved only to the
extent that the symptoms experienced by the deceased could be
shown to be consistent with poisoning. The sole test for poison,
employed only sporadically, was to feed some of the suspected
food to an animal, or, lacking that (poisoners, naturally, usually
discarded the contaminated food), some of the victim's vomit. If
the test animal died, poisoning was proved.[33]

By 1752, the year of the Blandy trial, chemistry had moved well
along in its evolution from the arcane medieval art of alchemy and

its obsession with the mythical philosopher's stone into a science capable of investigating the material structure of the natural world. Chemists had become familiar with the properties of hundreds of different natural substances, especially minerals, and had learned much about how those substances interacted with one another. Although they had as yet no valid theoretical understanding of what was going on at the molecular level, they had discovered through trial and error experimentation that when mineral A was added to a solution of mineral B, the solution turned blue, or a yellow precipitate formed, or some other striking transformation occurred. Chemists could, in short, identify certain compounds by running various laboratory tests on them, and so it was inevitable that sooner or later chemistry would be introduced into the court-room to prove the identity of a suspected poison.

Where arsenic was concerned, it would have been better had that introduction occurred later rather than sooner. By 1752, white arsenic could be identified by a combination of colour tests—several trials were needed to distinguish it from other minerals that might produce a similar colour if only one or another of the tests was performed. But successful identification required that the arsenic not be mixed with any organic materials. The presence of organic matter such as food or vomit, commonly the fact in crimi-nal incidents, interfered with the reactions, masking the colour of precipitates, for example, or even preventing their formation. In the words of Christison, organic matter rendered the tests 'absolutely useless', and as late as 1832, he was still advising that in the large majority of arsenic poisonings, identification of the substance was 'enveloped in much difficulty and uncertainty'.[34]

Dr Addington, the medical man who examined the sediment found in Mr Blandy's gruel, clearly did not realize that. To begin, he testified at the trial, the powder had 'a milky whiteness', and so does arsenic. It was gritty and essentially tasteless, like arsenic, and did not dissolve in cold water, again like arsenic. Thrown onto a red hot iron, it released 'the stench of garlic', and when put through five different tests (such as being mixed with a few drops of ammonia, or with syrup of violets) gave in each case colours or sediments visually identical to those produced by white arsenic subjected to the same tests. 'There was an exact similitude', Addington summed up, between the results in the tests done with the sediment from the gruel and those with arsenic purchased from the druggist. 'They corresponded so nicely in each trial that I declare I never saw any two things in nature more alike.'[35]

The powder probably was arsenic. But there are other substances that are white and tasteless and insoluble, or that produce similar precipitates or colour changes in the tests employed—Addington's tests were not specific for arsenic alone. Nor was his 'stench of garlic' test conclusive. That 'the Fumes or Steams of Arsenic...distinguish themselves by an abominable stinking Smell like Garlic' had been known since the tenth century, but that applies to arsenic the element, not the white arsenic (arsenious acid) that Addington would have burned. Although under the right conditions of temperature white arsenic can be reduced to the element, which can then undergo sublimation (direct transition from the solid to the gaseous state) to release a garlic odour, it is an unreliable process. Add to that the subjectivity of people's sense of smell, and one has a test that could be nothing more than suggestive. Many physicians (Orfila among them) would continue to endorse the garlic test on into the nineteenth century, but opposition to it grew steadily, until by the 1830s London students of medical jurisprudence were being instructed that, 'every test depending on the senses of taste, or of smelling, should be viewed with suspicion'. The most solid proof of arsenic in the Blandy case was the combination of the old man's symptoms and the pathology discovered at his autopsy. The chemical evidence adduced by Addington was rudimentary and inadequate, and, in the estimation of a twentieth-century medico-legal expert, 'would not be countenanced in court today'.[36]

Additional chemical tests that could identify arsenic as a possibility were developed after the Blandy trial, but still into the early nineteenth century arsenic analysis remained a confused endeavour. A particularly compelling demonstration of analytical uncertainty was given by the 1815 trial of Eliza Fenning, a servant girl who became a cause célèbre through being executed for attempted murder. Daughter of a London potato seller, Eliza was put out as a maid-of-all-work at the age of 14. From there, she gradually made her way up to cook, then, early in 1815, at the age of 21, took a job in the household of London law clerk Orlibar Turner. Less than two months later, she was arrested after Turner, his son and daughter-in-law, and an apprentice became acutely ill with apparent arsenic poisoning presumably acquired from yeast dumplings Eliza had prepared for dinner. The qualifiers 'apparent' and 'presumably' are in order because arsenic was never established as the cause of sickness with chemical certainty. That missing bit of proof, however, did nothing to save Eliza from the gallows, for in the minds of the authorities and the jury the circumstantial evidence was more than adequate for a conviction. First, Fenning had made the dumplings, and all who ate of them soon experienced vomiting, purging, and severe abdominal pain. Second, a packet of arsenic purchased by Mr Turner to poison mice disappeared from the desk drawer in which it was kept several weeks before the poisoning incident, about the same time the cook was reprimanded by her mistress after being seen one night going 'partly undressed' into the room of two teenage male apprentices who lodged in the house. Third, a fellow servant claimed to have overheard her vow shortly after the reprimand that she could never again like her employers. Fenning, in short, appeared to have motive, means, and opportunity, and to be of debased character in the bargain.[37]

The only fact in her favour was that she had eaten the dumplings too, and been made as ill as anyone in the house. Even that could be turned against her, though, for one could argue that whether out of guilt or fear (knowing that her crime would probably be discovered and she be punished) she decided to take her own life as well. She recovered, as did the rest of the household, but only to be jailed, given a hasty trial shot through with irregularities, and pronounced guilty by a jury that 'retired for a few minutes' only before delivering its verdict. Nineteenth-century juries did not dawdle, often making their minds up within half an hour, not infrequently within a quarter of an hour, and occasionally on the spot: in 1821, a Chelmsford man accused of using arsenic to kill a young woman he had seduced and made pregnant was tried and 'the jury immediately found the prisoner guilty'.[38] Not for them the hour upon hour of anguished wrangling of *Twelve Angry Men*.

Had the trial taken place only twenty years earlier, the verdict would not have been that upsetting, since when intended poisoning victims did not die, the crime was treated as a misdemeanour and punished with nothing more than a fine or limited jail time. But sadly for the ill-starred Eliza, an act passed in 1803 had made the administration of poison with intent to kill a capital offence. On hearing the pronouncement of guilt, then, the young woman, who had stoutly maintained her innocence all along, 'instantly fell into a fit, screamed and cried aloud most bitterly'. She was removed from the court 'convulsed with agony'.[39]

The verdict was perceived by many to be a miscarriage, a decision that rested entirely on loose interpretations of circumstantial evidence and ignored the possibility of someone else having tampered with the dumplings or of arsenic having got into the dough by accident, the sort of mishap that occurred often enough in other kitchens (a recent evaluator of the trial concludes that there was 'not enough evidence to hang a cat'). The jury was much influenced, for example, by the discovery in the prisoner's belongings of 'an infamous book' that, because it included instructions on abortion, clearly 'shews the depravity of her morals'. Appeals to reverse her sentence were issued to officials all the way up to the Home Secretary, but efforts were futile. On 26 July 1815, Eliza Fenning was escorted to the scaffold with the hangman's rope wound round her waist and the noose held in her hand. She denied the crime to the last, both in tear-stained letters from her cell to family, friends, and officials, and in her final words at the gallows.[40]

Newspaper accounts of her execution describe a mood quite different from the jollity that normally prevailed at hangings. Most in the crowd felt certain she had been horribly wronged, and 'the most heartrending sensations pervaded the minds of the thousands' (the tens of thousands, actually) in attendance, attending even though the morning was wet and gloomy: 'a thrill of agony ran through the hearts of that vast crowd when the bolt fell, and the slender form in white swayed in the wind and rain'. Thousands also accompanied her funeral procession five days later, several of them dealing 'rather roughly' with a man who dared speak against her at the graveside. Perhaps the most telling demonstration of the depth of public sympathy for the unfortunate woman was the respect shown her corpse. In Chapter 1, it was mentioned that by a law enacted the same year as Mary Blandy's hanging, the bodies of executed murderers were to be immediately turned over to London's surgeons for dissection. Everything has a price, of course, and it was possible to be spared from the mandated dissection by paying an adequate amount to the authorities: Mr Fenning was charged 14 shillings, no inconsiderable sum for a potato dealer, to keep the remains of his daughter. Nevertheless, her body was still exposed to the risk of being exhumed by 'resurrectionists', professional grave robbers who sold their quarry to medical schools and anatomy teachers. Yet no sooner was she interred than one of the city's most eminent surgeons, a generous patron of the resurrectionists, issued 'especial orders' that the body of Eliza Fenning, 'however desirable to possess, should on no account be brought to him', for he firmly wished 'to avoid an outrage upon popular feeling'.[41]

Denunciations of her trial and affirmations of her innocence would carry on for years. One can even mount a persuasive argument that a fictional character, Justine Moritz in *Frankenstein* (published three years after the execution), was modelled on Eliza Fenning, and for the very purpose of denouncing slapdash justice meted out to the lower classes. Justine, an attractive young servant girl hanged purely on the basis of circumstantial evidence for a murder actually committed by Dr Frankenstein's monster, bears too many similarities to Eliza for coincidence to explain. As late as 1867, no less a notable than Dickens professed that he 'never was more convinced of anything' in his life than that Eliza Fenning had been free of guilt. He believed the true culprit to be one of the apprentices. From other sources came reports of deathbed confessions made by Turner himself, or by his son Robert, or even by the baker who had supplied the yeast for the dumplings (one bit of information not elicited at the trial was the report of an apothecary that Robert Turner 'did on one occasion [shortly before the incident] betray symptoms of insanity' when attempting to purchase arsenic in his shop, and for that reason was refused the sale).[42]

Identification of the true murderer is now beyond reach, but very probably Eliza Fenning was wrongly convicted, if not actually framed. Certainly a key contention of the prosecution—that it was arsenic that she had employed against the family—was never conclusively demonstrated. The physicians who attended the victims suspected arsenic from the outset because of the symptoms exhibited, and the news of the missing packet of the poison. But for the circumstantial evidence to carry full weight it was necessary to chemically confirm that there was in fact arsenic in the dumplings, or in the victims' evacuations. No one thought to save the vomit and stools for examination, but there were dumplings left over, and one of the doctors involved, John Marshall, set about searching for arsenic there. Cutting the dumplings into thin slices, he performed several tests on them, some repeats of the experiments done in the Blandy case (including the garlic test), others chemical assays that had been developed in the interim but which were no more certain. His belief that he had found poison in the dumplings—the 'experiment infallibly proved' the presence of arsenic—can therefore hardly be accepted as infallible. Arsenic in some amount probably was present, given the victims' symptoms, but Marshall's experiments did not demonstrate it to any degree approaching certitude.[43]

The confidence with which a learned medical man presented those findings, however, must surely have impressed a jury of laymen that the circle of evidence was closed: a package of arsenic had disappeared from a desk drawer, people who ate dumplings got sick with the symptoms of arsenic poisoning, and arsenic was reported to be present in the dumplings. Ergo, the person who had cooked the dumplings must have intended to poison the family. Nor could a lay jury have been expected to question two other 'proofs' presented by Marshall. A knife used to cut the dumpling dough had turned black, he posited, because of the action of arsenic, which had also prevented the dough from rising fully.

Outside the courtroom, however, there was no shortage of sceptics to challenge those claims. One chemist joked about keeping his family 'in a state of agitation for several days, by making culinary experiments with arsenic', through which he found that the assertions that 'arsenic would blacken knives!' and 'that arsenic would prevent dough from rising!' were 'assumptions . . . even without the shadow of truth'. But when he brought his experiments to the attention of the judge during the interim between the trial and the execution, 'I received for an answer, "That he would ask his Cook!!!"' If a cook's guess was as good as a chemist's, arsenic analysis was surely in a muddled state. In any event, several experimenters confirmed that the darkening of the knives was due to vinegar in the ketchup used in the sauce served with the dumplings, and that dough would still rise when arsenic was present (arsenic inhibits the action of the yeast that causes dough to rise only after prolonged contact). These demonstrations quickly found their way into forensic medicine textbooks, and though it was no consolation to Eliza Fenning, the debacle of the dumplings had laid bare the confusion surrounding the detection of arsenic still at the beginning of the nineteenth century. Soon, however, the challenge of identifying the poison in food or other organic mixtures would be overcome, and toxicologists given a potent new weapon in their pursuit of poisoners.[44]

4

'The Chief Terror of Poisoners'

At the beginning of the 1840s, the decade during which arsenical homicide seemed to be surging beyond all bounds—'a moral epidemic more formidable than any plague', remember—the *Pharmaceutical Journal*, the professional voice of Britain's druggists and chemists, issued a wildly non-prophetic statement. This 'most execrable of crimes', it announced, this horror which had so recently seemed 'to threaten the destruction of the very bonds of society', had now 'happily been banished from the world'.[1]

What could the *Journal*'s editors have been thinking? How could chemists, of all people, draw the conclusion that the poisoner's favourite weapon was suddenly a threat of the past at the very moment it was coming into more vigorous employment than ever? The explanation is that they *were* chemists, and therefore aware of a momentous recent advance in the ability to detect the presence of even very small quantities of arsenic in human tissues and other organic materials, the so-called Marsh test. So in theory, at least, arsenic poisoning should soon be eliminated, for did it not stand to reason that if would-be killers knew that a simple laboratory test could demonstrate arsenic in their victim's food or stomach or vomit, they would reconsider and turn to some other agent, if not forgo the deed altogether? The tables had been turned. Heretofore, arsenic had been the most dangerous poison to the public.

Now, 'there is none so dangerous to the criminal'. His life had been made 'hell upon earth', for he must henceforth live in constant terror of the day when 'the very dead shall be drawn up out of the grave to bear witness against him'. Dead men tell no tales? *Au contraire*. The dead 'are now become the witnesses whom poisoners have most to fear', the dead, that is, and the chemists who took their posthumous testimony.[2]

The threat of arsenic poisoning was not, of course, about to be banished from the world altogether. Nevertheless, the Marsh test, introduced in 1836, would ultimately encourage a significant decline in the use of arsenic for murder. It would also contribute to the poisoning panic that gripped the public in the 1840s, since it made possible the discovery of crimes that previously would have gone undetected and thereby bolstered the perception of sharply increased frequency. Further, quite apart from its applications to crime, arsenic analysis had important bearings on the recognition and evaluation of the multiple sources of the poison in the Victorian domestic environment. Whether in wine, wallpaper, or women's gowns, arsenic could not be identified and measured without sensitive chemical tests. Familiarity with the evolution of the science of arsenic detection is thus essential to appreciating the full scope of the poison's threat to health in the nineteenth century.

The impact of the Marsh test can be demonstrated by a before-and-after comparison of cases, the Donnall trial of 1817 and the Lafarge trial of 1840. Falmouth surgeon Robert Donnall was charged with murdering his mother-in-law with arsenic. She was a woman of means, he a man lately fallen into debt, and on two occasions in the autumn of 1816 she took ill after drinking tea served by him; the second time she expired after fourteen hours of vomiting. Donnall the medical expert demanded she be buried quickly, else her body would swell and 'unpleasant circumstances might occur'. Before she could be interred, however, an anonymous letter to the authorities accused the surgeon of murder; when the letter was shown to him, 'his hands trembled, and...it dropt from his hands upon the floor'. Suspicions aroused, an autopsy was performed, despite Donnall's 'unwillingness to have it done': the woman's stomach was found to be inflamed in a way consistent with irritant poison. Then, when the stomach was removed for chemical examination, Donnall 'accidentally' dropped the organ into a partially filled chamber pot, conveniently compromising the analysis. Arsenic was found anyway. There seemed every reason to suppose Robert Donnall was guilty as sin.[3]

His trial in April 1817 drew a huge, agitated crowd that, despite the sheriff wading in with a wooden staff 'with the utmost fury', broke through the bolted doors of the courtroom and packed it to overflowing. They got the entertainment they had come for. Dr Edwards, the physician who had done the autopsy and expressed 'no doubt' that death was due to arsenic, was at once made a butt of forensic impertinence, badgered by defence counsel to acknowledge that *cholera morbus* produced the same symptoms and pathology he had described for arsenic. No fewer than three expert witnesses were called to testify that the medical evidence indicated death more likely came from disease than poison.[4]

Edwards's chemical findings were challenged next. The last meal of the deceased, the stomach contents in which Edwards had detected arsenic, had been 'smothered rabbit' (smothered, that is, in onions, then stewed). A defence witness related an experiment in which he had put sliced onions and meat—but no arsenic—to stand in water for several hours, then performed the two chemical tests used by Edwards. In both cases, the colour of the precipitate produced indicated arsenic (it would afterwards be determined that the tests would give a false positive result for arsenic if even small amounts of copper were present in contact with onions; since cookware commonly contained the metal, copper could easily have leached into the smothered rabbit). The reliability of chemical analysis had been thrown into such doubt that the jury needed only twenty minutes to reach its verdict of not guilty. That may well have been the correct decision. But it is also quite possible that thanks to the imprecision of arsenic analysis a guilty man escaped the noose.[5]

Guilty women may have escaped under similar circumstances. In 1834, an inquest was held for Penelope Bickle on suspicion of murdering her husband. The man's symptoms and pathology were congruent with arsenic, his wife had recently purchased arsenic (to poison rats, she said), and she had prepared the dinner that preceded his attack. But even though chemical tests run on his stomach contents indicated the presence of arsenic, defence witnesses attacked the tests as 'very unsatisfactory', and the jury took only a few minutes to decide they were 'not satisfied that the deceased died from poison'. Clearly there was need of an analytical method for arsenic that all could agree was satisfactory.[6]

Progress towards that goal was already underway when Bickle was acquitted. In 1833, an elderly farmer in a Kent village died suddenly from apparent poisoning. Circumstances implicated the man's grandson, who was arrested and eventually tried. At both inquest and trial, testimony was given by James Marsh, a local chemist, that arsenic was present in coffee the grandson prepared for the victim. The jury seems to have agreed that arsenic was the cause of death, but found the remaining evidence inconclusive and voted for acquittal. Twelve years later, the grandson, facing transportation to Australia after being convicted of attempted blackmail and with nothing to lose, finally came clean and admitted that he had in fact murdered his grandfather.[7]

Some good came of the trial nonetheless, as the experience opened Marsh's eyes to the need for a more reliable analytical method for arsenic. The ideal, he appreciated, was a method that would isolate the pure element from organic materials; the element could then be definitely identified through additional reactions. It took until 1836 to develop such a procedure, but once the Marsh test was announced it was immediately recognized as conclusive, and, backed by another test introduced just a few years later, would reign as the standard of arsenic analysis until the 1970s, when more sophisticated chromatographic and spectrophotometric methods became available.[8]

The Marsh test was designed to isolate even minute quantities of arsenic from organic mixtures such as coffee, soup, gruel, and other vehicles for poison. It was constructed on the readiness of arsenic in any form to combine with hydrogen to form the gas arsine (AsH_3). The test involved introducing either sulphuric acid or hydrochloric acid to the material to be tested, followed by the addition of zinc. The acid–zinc reaction generates hydrogen, any arsenic present bonds with the hydrogen to form arsine, and the arsine gas bubbles out of the solution. Marsh found that by passing the escaping arsine through a glass tube with a fine nozzle at the end and igniting it as it exited the nozzle, he could get metallic arsenic to precipitate as a black mirror on a sheet of glass held next to the flame (Fig. 1). The test was, moreover, extraordinarily sensitive, capable of detecting the presence of as little as two parts of arsenic per million in a solution. Through the Marsh test, arsenic was detected in human remains that had been buried for sixteen years in one case, and for as long as twenty-two years in another. Sensitivity to very small amounts of arsenic would acquire particular significance as the fear of slow poisoning took hold at mid-century. Unlike the victims of large quantities of the poison,

1. Marsh test apparatus

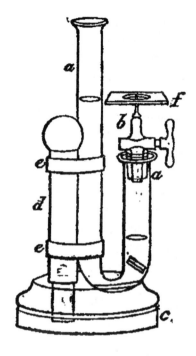

those killed by small and slow doses could be expected to have only traces of arsenic in their bodies. One of the most unsettling aspects of slow poisoning was that it might, in fact, leave no evidence of arsenic at all.[9]

As with any technical innovation, there were kinks to be ironed out. As a one-time chemistry major who moved on to other fields in part because of inaptitude for the laboratory, I can attest that chemistry is very much an art as well as a science. Marsh at first downplayed the art. So exuberant was he over the power of his discovery, he proposed that anyone could master the method, exclaiming that so long as zinc and sulphuric acid could be obtained, 'every house would furnish to the ingenious experimentalist ample means for his purpose'. Everyone could fend off assassination by becoming a do-it-yourself chemist and applying the Marsh test to suspect victuals.[10]

In less enthusiastic moments, Marsh acknowledged the procedure was not to be entrusted to the hands of just anyone. If the glass were held too close to the flame, for example, it 'might sometimes fly to pieces'. Worse, if the experimenter failed to burn the escaping arsine completely and managed to inhale the gas, he would be in for a much more jarring experience than having to dodge flying glass. Arsine is extremely toxic. A renowned chemist of the eighteenth century, Otto Tachenius, accidentally breathed the gas during an experiment, sucking in 'so grateful and sweet a Vapour that he greatly admired it': for half an hour. By the end of that time, though, his stomach was burning, his limbs convulsing, and he was passing bloody urine; he was lucky to survive. Not so the prominent Munich chemist Adolph Gehlen, who in 1815 was killed when, suspecting a leak in his apparatus, he 'smelt strongly at the joints'; his death came only 'after nine days of unheard-of suffering'. By 1900, eight fatalities would be recorded among analysts inhaling arsine during the Marsh test.[11]

Those dangers avoided, there remained purely chemical problems. If the sample being tested was comprised primarily of organic materials, as would generally be the case, the viscous fluid could be expected to foam and froth in such a way as inhibited the release of the arsine. It also became evident that if any antimony were present in the sample it could be deposited on the glass in a film quite similar in appearance to the arsenic mirror (the practised eye could distinguish between the two, arsenic having a blackish shade, antimony more of a blue coloration, but the difference was subtle). Since physicians often administered a compound of antimony to induce vomiting in poisoning cases, as well as to treat other conditions, it was vital that the test be able to distinguish clearly antimony from arsenic.[12]

The arsenic/antimony question was soon resolved by Orfila, as was the problem of organic samples foaming. Marsh had approached the frothing difficulty mechanically, by filtering out the larger pieces of animal matter. Orfila recognized it was desirable to separate all the animal material, not just the chunks, and for that chemical measures were needed. The addition of nitric acid and heat, he found, destroyed the organic matter (reducing it to carbon), eliminated the foaming, and allowed free formation of the arsenic mirror.[13]

But no sooner is one problem overcome than another appears in its place. In working on the Marsh test, Orfila was surprised by sometimes obtaining positive results from a control solution to which no arsenic had been added. Where had it come from? The answer, he determined, was that both zinc and sulfuric acid were themselves often contaminated with traces of arsenic during the process of their manufacture. One therefore had to first employ non-Marsh methods to the zinc and acid to be certain they were pure before proceeding with testing the sample from the crime scene: one would not want to accuse a person of murder when the only culprit was a lax sulfuric acid producer. The presence of impurities in test reagents would interfere with arsenic analysis for years to come and, as will be seen in the Smethurst case below, to embarrass even the most skilled chemists.[14]

*

Orfila was also at the very centre of the murder trial that served to establish the Marsh test as the state-of-the-art procedure for identifying arsenic in criminal cases. In the summer of 1839, Marie Cappelle, a cultivated Parisian woman in her early twenties, was pushed by relatives into marriage with Charles Lafarge, an iron manufacturer from the provinces who presented himself as a wealthy businessman possessed of a luxurious chateau. As has been known to happen in arranged marriages, she ('delicate, refined') and he ('coarse in his habits, and rough in manner') were ill-suited to one another. Nor was life at his home in the Limousin quite what Marie had been led to expect. The chateau a dilapidated hulk, the forge near bankruptcy, Lafarge's vaunted estate, she discovered, was a fraud. Add to that frequent unwanted sexual advances from her boorish and older, homely husband, and one can understand that Marie felt betrayed and trapped. Beginning in November 1839, Monsieur Lafarge began to experience attacks of vomiting and diarrhoea. He came through each alive, but Marie was nothing if not persistent and he nothing if not a slow learner, accepting one dose after another of doctored food and drink from his wife. Only as the end neared did he at last see the light: he 'shuddered at the sight of his wife, and would take no food from her hands'. He had, unfortunately, figured out the situation too late.[15]

Better too late than never. By the time Lafarge died, other members of the household had also begun to suspect Madame Lafarge. It was known she had purchased arsenic, ostensibly to poison rats, and on more than one occasion she was seen adding a white powder to drinks she served him. She had even been so careless as to enquire, well before her husband showed any signs of sickness, as to the customary period of mourning for widows in the region, declaring she simply would not wear widows' weeds a day longer than the year prescribed by custom in Paris. Not surprisingly, she was arrested soon after Lafarge's death, and eventually found guilty. And the factor that clinched the case was Marsh's test.

Recognizing the importance that chemical evidence could have in the determination of guilt or innocence, local authorities seized both a sample of Lafarge's vomit and some egg punch into which

Marie had been seen to stir a powder. It was ordered that the dead man's stomach be removed for analysis as well. The chemists given the job, however, were not *au courant* with their science and used a test dating to the eighteenth century. With it, they detected arsenic in the stomach and the punch; with the vomit, the amount was too small to allow a conclusion. This did not bode well for Madame Lafarge, but her attorney was a clever gentleman: 'knowing that in such affairs M. Orfila is the prince of science, I wrote to him' to ask if the test used by the local chemists was reliable. By no means, came the reply; only Marsh's test would do. Presented with that dictate from the ultimate authority in matters toxicological, the judge ordered the analysis be redone *à la* Marsh. This time, no arsenic was found. Marie Lafarge appeared to be off the hook.[16]

Now it was the prosecutor's turn to recruit Orfila. He pointed out that the father of toxicology had written that arsenic was sometimes eliminated entirely from the stomach by the repeated vomiting it produced. Yet because the poison acted only after being absorbed into the circulation and carried through the body, one might expect to find it in organs even when missing from the stomach's contents. While perfecting the Marsh test, Orfila had given the theory a trial by poisoning more than 200 dogs and analysing their viscera. Arsenic indeed was found throughout their organs, and analysis of the liver, heart, and all the rest had since become standard practice in Paris. 'All the rest' is emphasized because only very small quantities of arsenic might be deposited in any one organ, so to be sure of having enough poison to yield a positive result, the analyst had to subject the entire cadaver to the Marsh test ('in some recent French trials', a London toxicologist laughed about that perverse race on the other side of the Channel, 'the medical witnesses have not hesitated to boil up and evaporate the whole of the human body with many gallons of water and acids in large iron cauldrons'). So, the prosecutor argued, to be absolutely certain Lafarge had not died by arsenic, it would be necessary to exhume the man's body and apply the Marsh procedure to the organs that remained.[17]

A sizeable throng gathered to witness the disinterment, and though Lafarge had not been that long in the ground, his remains were found to be 'ghastly...in a loathsome state of decomposition', a 'species of paste, rather than flesh', a mockery of the rule that arsenic preserved the cadaver. The 'paste' was conveyed to the Palais de Justice, where the court-appointed chemists had set up a laboratory outdoors, a lab already surrounded by spectators. The gawkers were all male, of course. Two women applied to be onlookers, but were denied, and should have counted themselves fortunate, for not only were the chemists' flasks invisible behind the dense fumes emitted, the fumes were a 'foetid vapour' so foul that consideration had to be given to cancelling the afternoon session of the trial. Proceedings nevertheless went ahead, and ladies in attendance 'sustained the annoyance with astonishing resolution.... Everyone was holding a handkerchief to the nose with one hand, and a smelling bottle in the other.' It was rumoured that upwards of 500 bottles of smelling salts were sold in that single day. At the end of the day, the results of analysis were announced: arsenic was nowhere to be found. At the news, the defendant betrayed 'a deep state of emotion...tears fell from her eyes, [and] an indescribable smile played on her lips'; her attorney 'wept tears of triumph'; and 'loud bravos were uttered in every part of the court...almost every female present was in tears, and many men displayed their...emotion in a similar way.'[18]

Their relief was to be short-lived. The prosecuting attorney, realizing the only hope remaining was that the local chemists had blundered in their analyses (they had, after all, never performed the Marsh test before the trial), requested that Orfila, the man who had perfected the test and carried it out countless times, be called in to double-check the initial findings. If this were done, he predicted, 'the prisoner might have occasion to repent the applause she had excited'. Madame Lafarge's attorney could hardly object, as it was he who had brought Orfila into the case to begin with, building his plan for acquittal by insisting that the top expert in the field be consulted. Now he was to be consulted again. A telegraph to Paris brought the great man to town by express stage just three days later. Promptly setting about his work, Orfila took what material was left—'liver, a portion of the heart, a certain quantity of the intestinal canal, and a part of the brain'—and macerated the giblets into a sort of human haggis (again, the 'exhalations were fetid beyond description'). The Marsh procedure was then applied to the mix, and in short order a black mirror appeared. The local experimenters had indeed committed an error. The Marsh test, for all the certainty it could provide, was a tricky operation, one that took experience to master. The provincial chemists did not have that experience, and, Orfila suggested, must have used too powerful a flame, the most common mistake, or by some other error of technique botched the trial. In any event, Marie Lafarge's rollercoaster ride had been brought to an end; 'the public withdrew [from court] in a feeling of stupor and amazement'. As a newspaper story summed it up, 'within two days the accused was declared innocent by the verdict of science, and now she is judged guilty by the verdict of that same science'. She was sentenced to hard labour for life. There quickly grew something of a cult following of young people who believed in the innocence of *la pauvre calomniée*, 'the poor slandered one', as she had taken to calling herself. This of course included the obligatory young men who, having learned nothing from her husband's example, showered her with proposals of marriage. The life sentence turned out to be rather brief. As the prison regimen broke down her health, she became even more an object of pity, and was finally pardoned by Louis-Napoleon in 1852. She died just a few months after being released.[19]

While in France, another case might be briefly considered. In 1846, the body of a man was discovered in the pit of an outdoor privy, his stomach slashed open and internal organs removed. There was, however, reason to suspect his wife of having poisoned him, and enough organ tissue still clung to the body to allow a test for arsenic. It came out positive. When it was also determined that the abdominal wound had been inflicted after death, the wife's scheme became clear. She apparently had read just enough about forensic toxicology to presume that if she eliminated his viscera the poison would be eliminated as well and his death would be registered as a brutal mutilation killing. Her little learning was a dangerous thing, though Alfred Taylor drew a different moral. To him, it was a compelling demonstration of the power of the new arsenical analysis. Poisoners' backs were now to the wall, he crowed: only through 'the entire destruction of the body' could anyone killing with arsenic any longer hope to get away with the deed. Had it not been for 'the newly discovered processes of detecting arsenic in the tissues,' he concluded, 'this crime must have passed undetected and unpunished'.[20]

Such encomiums to the Marsh test were commonplace in the aftermath of the Lafarge trial, which was seen by forensic toxicologists as a watershed, the event that established that they now held the upper hand. But note that Taylor referred to newly discovered 'processes', plural. By 1846, the Marsh test no longer stood alone; it had been joined by the Reinsch test. Marsh's process, after all, was not exactly foolproof. Though the test was sound, it required more than ordinary experience and skill to perform properly. In untrained hands, it was open to erroneous or misleading results, as chemists in the Lafarge trial had demonstrated only too well. Lawyers were aware of its difficulty too, of course, and used it to put medical witnesses in the bind of being damned if they didn't and damned if they did. If they didn't use the Marsh test, they were sure to be attacked for employing outmoded methods; but if they did use it, physicians complained, the counsel for the defence was just as certain to object: 'In what estimation are we to hold these results', he would ask, 'obtained by means of a method liable to every possible deception and error?'[21]

In 1841, the German chemist Hugo Reinsch published a description of an arsenic test that required much less manipulative skill. It involved simply cutting the solid organic material, such as a stomach, into thin strips, adding water and hydrochloric acid, boiling the mixture for half an hour, then immersing a sheet of copper foil into the liquid. Any arsenic present would form a gray-to-black metallic coating on the copper. Although not as sensitive as Marsh's test, it was simple and quick. With the Marsh test, destruction of the organic components of the mixture took several hours of boiling; the Reinsch test could be done without eliminating the organic matter. Toxicologists embraced it at once, Christison proclaiming from Edinburgh that 'nothing can be more easy than the method of Reinsch'. He was the first to employ it in Britain, in the 1844 trial of an Edinburgh woman who was convicted of murder by Christison's 'irrefragable evidence' of arsenic in her husband's liver.[22]

It was the introduction of these two methods of arsenic analysis so close together that enthused both the medical and legal professions with the vision of a poison-free utopia with which this chapter opened (in which arsenical murder would be 'banished from the world'). Thanks to chemistry, poisoning was now in the same category as stabbings and shootings, a crime that 'always leaves behind it complete and incontestable traces of guilt'. That point would echo through the rest of the century: when the sentence of death was read to Mary Ann Cotton in 1873, the judge could not refrain from reminding the prisoner how she had been caught, that poison now 'writes an indelible record of guilt'. Even at the height of the Essex poisoning outbreak, there were assurances that such an event would never happen again thanks to the certainty of detection, which meant an 'equal certainty that the culprit will pay life for life on the gallows'. The inevitability of being found out and executed 'will be sufficient to wipe out this stain from the land'. The tests developed by Marsh and Reinsch had become 'the chief terror of poisoners.'[23]

*

The Reinsch method was easy, but the Marsh procedure had the advantage of being more accurate quantitatively: conviction of a suspect was more likely if it could be shown that there was a lethal quantity of arsenic in the body. Reinsch's test, further, was not sensitive to every form of arsenic that might occur in organic mixtures. Since neither method was perfect, chemists felt free to choose according to individual preference, some opting for Reinsch, some for Marsh, and some—those set on thoroughness—adopting both (in 1879, the Gutzeit test, a variation on Marsh's procedure, was added to the options). Whatever their preferred method, and despite each test's shortcomings, analysts oozed confidence they could uncover arsenic anywhere it was to be found and were patently eager to demonstrate their skills. Puffed up with chemical esoterica, they opened themselves to the same sort of ridicule as is heaped on computer geeks today. Thus in a popular novel of the time, an elderly physician exclaims about 'these new-fashioned chemists' that they 'will find arsenic ... in your walking-stick; they will indeed. I'll lay my life, sir, that they would extract arsenic from my hat.' (As a later chapter will show, they might well find arsenic in anyone's hat, and even in his walking stick if it were painted green.) A Daumier lithograph stretched the theme further, depicting a chemist giving a demonstration on arsenic and informing his audience that if they desire, he will poison the friend standing beside him and then recover the arsenic from his eyeglasses. Below the demonstration table can be seen the carcasses of animals he has poisoned in experiments, twisted faces showing their final suffering. The title of the piece? *L'Amitié d'un grand chimiste n'est pas un bienfait des dieux*: the friendship of a great chemist is not a blessing from the gods.[24]

For arsenic to be detected in top hats and eyeglasses, it was necessary that the person conducting the tests be a true *grand chimiste* and master the requisite skills. It appears that few did, at least during the first half of the century. Even before the introduction of the Marsh test, a physician had alleged that 'scarcely one in fifty' of his medical brethren possessed the ability with the old, simpler tests to determine 'whether a pudding or a mess of pottage be contaminated with arsenic or not. Even the whole medical staff of our great metropolitan hospitals are often incapable of clubbing together a sufficient degree of chemical knowledge' for the task. Appearance of the more complicated Marsh procedure only exacerbated the situation. As one English chemist saw it, the Marsh method gave 'very correct indications' when placed 'in scientific hands'; but it was 'wholly unfit to be entrusted to those unaccustomed to careful chemical manipulation'.[25]

By the end of the Lafarge trial, it was clear that the new analytical method had great potential for detecting arsenic poisoning, but only if carried out by a knowledgeable and experienced chemist. The time-honoured procedure of leaving chemical analyses to the abilities of whatever neighbourhood physician or surgeon or apothecary happened to be the one called to treat the victim of poisoning would no longer do (as late as the sixteenth century, physicians, surgeons, and apothecaries were distinct groups, each with its clearly defined duties; as time passed, however, surgeons and apothecaries took on the role of general medical practitioners, especially among the lower classes, so that by the nineteenth century when a case of poisoning occurred the family was as likely to summon an apothecary or a surgeon as a physician). From the 1840s on, arsenic trials would require the services of expert chemical witnesses.

The term 'expert witness' had come into use in the later eighteenth century to denote a physician or other person of specialized learning who could give evidence in court that included not just facts, the type of testimony to which ordinary witnesses were restricted, but also opinion about the meaning of those facts so as to assist judge and jury in reaching correct decisions. As it became apparent that doctors who were expert in interpreting symptoms and pathology were usually not expert at performing the Marsh (and later the Reinsch) test, courts began insisting that all arsenic analyses be conducted by qualified chemists. Expert chemists were called upon frequently: during the mid-1800s, very nearly half of all trials at which medical evidence was solicited involved poisoning. By happy coincidence, several factors were at that time promoting the expansion of chemistry as a profession, bringing about a marked increase in the number of chemists in both academic institutions and medical schools who could be tapped to carry out dependable analyses for arsenic. Throughout the country, individual chemical practitioners established local reputations as expert witnesses for poisoning trials held in their town or area, and at least four—Alfred Swaine Taylor and Henry Letheby in London, Robert Christison in Edinburgh, and William Herapath in Bristol—achieved national recognition as forensic analysts. Henceforth, rank-and-file physicians, the men who would be first on the scene of a possible poisoning crime, would be trusted to record symptoms and perform the post-mortem, if necessary, but expected to turn over samples of food, evacuations, or organs to the chemical expert.[26] (Figure 2 shows Alfred Taylor, left, performing an analysis with colleague George Rees.)

Expert toxicologists often ran both the Marsh and the Reinsch tests before drawing conclusions. For their findings to be trusted, however, one had to ensure that the material to be tested was kept

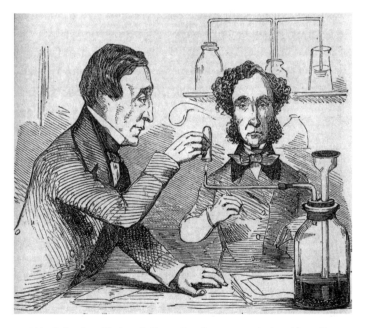

2. Alfred Swaine Taylor (left) performing an analysis with colleague George Rees

safe from external contamination. Placing a stomach in a chamber pot, as Robert Donnall had done, could not be allowed. Medical practitioners thus had to be instructed in the fine points of collecting and protecting samples so that analyses would stand up in court. In arsenic cases, vomiting and purging were usually still going on when the medical attendant arrived and ejected material could simply be transferred to a clean jar and sealed from the atmosphere—the recommended method was to insert a cork, wrap the cork with tin foil, then cover the foil tightly with leather. If the patient was no longer eliminating vomit or stools, there might still be material in a chamber pot, though family members often threw the offensive material out at the first opportunity. Quick disposal, of food as well, was especially likely if one of the household was attempting murder. And even if everything had been discarded, there still could be traces of vomit or faeces on the victim's clothing or bedding, or on the carpet, and the soiled section of the fabric be cut out and preserved. Did the vomit fall onto a wood floor? Scrape up the affected section of the wood. Did it fall upon a stone floor? Use a clean rag soaked in distilled water to wipe it up.[27]

There were exceptional instances in which no trace of food or evacuations could be found for testing, but that did not necessarily defeat the analyst. A woman who poisoned her husband with arsenic in soup emptied the uneaten portion into the barnyard, thinking thereby to have eliminated the critical evidence. But as it happened, a pig and several chickens came upon the soup and ate it. They all died, and even though the husband's evacuations were similarly disposed of, and no arsenic could be found in his stomach, analyses of the animals revealed arsenic throughout their viscera. The wife was convicted and executed. In a similar case, a Bedfordshire woman was convicted of killing her husband partly on the evidence of arsenic in an animal that consumed some of the dying husband's vomit.[28]

This process of drawing on animals for evidence could work in reverse. In the case of a Warwick woman who poisoned her uncle with arsenic, she explained her possession of arsenic with the usual excuse, that she had purchased it to destroy vermin, and even brought forth a dead mouse to confirm her alibi. When analysis could turn up no arsenic in the mouse, she was found guilty of murder. Negative findings could lead to convictions in other ways. A wealthy man in Sheffield in the 1880s developed an attachment to his much younger maidservant. One night they both fell sick with vomiting after dinner. She survived, he died; arsenic was found in his vomit, none was present in hers. Chemistry thus was able to demonstrate that the maid had poisoned the master with arsenic while attempting to deflect suspicion from herself by inducing her own vomiting through some non-toxic means. She was sentenced to penal servitude for life.[29]

Organs removed from the deceased were also to be placed immediately in a clean container and sealed; both stomach and intestines had to be ligatured at both ends to prevent loss of contents (spills happened all too easily, as occurred with the man whose skull was opened for analysis and his brain found to be 'so diffluent that it poured out on the floor, and no further attention seems to have been paid to it'). 'Immediately' and 'clean' were both key procedures. In perhaps the most egregious violation of this commonsense precaution, the stomach of Monsieur Lafarge was stored in a magistrate's desk drawer for several days before being analysed. Had the Marsh test revealed any arsenic in the stomach, the defence would have been able to argue that the poison must somehow have been picked up from the drawer. In another case, an analyst's finding of arsenic in a stomach was thrown out of court because in his haste he had stored the stomach in a jar obtained from a neighbouring grocer who also stocked arsenic in his shop.[30]

Finally, the clean containers had to be accurately labelled with respect to the name of the deceased and the date of removal, and zealously guarded by the physician: 'The suspected substance...should never be let out of his sight or custody,' Taylor instructed, and must be 'locked up while in his possession, in a closet to which no other person has a key'. In an arsenic trial in Scotland in the 1820s, the physician in charge of containers of intestines, stomach, and stomach contents made the point in his testimony that he not only kept the materials in a locked room, but 'the morbid parts...were afterwards taken along with me to my bed-room, when I went to bed'. More than once a case with strong circumstantial evidence of guilt was lost because vomit or organ samples were entrusted by the doctor to people who did not protect the containers from access by others (let alone sleep by them).[31]

But, of course, even the experts could err, and as excitement built over the deterrent power of the chief terror of poisoners, a new anxiety grew in parallel, that false positive findings through the Marsh or Reinsch tests could lead to wrongful convictions. If 'we must needs pin our faith upon the conclusions of chymists', *The Times* warned, there was a constant danger we might 'hang a fellow creature because a small crystal...is exhibited on a scrap of copper wire'. Chemists must be exceedingly careful lest they commit an error that resulted in 'judicial murder'.[32]

*

We do not know if any judicial murders were indeed committed by a clumsily done Marsh test. But there was one trial that came very close, and it involved an error by the most trusted expert of all, Alfred Swaine Taylor. Educated in medicine, Taylor was first a lecturer in medical jurisprudence, then professor of chemistry at Guy's Hospital in London. Author of respected textbooks on medical jurisprudence and toxicology, Taylor played second fiddle to no one as an expert witness. At the height of his fame, samples of vomit, faeces, and stomach contents were shipped to him from all over England, and his analyses provided important evidence at more than thirty trials for poisoning. It was Taylor who found the arsenic in Sarah Chesham's husband's stomach (and who at her earlier trial had discoursed on the properties of arsenic and so alerted her to the advantages of slow poisoning). Taylor fully deserved his reputation as the 'gentleman whose test-tube has brought many a man to the gallows'. So great was his stature, on at least one occasion the *accused* appealed to have Taylor do an analysis of the victim's stomach, hoping in desperation he would find no arsenic, and knowing that if he did not the testimony of lesser chemists that it was present would be overridden (as the court commented on the request, 'Dr. Taylor's evidence would be above suspicion'). Fortunately for the two women making the appeal, there was so little supporting evidence that they had poisoned the infant daughter of one (and granddaughter of the other), they were acquitted after a brief trial and before Taylor could get to an analysis.[33]

But then Taylor became involved in the Smethurst case, one of those life-is-stranger-than-fiction sagas that would be presumed too outlandish to take seriously were it a novel or movie. Thomas Smethurst was a London physician married to a woman twenty years his senior. In 1858, at the age of 53, he met Isabella Bankes, a lady in her early forties who took rooms in the same Bayswater boarding house where he and his wife dwelt. The two quickly fell into an amour, displaying their mutual affection so openly that the landlady felt compelled to give the new boarder the boot for 'improper familiarity' with a married man. Within two weeks, Smethurst left the house as well and promptly married Isabella, bigamy laws be damned. The newlyweds settled in the Thames-side town of Richmond, and almost at once the bride began to suffer with 'violent retchings which almost shake the very life out of her' and frequent bloody stools. Smethurst, who had retired from medical practice some years before, called in a respected local physician who diagnosed his wife as a simple case of diarrhoea and treated her accordingly with chalk. Her condition worsened, though, and she began to complain of burning pain in her throat and abdomen, leading her doctor to entertain the notion of irritant poison.[34]

At the end of April 1859, as the poor woman lay in bed only two days from death, her husband approached her with a lawyer and a will he had drawn up granting virtually all her possessions to 'my sincere and beloved friend, Thomas Smethurst'. She approved and signed the document. In the meantime, her physicians (she now had three) came to believe they saw signs of slow arsenic poisoning: it was they who recorded that 'strange look of concentrated terror' noted in Chapter 3. The physicians sent a specimen of her bowel evacuations to Taylor for analysis—and he found arsenic. Being a doctor himself, Smethurst had been under no pressure to call in other medical attendants. He had done so, it was now speculated, merely to put on a display of concern for his failing wife and place himself above suspicion. 'He overacted his part,' a newspaper commented. 'He was so sure of his ability to baffle detection that he was detected.' Dr Smethurst was arrested as soon as Taylor reported finding arsenic in the bowel fluids, then released on his own recognizance, then taken back into custody the following day when Isabella Bankes died. The post-mortem found extensive inflammation of the intestines, but Taylor's analysis of stomach, intestines, liver, spleen, uterus, and gullet turned up no arsenic in her organs. Nevertheless, on the basis of the will, the inflamed intestines, and—not least—Taylor's finding of arsenic in her stools and in one of several dozen bottles of substances taken from Smethurst's bedroom—the inquest jury returned a verdict of guilty.[35]

When Smethurst came to trial in July, he entered a plea of not guilty, then demanded a new judge on the grounds that the present one was a close friend of one of the prosecution's chief witnesses, Alfred Taylor. He was summarily overruled, however, with the observation that since the expert witness was a legal celebrity, well known by all the London judiciary, one judge could be no more biased than another (besides, Lord Chief Baron Pollack added, he had not seen Taylor for 'a considerable time' unless one counted his attendance at a party at the judge's home a few days previously). The trial then proceeded normally, through the opening speech for the Crown and the examination of witnesses until, early the second morning, a juror was taken suddenly ill while listening to the details of the post-mortem and determined by medical witnesses to be unfit to continue his service. With that, Smethurst's trial was halted and the jury discharged until the proceedings could be started anew the following month.[36]

The revived trial was largely a contest between medical witnesses for the prosecution testifying that the dead woman's symptoms and internal lesions were indicative of arsenic poisoning and medical witnesses for the defence insisting that symptoms and pathology were more in line with death from natural causes, either dysentery or some other intestinal condition. Many of the symptoms were consistent, furthermore, with pregnancy—the post-mortem on Bankes had revealed that she was seven weeks with child, and one doctor averred that chronic vomiting from that condition was itself sufficient to cause death in extreme cases. There was, in effect, a stalemate between the two sides with respect to the medical evidence. But even so, one would anticipate, any supposition of natural death would be obliterated by the toxicological evidence: arsenic had been found both among Smethurst's possessions and in the victim's evacuations. Case closed![37]

It probably would have been that simple a matter had not Taylor made a startling discovery in the interim between inquest and trial: the copper foil he had used in the Reinsch test, his preferred assay for arsenic, was itself contaminated with arsenic and had been the source of the positive results of his analyses. Under the right chemical conditions, some of the tainted foil would dissolve in the tested liquid, releasing its arsenic to be visibly deposited on the remaining foil. Taylor at once notified both the prosecution and the defence of his error, and freely admitted at the trial that he had been mistaken in testifying before the inquest jury that he had found arsenic. But the damage had been done.

First, there had been heavy pre-trial publicity of alleged poisoning, so heavy that one juror admitted before testimony even began that he had already determined on a guilty verdict (his request to be excused from duty was nevertheless denied, on the grounds that he had been sworn in and it would be too disruptive to start over a second time). And even without such prejudice, Smethurst was a far from sympathetic figure, having jilted his ageing wife of thirty years for a much younger woman. There was still the troubling matter of no arsenic being found in the victim's organs, but according to the prosecution that was because Smethurst was 'a very skillful chymist' as well as physician, and had used his chemical knowledge to administer the arsenic in combination 'with such other ingredients so as to cause it to be removed from the system and to render its discovery in the body...almost impossible'. The theory was not even half-baked, but the jurors, none of them 'skillful chymists', bought it. Eleven were persuaded of the defendant's

guilt by the time closing arguments ended; it took only forty minutes of deliberation to convince the twelth.[38]

Smethurst was sentenced to hang a fortnight hence, but almost
at once the press began to circulate rumours that the execution
would never take place. Although the jury had been quick to decide,
outside observers saw too much ambiguity in the medical evidence
to justify the irrevocable act of hanging. After all, seven of the
seventeen expert witnesses had deposed that the victim was more
likely to have died of disease than poisoning, and if one figured in
as well the confusion caused by the Reinsch-test red herring, it was
difficult to disagree with the position taken by a leading London
medical journal: 'Is the prisoner guilty? We believe he is. Was he
proved guilty? Certainly not.' Though one might feel no sympathy
for the man (and it appears few did, *The Times* describing him as
'a liar, a cheat, a scoundrel of the blackest dye in every relation of
life'), there was sufficient reason to believe he might be innocent to
demand revocation of the capital sentence lest the state commit
'judicial murder'. The judge appeared to share those reservations,
for in passing sentence he had omitted to tell the prisoner 'that
there was no hope, and to prepare to leave this world'. Such a mal-
ediction was always pronounced if the judge truly intended that
the death sentence should be carried out. Hence there was reason
to expect that a royal reprieve would be forthcoming and death
replaced by life imprisonment or transportation.[39]

In the end, Smethurst did even better than that. Within days
of the verdict, not only his lawyer but groups of both physicians
and barristers submitted petitions to the Home Secretary to over-
turn the death sentence. Newspapers were 'inundated' with letters attacking the verdict as unproven. Even his first wife issued
a plea for leniency, maintaining that as he had always shown her
'the most uniform kindness and attention', it was inconceivable he

would kill anyone. True, he had deserted her for another woman, but he had been seduced: 'the first advance came from her', the wife charged, 'although unhappily', she had to concede, Isabella Bankes's temptations 'met with too ready a reciprocity on his part'. The Secretary, in turn, passed these appeals to one of London's brightest medical luminaries, surgeon Sir Benjamin Brodie, for review and recommendation. While that process crept forward, of course, the appointed day sped closer, yet the condemned man remained remarkably calm in his cell in Horsemonger Lane Gaol. Journalists informed the public that even as he stared eternity in the eye, the prisoner could joke that he would hardly cut a natty figure in Madame Tussaud's chamber of horrors if he were recreated in his prison garb.[40]

Smethurst's composure was to be vindicated. On Friday before the scheduled Tuesday execution, as the sounds of gallows under construction rang through the gaol, the message of a reprieve was delivered. Sir Benjamin had determined the medical evidence to be inconclusive, the Home Secretary had relayed this opinion to the Queen, and the capital sentence had been commuted. Eleven members of the jury that had convicted Smethurst immediately protested in a letter to *The Times*, but the majority of the public applauded the decision, though just what punishment would be substituted for death was still unclear. Two months later, on 14 November, Smethurst learned that Victoria 'was graciously pleased to extend our grace and mercy unto him... and to grant him a free pardon'. There would be no punishment at all.[41]

There would be no punishment, that is, for the *death* of Isabella Bankes. The *marriage* with Isabella Bankes was another matter, however—the free pardon did not extend to his commission of bigamy. Smethurst thus remained in his cell another two weeks, until he could be brought to court to face that lesser charge.

Entering a plea of not guilty, his lawyer sought to save him with the argument that he had never truly been married to his first wife, Mary Durham, because she was already married to another man, a Mr Johnson, at the time she wed Smethurst. The person who had committed bigamy, in other words, was Mary Durham, and since that effectively annulled her marriage to Smethurst, Isabella Bankes was technically his first—and only—wife. The prosecution countered with evidence that Mr Johnson had in turn been married to another woman before taking Mary Durham as his bride. That meant Durham was never legally married to Johnson, thus did not commit bigamy when marrying Smethurst, and since that marriage was therefore legal after all, Smethurst *was* guilty of bigamy when he married Bankes. The jury at least pretended they could follow all that, and convicted Smethurst. But the year of hard labour to which he was sentenced was still preferable to dangling at the end of a rope. He would not be well paid for his hard labour, however. A final irony for Smethurst to contemplate was the legal provision that those convicted of bigamy forfeited all claim to any property associated with the illicit spouse. The will he had so carefully drawn up for Bankes was now a meaningless document. Her property passed instead to her family, with Smethurst precluded, a reporter noted with unconcealed glee, 'from obtaining a single farthing'.[42]

There was nevertheless some satisfaction to be had by Smethurst from the embarrassment suffered by Alfred Taylor, the man he blamed for his wrongful conviction. The erroneous report of arsenic presented by Taylor at the inquest, he believed, had created a 'universal prejudice...in the public mind' that 'rendered it impossible...to permit a fair trial in [my] case'. So if there was any justice in the whole messy proceeding, from Smethurst's viewpoint, it was in the scorn heaped upon Taylor by his peers in the

aftermath of the trial. Indeed, the eminent toxicologist had practically invited scorn by his haughty demeanour on the witness stand.
'Have your tests been disputed...before this occasion?' he had
been asked. 'Yes; but no instance has ever occurred where I was
proved to be wrong.' Well, it had occurred now. 'In the face of all
England,' rival analyst William Herapath proclaimed in *The Times*,
'I say [that] the whole set of operations were [*sic*] a bungle.' But,
he hastened to add, the bungling did not end there, for Taylor had
acknowledged using the same sample of impure copper gauze in
his Reinsch analyses for nearly twenty years: 'what shall be said
of the justice of the convictions and executions which have taken
place during those years upon Dr. Taylor's evidence!'[43] Incorrect
analyses, Herapath implied, had probably led to judicial murder.

Others piled onto the downed Taylor, including the editors of
the *British Medical Journal*: 'If ...the man who holds in his hands the
keys of life and death will not insist upon purity in his tests', then
we were returned to 'the days of witchcraft, when human life hung
upon the lips of any old crone'. Alfred Swaine Taylor any old crone?
Yet this was the same man who a decade earlier, in his authoritative
textbook of toxicology, had written of the old days before reliable
chemical tests for poison had been developed that 'innocent persons charged with the crime of poisoning, incurred great risk of
their lives, in consequence of the chemical mistakes into which the
medical witnesses of those days were so apt to fall'.[44]

Taylor certainly fell in the estimation of his contemporaries both
medical and legal, but he hardly withdrew into the obscurity urged
upon him by his assailants. Instead, he counter-attacked, issuing
a lengthy series of articles defending his work, describing ways of
getting around the impure copper problem, and pointing out that
the copper used in the Reinsch test by other analysts—William
Herapath, for example—must also have been contaminated with

arsenic. Hence they too had committed 'chemical transgressions', they too were responsible for questionable convictions and executions, and so on. He even proposed that Herapath ought to give him thanks for having discovered the problem of impure copper and saved him from further transgressions. To unbiased medical observers, meanwhile, the whole proceeding was an embarrassment that threatened to undo all the progress that had been made against the crime of poisoning. The *British Medical Journal*, for example, outraged by the spectacle of reputable scientists 'throwing as much polite mud at each other as they think will stick', demanded an end to the 'farce' of the 'most celebrated toxicologists of the country contradicting each other in matters where there should be no possibility of doubt'. The public were 'scandalized' by their antics, and the only outcome could be that in future 'very little dependence will be placed on their science as a handmaid of justice'. From being the chief terror of poisoners, chemical analysis would be so discredited as to encourage even more people to turn to arsenic on the supposition that juries would disregard the testimony of chemists.[45]

But though the Smethurst fiasco temporarily threw the reliability of toxicological analyses into question, once the waters calmed it was accepted that as long as the analyst assured the purity of his starting materials and conducted the tests with care, the Marsh test and the Reinsch test could be trusted and thereby be expected to inhibit the resort to arsenic for murder. They could never be counted on to banish the crime from the world entirely, as the writer who opened this chapter had so confidently predicted, but by making the act a great deal riskier for the perpetrator than it had ever been before, the tests did decrease its frequency. As for Smethurst, he truly does seem not to have been a poisoner. Recent interpretations of the autopsy report on Isabella Bankes have directed attention to lesions in her intestines that appear to be those of Crohn's disease (so-named for the author of a pathological characterization published in 1932). When the vomiting of pregnancy is added to the common symptoms of Crohn's, there is formed a clinical picture essentially identical to the illness of Bankes. Had she only been autopsied by her physician husband, gastroenterologists today might well be diagnosing Smethurst's disease instead of Crohn's.[46]

5

A Penn'orth of Poison

In the winter of 1851, a hunter who had gone into a rural grocery to restock on gunpowder chanced upon a disturbing transaction. 'A little girl' placed an order for tea, sugar, flour, currants, red herrings, and several other culinary items that ended with a request for two ounces of arsenic to deal with rats. The order was promptly filled, and the child 'jumbled them all into her apron, and went her way'. Surprised the grocer could be so cavalier about dispensing poison to one so young, the sportsman observed that some of the ingredients might be intended for a pudding. 'Loikely,' the grocer acknowledged in his thick Derbyshire accent. What if the paper packet holding the arsenic were to tear, the hunter asked, might not the girl's 'whole family . . . be poisoned?' Quite possibly, the grocer agreed, and therefore—obviously—'they should moind what they're at'. The hunter persisted, reminding the shopkeeper of several instances of accidental arsenic poisoning that had recently occurred in the area: 'They should moind what they're at,' the grocer repeated.[1]

Laissez-faire with a vengeance was the practice with regard to the sale of arsenic throughout the first half of the nineteenth century in Britain. The regularity of offhand references to 'the common white arsenic of the shops' is a measure of how unexceptional a purchase it was (the arsenic came in fine powder form or, less commonly, in blocks that could be easily reduced to powder). As the phrase suggests, it was common to shops in general, not merely druggists' shops (the professionals that today we call pharmacists were at that time more frequently identified as 'druggists' or 'chemists'). For most of the century, at any rate, one did not have to be a trained chemist or druggist in order to vend drugs and poisons. Medicines and other chemicals were readily available from grocers, from chandlers (candle sellers), paint dealers, oilmen (purveyors of lighting oil), and an assortment of other tradesmen frequently lumped together under the heading of 'hucksters'. In short, anyone could sell it. Likewise, anyone could buy it, and nothing more was expected of buyers than that they mind what they were at in using it—caveat emptor.

The consequences were predictable. The retail sale of arsenic for rat poison, the leader of the English pharmaceutical profession declared at mid-century, was 'the most fertile source of accident'. Vigilance, after all, is never eternal, and no matter how much people intended to mind their arsenic, some would sooner or later suffer the consequence they had intended for rats and mice. Time after countless times arsenic meant for vermin, or for steeping wheat seeds, or relieving sheep of insect infestations, somehow ended up on the dinner table. 'Arsenic becomes as much a part of the stores of a farmer's, shepherd's, or cottager's cupboard as his family's food,' the hunter noted, and since it looked so much like that food, like sugar or flour or baking powder, mistakes were inevitable. A jar of the poison would be put away on a shelf and forgotten, until one day a child falls ill and its mother 'fancies she has some cream of tartar somewhere, and that is good for a fever'. She doles out the supposed medicine from 'the fatal jug' and her innocent child dies. The woman would not be punished by the law, for the death was accidental. But she would be condemned nonetheless, doomed to an 'embittered life' as a victim 'to the want of legislative enactments to prevent such catastrophes'.[2]

The want of legislative enactments to prevent the frequent accidental poisonings with arsenic became the subject of intense discussion by the 1840s, discussion that eventuated—in 1851, less than three months after the little girl was so casually handed arsenic along with her sugar and red herrings—in a national law to regulate the sale of the poison. The context and aftermath of that law, the Sale of Arsenic Act, form an essential element of the story of the poisoning of Victorian Britain.

In suggesting above that the instances of accidental poisoning with arsenic were countless, I am guilty of only slight exaggeration: in the two-year span from 1837 to 1839, for example, 506 such accidental deaths were recorded in England and Wales, and surely many more went unreported. Again and again, despite the most forceful warnings to be careful and newspaper reports of yet another case of lethal negligence, people simply failed to mind what they were at. 'Perverse carelessness' was the way the *British Medical Journal* described the actions of a woman who found white powder left in a trough by the farm's previous tenant, presumed it must be baking powder, used it to make a cake, and killed her husband; the powder was subsequently determined to be residue from sheep dip. 'Almost incredible carelessness' was the way that same journal described the case of a Surrey shepherd who outfitted his well with a bucket he had been using for sheep dip mixture and had only cursorily rinsed; he died along with his wife, his son, and two daughters. The wife of a Lincolnshire shepherd (being a shepherd's wife was a position fraught with peril) made cheesecakes using what she thought was rice flour in the batter. It was in fact sheep dip powder that her husband had stored in the same cupboard as the flour and in an identical tin (what adjectives can possibly do justice to this degree of carelessness?). The woman died only hours after eating a cake, and nearly a dozen neighbours who had also partaken were made gravely ill.[3]

Sheep-dip stories could be recounted till the cows come home. But they were only one category of carelessness with arsenic. At least as common was the consumption of arsenic meant for household pests. In an incident reported by Christison, four people in a travelling group were suddenly stricken with vomiting and purging. They immediately suspected their luncheon soup, since a fifth member, who had not taken that course, was unaffected. But the person who had eaten most heartily of the soup was experiencing the least discomfort while the one who had consumed the smallest amount of the dish was hardest hit. There was then noticed a direct correlation between the quantity of cheese each had added to the soup and the severity of his or her symptoms. After all recovered, the innkeeper who had served them was told of the events and came to realize that he had mistakenly served his guests cheese seasoned with arsenic to poison rats.[4]

Similar episodes abound. Rat poison stored in a cabinet was assumed to be flour; a New Year's Eve pudding made by a woman killed both her and her son within hours (he in 1857, she in 1858); her husband followed two days later. Five children from a family of nine died from rat arsenic incorporated into their rhubarb pudding. A farmer hid leftover rat poison inside a clock case, thinking it would be safe from misuse there. Unfortunately, he stored it in a spice box, so when a servant somehow came across it four years later she put what she thought must be baking powder into the evening dessert; she died and the rest of the family came close. Two young sailors assigned to clean a shipboard cabin discovered a jar of what looked like tartaric acid powder, popularly used to make an imitation lemonade. They stirred some into water, drank it, and died. And at a funeral in Lincolnshire, the rice pudding offered guests before the ceremony created a ghastly procession to the burial ground: 'Some of them fell down, some staggered... and others had to be immediately put to bed.' It was only because appetites are not all that keen before a funeral that no one consumed enough pudding to join fates with the event's guest of honour.[5]

Even when arsenic was given a different colour by being mixed with other materials in commercial products, it could be mistaken for food. Hammond's Rat-cake Poison so nearly resembled 'common brown cakes' that a schoolboy died after taking a cake from a friend's jacket pocket. A labourer picked his supervisor's coat pocket to get a piece of cake, which he shared with two mates: 'the repentance of the trio was... as complete and sincere as their sufferings.'[6]

In 1857, an international incident was threatened when Chinese bakers in Hong Kong were accused of intentionally poisoning the British residents of the city with arsenical bread. Ten were brought to trial, with every expectation they would be found guilty of participation in a broader conspiracy against Europeans that included a 'gang of ruffians' who had raided HMS *Thistle* in Hong Kong harbour and murdered all the crew. Their bread was demonstrably arsenical, containing as much as fifty grains to the pound. But to the deep disappointment of many, it was determined at trial that the poison had been introduced by accident, the flour having been shipped from America in barrels previously used to store arsenic.[7]

A family was poisoned by eating a roast that had been coated with 'flour' that had spilled from a bag of arsenic intended for steeping wheat—the arsenic had been put on the shelf above the one on which the roasting pan was stored. There were even fatalities from eating the treated wheat seed itself. One such case involved a farmer who mistakenly sent steeped wheat to a mill for grinding; the resulting flour killed one child and sickened a number more.[8]

It was just as easy to mistake arsenic for medicine as for food. Jars of arsenic were repeatedly supposed to contain magnesia (magnesium oxide), a common home remedy for headache, nausea, and diarrhoea that unfortunately came in the form of a white powder. Thus a small boy was killed in 1870 when an illiterate servant dosed him from a bottle clearly labelled arsenic. People also regularly confused arsenic with sulphur, which was a standard treatment for sore throat and some skin conditions. Such a mistake seems unlikely on first consideration, given that sulphur is yellow and arsenic white. But the two were combined in some sheep-dip preparations, resulting in a pale yellow tint mistakable for pure sulphur. A farmer and his son died after his wife gave them 'sulphur' from a can of Cooper's Sheep Dipping Composition someone had foolishly stored on the medicine shelf. Yellow sheep dip also looked very much like powdered mustard and surely found its way sooner or later into someone's Welsh rabbit.[9]

Sometimes even meticulously minding what they were at was not enough, as it was all too easy for conscientious people to be poisoned through the irresponsibility of others. Druggists and grocers were the greatest offenders, time and again wrapping up arsenic instead of whatever white powder the customer had requested. In 1848, a woman purchased magnesia to give to her 7-month-old child. On opening it at home, she decided it looked different from magnesia she had used before, so she returned to the chemist to air her suspicions. He assured her it really was magnesia, she gave it to her baby, and the child died of arsenic poisoning a few hours later. In the 1850s, a rector died from arsenic sold to him by his grocer as arrowroot. In the 1870s, a woman who often took chalk powder to relieve heartburn was killed by arsenic given her in error. In 1857, a

Worcester mother purchased white lead to be used as body powder on her 6-week-old. White lead is hardly a desirable substitute for talcum, of course, but it is still preferable to white arsenic. Shortly after being dusted, the infant's skin showed signs of irritation, 'a wound formed, and the child died in great pain...of a slow burning, and must have suffered fearfully'. Investigation revealed that the druggist's new apprentice had noticed the white lead drawer was empty and, eager to demonstrate his dedication to duty, had refilled it—with white arsenic.[10]

The last case was a preview of sorts of an outbreak of poisonings—the 'arsenical violet powder' incident—that horrified the nation in the spring of 1878. Violet powder was the name applied to a broad range of preparations of baby powder. The most popular formulations were based on either cornstarch or potato flour to which violet-scented perfume was added. It was the usual practice after washing a newborn to dust it with the powder, using a puff, and to regularly repeat the applications with the changing of napkins. Towards the end of May, a baby girl was born in a village on the northern fringes of London. The family's nurse cleaned the baby and applied violet powder to her entire body; later in the day, more powder was dusted over the genitals. When the infant was undressed the following day, her skin was seen to have turned bright red; the nurse treated the inflammation with more powder. Soon the baby's skin began to blister and peel, until finally, ten days after birth, the infant died. Her body was cut into pieces, boiled, and analyzed: more than six grains of arsenic were found. An analysis of the violet powder determined it to be only 55 per cent potato flour; most of the rest was arsenic. The poison had been absorbed through the baby's skin, especially after it ulcerated, as well as through the vagina, and no doubt had been inhaled every time she was dusted.[11]

This child was but one of a number (most in villages in Essex!) affected by violet powder. Eventually, more than thirty cases would be recorded and at least thirteen deaths, most within the first ten days of life: one infant 'swelled up like a bladder of water' before expiring, another 'gave out from its nose and mouth a kind of black blood. Its agony was awful, and during the night before its death it screamed continuously.' In one case, the powder was applied just a single time, then discontinued when the mother read of another child dying after being powdered; her child died anyway. In at least one other case, the infant was poisoned by sucking on the puff used to apply the powder. The violet powders involved, most of which were around 25 per cent arsenic by weight (though one sample exceeded 50 per cent), had been purchased from as many different shops, but the retail outlets had all obtained their powder from the same manufacturer, Henry King, who swore he had not put arsenic into his product. The fault, King protested, must lie with his supplier of starch—another case of mistaken chemical identity. He was charged with manslaughter nevertheless, though at his trial—*Queen* v. *King*—the jury agreed he had not known of the arsenic in the powder and was therefore not liable. The chemists from whom he had bought his starch, furthermore, all swore they had not delivered arsenic, and as it was impossible to prove otherwise, no one was held responsible.[12]

Accidental poisoning by arsenic was, clearly, an all-too-ordinary occurrence, so common an event that any lawyer preparing a defence for an accused killer would automatically look for some way to attribute the death to accident. In the trial of Mary Ann Cotton, for example, defence counsel argued that one child died from arsenic released from a poisoned soap mixture the loving mother had applied to his bedstead to destroy bugs. As the mixture dried, it was subject to crumble and fall to the floor, with the result that every time the child moved about the room 'a cloud of these poisonous atoms must have arisen and been inhaled by him'. It was a clever enough try, but a too-transparent clutching at straws for the jury to be taken in.[13]

*

The great majority of people poisoned by arsenic ingested the substance unwittingly, the victims of carelessness or malice. There were, however, those who took the poison by design, for its reputation for certain death made it an appealing choice for anyone bent on suicide. It was not the most popular option for self-murder: according to a survey done in the 1850s, 80 per cent of suicides were accomplished by physical measures such as hanging, drowning, jumping, or severing blood vessels. And in the 20 per cent carried out by poison, opium, which painlessly plunged people into interminable sleep, was most frequently the drug of choice, being used by 40–50 per cent of self-poisoners. Fewer than 10 per cent selected arsenic (the proportion seems to have been much higher in the United States, towards the end of the century at least, when some physicians wondered if Americans had adopted that form of suicide 'as a national peculiarity').[14]

Those who purposely swallowed arsenic were the ones who had been taken in by popular lore that not only was arsenic most sure to do the job, it acted so quickly as to bring about a relatively easy death—this despite all the chilling accounts of arsenic victims' agonies in newspaper stories and, after 1857, the harrowing passages recounting the torture endured by Madame Bovary (merely writing about his character's anguished demise caused Flaubert to throw up his dinner on two separate evenings). Medical writers thus accepted that disabusing the public of its arsenic mythology was an important professional responsibility. 'Were the awful symptoms and horrid sufferings, arising from the actions of this poison more

generally contemplated [by] the unhappy individual who aims at
self destruction,' a London physician opined in prose purple even
for that day, 'it possibly might have a tendency to appall such irre-
ligious and execrable projectors, who presumptuously attempt to
put a period to the inestimable blessing of human existence.' In
plain words, the object was death, not torment, and no person,
'however depraved', could be 'so callous as to seek or require such
additional pangs' as those brought on by arsenic.[15]

But self-destroyers were beyond depraved, at least in the eyes of
the law, which regarded suicide as 'the most heinous description
of felonious homicide'. It was a double offence, in one instance an
act against the Crown, which had an interest in the lives of all its
subjects, in the other an insult to the Almighty (the only legitimate
arbiter of life and death) by 'rushing into His presence uncalled
for'. In former centuries, the perpetrator of the act of *felo de se*
(felon upon himself) was buried at a crossroads with a stake in
his heart. That bit of medievalism had been abandoned by 1800
(though it was not officially outlawed until 1823), but it was still
Church of England policy not to perform the Burial Office, the
service promising salvation and resurrection to the deceased, for
those who had taken their own lives. Suicides were also commonly
buried 'on the backside of the church', that is, on the shaded north
side. If all that weren't discouraging enough, life insurance policies
were made null by the commission of suicide.[16]

The deterrents nevertheless often failed, life's trials and disap-
pointments being too much for some to bear. Those who chose
arsenic as the way out (a higher percentage of female suicides than
male) did so for all the same reasons as those who elected less painful routes. 'Lunacy' was the most frequently assigned explanation,
followed by a category filled with 'young woman, married unhappily', 'girl, seduced and deserted by a married man', 'pregnant

girl, deserted by her lover', and like casualties of what one doctor described as an epidemic 'peculiar to some young women, known as an "hysterical love-fit"'. Men were subject to their own fits. A tailor of 'dissipated and debauched habits' killed himself because he had made a maiden pregnant. A farmer who inherited a sum of money 'spent it in riotous living, got into debt, and took poison to escape his creditors'. A 'notorious drunkard' of a butcher swallowed arsenic after being treated unkindly by an aunt from whom he had hoped for an inheritance. A Birmingham man poisoned himself after being treated unkindly by a horse on which he had placed a heavy bet. Finally, a young girl who had been caught stealing by her father took arsenic to escape the beating she knew would follow; 'she vomited during the flogging, and died in convulsions', yet even though 'marks of violent treatment were found' all over her body, poison was designated the cause of death and the father was excused.[17]

The poison didn't always work, of course. One young woman who tried to kill herself with arsenic failed on the first attempt, tried again with a larger dose, failed, and then, despite having twice experienced wretched suffering from the poison, took a still larger dose and succeeded at last. A young man who attempted suicide with arsenic was more imaginative. When it failed to kill him as promptly as expected, he slashed his arm; then when the bleeding proved too slow to meet his needs, he hanged himself. On occasion, arsenic taken for suicide failed because it wasn't actually arsenic. Druggists, cognizant of the popularity of the drug for self-destruction, sometimes sold some innocuous white powder in the guise of arsenic to buyers they suspected of being suicidal. The hope was that not only would the immediate attempt be foiled, but in the process the fear of dying provoked by the illusion of arsenic in the system would destroy the impulse towards self-murder altogether. Cream of tartar was the usual substitute, though any harmless white powder would do. In 1849, when a depressed Nottingham tailor informed his mates at the pub he had swallowed arsenic, they rushed him to a dispensary run by the ominously named Dr Stiff, who applied the stomach pump and brought up several quarts of fluid found to contain nothing more noxious than flour, the staff of life rather than the powder of death.[18]

Mention of the stomach pump is a reminder that whether a person ingested arsenic by accident or by intent, or by an assassin's intent, all was not lost, for treatments were available. Prompt removal of the poison from the stomach offered the best hope, with odds highest for those who cooperated with therapy. Those attempting suicide, naturally, often resisted help, though few so strenuously as the man who, jilted by a lover, tried to kill himself with his bayonet, then, failing to hit a vital spot, turned to arsenic in a pint of porter. When a doctor tried to force an emetic down his throat, the man bit off the bowl of the spoon. He died.[19]

Eighteenth-century physicians had induced vomiting with emetic drugs, warm water, olive oil, or a finger down the throat. From the mid-1800s onwards, however, practitioners turned increasingly to the stomach pump or, as they also called it, the stomach tube or the siphon tube. Arsenic, it will be recalled, often adhered to the walls of the stomach in spite of heavy vomiting, but the stomach tube provided a vigorous lavage that dislodged particles of the poison much more thoroughly. The device was as simple as it was unpleasant. A flexible rubber tube half an inch in diameter and five feet long was lubricated with oil, then passed over the tongue (held down by a finger) to the back of the mouth and down the esophagus to the pit of the stomach. Next, a funnel was inserted into the exterior end and held above the patient's head while a liberal quantity of warm water was poured into it. Then the tube was pinched shut and lowered to a position below the stomach. When the pressure on the tube was released, siphon action brought the contents of the stomach gushing forth.[20]

But it was not enough to bring the stomach pump into play promptly; it also had to be employed carefully. The end of the tube could produce tears of the oesophagus or stomach and less frequently, though often enough, the tube was pushed into the trachea instead and fluid poured into the lungs. Even without such mishaps, the stomach pump caused great discomfort, and patients can be forgiven for fearing it. So dreaded was the experience that physicians joked that often just the sight of the tube being readied for action was enough to provoke vomiting (the design of the pump would become technically more sophisticated in the twentieth century, but as effective antidotes were discovered for many poisons, the pump fell into disuse and today is employed only in rare situations).[21]

Much hope was also placed in chemical antidotes that might neutralize the poison, most particularly the compound hydrated sesquioxide of iron, introduced in 1834. Its efficacy seemed corroborated by extensive experiments done by Orfila the same year, and it was soon in general use under the name 'Orfila's antidote'. The sesquioxide worked by forming a highly insoluble compound with any arsenic in the stomach, thereby preventing the poison's absorption into the system. Such was the theory, at least, and Orfila's antidote held sway as the standard therapy for arsenic poisoning into the early 1900s. Eventually it was determined that the compound merely delayed the absorption of arsenic, and that its cure rate was minimal at best (all those people 'cured' by the sesquioxide, in other words, would probably have survived without it). The tried-and-true procedure of prompt emptying of the stomach through emetics or the siphon tube was actually the patient's best chance all the way down to the mid-1900s, when truly effective chemical measures were at last introduced.[22]

*

Even had the nineteenth-century antidote worked, one could argue that an ounce of prevention was worth a pound of sesquioxide and that inhibiting people from poisoning themselves or others in the first place was the preferred approach. The most powerful antidote for arsenic poisoning was to remedy that 'want of legislative enactments' bemoaned by the hunter who opens the chapter, that is, to pass a law to regulate public access to arsenic. Such legislation was already on statute books on the Continent. In France, for example, arsenic and other poisons could be sold only by licensed pharmacists, and only to persons known to them; with all sales, the purchaser had to sign a register and indicate the use for which the poison was needed. Similar rules governed commerce in many other countries. In Russia, furthermore, all poisons were sold in bottles of distinctively coloured glass, giving clear warning of their dangerous contents; in France and Germany, some colouring agent such as lampblack was mixed with arsenic before sale to prevent it being mistaken for flour or sugar.[23]

The British, of course, tended to regard such close regulation of the marketplace as paternalistic intrusions into people's personal lives: more than one champion of public safety despaired of his countrymen ever submitting to the 'despotic measures' characteristic of the Continent.[24] In general, there was good reason for despair, as will be seen with attempts at legislative control of arsenical hazards in food and domestic products. But with respect to the direct sale of arsenic, resistance turned out to be almost non-existent. So patent was the danger of criminal and accidental death from the poison, so nervous had people been made by the arsenic panic of the 1840s, that when a serious campaign to enact a law to control arsenic was finally mounted, it succeeded almost overnight, spurred onwards by the strange case of Henry Marchant.

On Saturday, 31 March 1849, the 28-year-old quarry worker from Bath came home around midnight after an evening of drinking with friends. He had his wife make him a cup of tea, drank it, went to bed, but soon awoke, 'seized with a violent retching'. He would vomit almost continuously throughout the next week, finally dying the following Saturday, some hours after a last wife-prepared meal of barley gruel. The surgeon who attended him registered the death as 'acute disease in the stomach', and the matter might have ended there had not his widow behaved with such glaring indiscretion. Only three days after his funeral, the woman who had been married to him 'in harmony' for seven years took a new spouse, a man 70 years of age. So brief a period of mourning, along with the thirty-eight-year age difference between the newlyweds, raised eyebrows, naturally. But rumours had already been circulating that something strange was going on between Charlotte Marchant and William Harris. The old man had been seen on several occasions lingering about the stall in the marketplace where the young woman sold oranges. A week before her husband's death, it was noticed, Charlotte went to Harris's house to have tea and 'was in his room a very considerable time'. Harris, furthermore, was a man of property, so what else could one think but that the orange-dealer was a gold-digger who had done away with her first husband so as to get her hands on a richer one?[25]

On coroner's orders, the first husband was exhumed two weeks after burial, and his stomach, intestines, and liver conveyed to William Herapath, who found arsenic in considerable amount in all three organs. Charlotte Harris, as she was now named, was immediately arrested. Her new husband just as swiftly cut her loose, exclaiming he hoped she would hang for having brought 'disgrace to me' (the disgrace was that he was arrested too, as a possible accomplice, since he had had three earlier wives die on him in the previous thirteen months; when their bodies were disinterred, however, no arsenic could be found and Mr Harris was set free). The fourth Mrs Harris was tried in August and convicted. There was, however, a final twist to the already improbable tale. Charlotte Harris, her attorney announced, was pregnant (by an unspecified source). Mercy was granted, and execution commuted to transportation for life.[26]

Although the Marchant case was undeniably bizarre in certain respects, for the most part it was much like any other incident of arsenical murder—except that it was the one that brought to a head the agitation for a legislative enactment that would impose controls over the sale of arsenic. Shortly before her husband's sudden illness, it came out, Charlotte Marchant had purchased from a pharmacist a 'penn'orth of arsenic for rat poison'. The poison typically sold for two pence an ounce at most, so a penn'orth—a penny's worth—was enough to poison a multitude of rats. It was enough to kill half a hundred people, for that matter. It was more arsenic than anyone needed for either rats or humans, but a penny's worth was the smallest amount druggists offered for sale, and a penny was affordable for just about anybody: it was the same as one would pay for a cup of coffee or for use of a public toilet. So no one baulked at the price, and by the 1840s, 'a penn'orth [or 'pennurth'] of arsenic for rat poison' had become something of a catch-phrase in conversation and in literature, understood by everyone to be code for 'enough arsenic to kill my brutish or old and rich husband, shrewish wife, exasperating child, cuckolding neighbour—fill in the blank'. Sarah Chesham poisoned her sons with arsenic purchased ostensibly to kill rats; when a teenage son not given poison testified against his mother at her trial and was asked if he had ever seen rats in the house, his sardonic reply was 'only one'. The trial transcript notes the jury reacted with laughter.[27]

Punch provoked a bit of laughter as well, with a cartoon published only a few months after Henry Marchant's death showing a small girl requesting of the druggist that he be so good as to fill her bottle with laudanum (opium in solution) and 'let Mother have another pound and a half of arsenic for the rats' (Fig. 3). The druggist replies; 'Certainly,' and offhandedly asks if any other articles are needed. A sign to the left of the pair announces 'all sorts of poisons constantly on sale', while on the right can be seen a drawer labelled 'arsenic'. Above the drawer a jug of arsenic solution stands on a shelf. 'Fatal Facility; or, Poisons for the Asking' is the title given the drawing.

Nearly as common an excuse for a penny's worth was to poison mice, or unwanted dogs or cats, or sundry bugs and insects (fleas in bedding and 'black beadles' seem to have been especially plentiful). Whatever the reason given, the fact that a penn'orth could be so easily acquired by a woman to add to her husband's tea and soup had provoked consternation for some time before 1849. But in the wake of the Marchant murder, a case whose scandalous details stirred national interest, consternation was at last crystallized into organized political action. At the beginning of August 1849, the Provincial Medical and Surgical Association (forerunner of the British Medical Association) appointed a committee to draw up for submission to the House of Commons a document that would expose the 'GREAT ARSENIC EVIL' in all its 'naked deformity' and lay down guidelines for bringing the evil under control. Committee members acted quickly, two months later presenting to Parliament a statement of their 'just alarm [over] the frequency of the crime of Secret Poisoning, and its increase within the last few years', their dismay that arsenic could be 'so easily procured under the

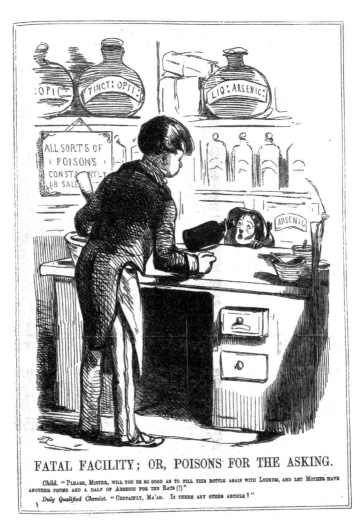

FATAL FACILITY; OR, POISONS FOR THE ASKING.

Child. "Please, Mister, will you be so good as to fill this bottle again with Lodnum, and let Mother have another pound and a half of Arsenic for the Rats (!)"

Duly Qualified Chemist. "Certainly, Ma'am. Is there any other article?"

3. 'Fatal Facility; or, Poisons for the Asking', *Punch* cartoon, 1849

most frivolous pretences', and their conviction 'that some check is necessary to restrict the indiscriminate sale' of the poison. And as Exhibit A of their argument, indeed the only substantive exhibit, they offered Henry Marchant's death, a case that, even 'if no other existed, calls loudly for the interference of the Legislature'.[28]

But just what form should that interference take? To prohibit the sale of arsenic altogether seemed too extreme, as the poison did have legitimate uses. While there were other compounds effective as rat poison, they were more expensive, and cost was no negligible consideration when on many farms hundreds, even thousands, of rats had to be killed each year (one farmer reported an unlikely 40,000 of the pests as his annual take). The majority of experts on rat control maintained that the animals could not be kept within bounds any other way. In addition, various tradesmen needed arsenic in their work—taxidermists utilized it to preserve specimens, for example, and jewellers in the process of bronzing items.[29]

One could nevertheless try to ensure it was not administered to people, the committee proposed, by requiring druggists to record the name and address of every purchaser of arsenic. It happened that even when circumstances were highly suspicious and arsenic was found in the victim's body, juries were reluctant to convict unless it could be demonstrated that the suspect actually had bought some of the poison ('the ends of justice are too frequently defeated', a Dorset coroner had complained in the 1830s, 'for want of a compulsory registration'). Written proof of purchase would plug that gap, and give pause to anyone considering murder by poison. Further protection could be provided by mandating that before sale arsenic be mixed with some harmless substance that would change its colour or give it an unpleasant taste: potential victims of murder or accident could thereby be saved, though suicides would remain undeterred (not even prohibition of arsenic could stop the self-murderer, it was accepted, for where there was the will to die, there were many ways, and if the poison way were removed, one would simply turn to the three Rs, 'the razor, the rope, or the river').[30]

Neither of the recommendations was original with the Association's committee. Among more conscientious druggists, at least, it had for some time been a common practice to refuse to sell arsenic to anyone not personally known unless he or she were accompanied by a witness to vouch for character and good intent, and in a few pharmacies a record of the sale was entered into a register and signed by all parties. But those measures were voluntary, and chemists often complained that less professional dealers in the poison, grocers and chandlers and hucksters, observed no precautions at all. So nonchalant a handling of the deadly material could hardly be countenanced when, in the busiest shops, a ton or more of arsenic crossed the counter each year.[31]

Likewise, much attention had already been given to methods of making arsenic 'self-detective', as physicians phrased it, by the addition of substances that affected its colour or taste. As early as 1844, a French chemist announced a system of adding small amounts of certain compounds of potassium and iron to arsenic so that when the poison was put into wine the liquid turned violet, when into flour dark blue, when into stew green, and so on for a total of twenty common food items. Green stew and blue bread were sure to put most people off their feed and thereby save them, and similar colouring schemes were being put forward by British scientists. One came up with four additives that would produce a green tint when introduced into food, eight that would give black, ten that gave blue, another ten that gave yellow, and no fewer than thirteen that produced red.[32]

On 11 March 1851, a bill to regulate the trade in arsenic was introduced into the House of Lords by the earl of Carlisle. The bill clearly was perceived by the public to be important, for the earl was quickly deluged by 'a vast number of communications from all parts of the country containing suggestions for its improvement'. Several of those suggestions were incorporated into a revised bill, including one that arsenic should not be sold to any one 'other than a male person of full age', so as to prevent the tragic accidents that had too often resulted from its sale to children and female servants. The fact that the Essex poisoners so recently prowling the countryside were women was a still more powerful motivation for restricting purchase to males, but the provision was soon deleted nonetheless due to protestations from women 'indignant at this aggression on their liberty'.[33]

The bill quickly moved through both houses of Parliament with few revisions and little debate. On 5 June, less than three months after its introduction, 'An Act to Regulate the Sale of Arsenic' became law, welcomed by expectations that the 'carelessness and villainy [that] have long held sway' would soon be relegated to the past. The Act provided, first, that a detailed record be made of every retail sale of the poison, the seller being required to register the name, address, and occupation of the purchaser; the date of the transaction; the quantity of arsenic purchased; and the purpose for which it was to be used. Both seller and buyer had to sign the record, and when the buyer was not personally known to the seller, a third-party witness who was known had to be present and sign the register as well. In addition, any quantity of less than ten pounds had to be coloured with soot or indigo to produce a black or blue colour that would prevent accidental ingestion of the poison. Ten pounds was selected as an amount far above what was needed for murder or suicide ('like buying an 80-ton gun to blow out his brains'), but lower than the quantities needed for legitimate uses in which coloured arsenic was undesirable: farmers, for instance, would not have welcomed black or blue sheep dip. Failure to observe the provisions of the Act was punishable by a fine of £20.[34]

The Act provided that purchasers of arsenic had to be 21 years of age, but could be of either sex (ladies were nevertheless patronized by wags unable to resist pointing out the delicate creatures would 'be in danger of soiling their fingers' with the colouring agent). Vendors of arsenic, on the other hand, had neither age nor other restrictions placed on them. It remained permissible for anyone to sell the poison, and even for anyone to designate himself a chemist or druggist. Both facts greatly vexed the nation's genuine chemists and druggists. As the head of the Pharmaceutical Society grumbled in 1848, 'any man, however ignorant—an individual unable even to sign his own name—half of whose shop is stored with butter, bacon, [and] cheese' was free to dispense the most deadly poisons from the other half. Trained druggists not unreasonably believed that those who dealt in dangerous drugs should have some knowledge of them, and that the public should be able to distinguish the qualified from quacks; ignorance inevitably led to deadly mistakes. In Continental countries, druggists had to be licensed, and could be so only after demonstrating mastery of their field. It was for the purpose of bringing about similar requirements in Great Britain that the Pharmaceutical Society was founded in 1841, and much of the Society's activity since that date had been aimed at achieving Parliamentary definition of the title 'Chemist and Druggist' and designation of licensed chemists and druggists as the only legitimate dealers in medicines and poisons. Much of the Pharmaceutical Society's support for the Sale of Arsenic Act stemmed from its desire to lift chemists out of such degrading associations and give them professional status; determination to protect the public from poisoning was not their only consideration.[35]

The petition presented to Parliament by the Provincial Medical and Surgical Association likewise included a request that no druggist be permitted to sell arsenic without a licence. The proposal was ignored by lawmakers, however, both because they were reluctant to strip grocers and other tradesmen of a lucrative part of their business and because there was as yet no legal definition of the term 'Chemist and Druggist': how could one grant a monopoly to a group that technically did not exist? A statutory definition would be provided the following year, when the Pharmacy Act of 1852 established a Register of Pharmaceutical Chemists, but that law did nothing to restrict the right to sell poisons. Not until 1868 and the passage of another Pharmacy Act were non-registered pharmaceutical chemists prohibited from trafficking in drugs and poisons.[36]

In contrast to pharmacists, parliamentarians initially believed that it mattered not who sold the poison. So long as vendors adhered to the requirements of the 1851 act, the incidence of poisoning deaths from both accident and murder must drop drastically. Such was the theory. The reality—as more than one correspondent complained to newspaper editors—was that arsenic vendors 'went on selling it in precisely the old way'. Within weeks of passage of the Act, two pharmacists were arrested for selling uncoloured arsenic to a woman who used it to kill her husband. She was executed, they got off with a small fine and a warning. The magistrate who fined them expressed the hope that the punishment 'would act as a caution to other dealers in poison', but it didn't. Although calls for stricter enforcement were loud and numerous, violations of the Act continued to be recorded. A full five years after the law had been put into force, for example, a 17-year-old druggist's apprentice in

Liverpool sold a quarter-pound of uncoloured arsenic to a customer he did not know, who then used it to poison her husband
(the husband survived, but several chickens who ate what he vomited in the barnyard did not). Thus in spite of the law, *The Times*
commented on the case, 'arsenic is freely sold and freely bought
in market overt. A bleareyed boy, domiciled amongst...invalided
leeches, freely dispenses it by the handful to the first ragged girl
or desperate matron who is anxious to deal.' It mattered not what
excuse for purchase was offered: 'Let her put forward the flimsiest
pretext of fleas, bugs, dogs with sore ears, or any domestic affliction
of that description, and the lethal commodity is actually forced
upon the reluctant customer.'[37]

'By such hands as these', *The Lancet* added in a protest against the
same incident, 'are poisons suffered to be distributed broad-cast
amongst the population.' Hands such as whose? Hands such as
those of the chemist who in 1860 sold uncoloured arsenic to a servant girl who used it to poison her master. Hands such as those
of the druggist who in 1863 accommodated a man who requested
uncoloured arsenic to kill rats, then killed himself instead. Hands
such as those of the pharmacist who was arrested in 1880 for having sold enough uncoloured arsenic 'to poison all the inhabitants
of the borough'. There were many more such hands, chemists and
druggists being arrested and fined on a regular basis for years after
passage of the Arsenic Act. To be fair, convictions were often for
relatively minor infractions, such as failing to record the date of the
sale or the occupation of the buyer. There nevertheless were all too
many cases such as the druggist from Louth who, when arrested for
selling a pound of arsenic without colouring, explained he was only
doing what all the other chemists in the area did. 'If a customer
could not get it in one place he could in another,' it was reasoned,
so why not give it to him in your place. 'The law was frequently

evaded in this way,' he testified. 'If customers applied for one or two pounds, and were told they must take ten pounds, they say "Well, enter me ten pounds and I will get it as I want it."...It was invariably the custom of the trade.'[38]

Most druggists maintained that if such was indeed the custom of the trade, it was primarily grocers and chandlers, not professional chemists, who made it so. Ignorant of the science of drugs and poisons, lacking any professional ethos, caring only about making the sale, it was those corrupt tradesmen who were the ones to be feared. Such was the argument pushed to impel passage of the 1868 Pharmacy Act, which at last designated registered chemists and druggists as the only legal purveyors of poisons. The grocers and other non-druggist vendors already in business were, of course, grandfathered into the law and allowed to stay in the business. But new unregistered tradesmen continued to enter into dealing in poisons, especially arsenic, for years after the law was enacted, and often did so with impunity. The law simply was not enforced with rigour, at least not enough rigour to satisfy the Pharmaceutical Society. As late as the 1890s, the Society still sponsored 'inquiry agents' to seek out and report non-registered vendors of arsenic, and even to incriminate them through sting operations such as sending obviously under-age buyers into their shops. Eventually the police turned to such tactics as well. In 1894, a Chester tradesman provided arsenic to a 17-year-old boy, who, as soon as he left the shop, handed his purchase to Detective-Inspector Gallagher, who promptly cited the seller. The seller just as promptly turned the tables. In the interim before his court appearance, he recruited his own teenage boy and sent him to five different shops run by registered chemists; in every one, he was supplied with the arsenic he requested. Apparently it indeed was 'the custom of the trade', whether the trade was that of grocer or druggist.[39]

To call it 'invariably' the custom of the trade, however, was to exaggerate, for clearly many pharmacists did abide by the Arsenic Act, and the incidence of arsenic poisoning did decline significantly during the last third of the century. It did not, however, disappear. If a person tried hard enough, he could lay hands on uncoloured arsenic, and arsenical murder and suicide, as well as accidents, continued on into the twentieth century. When the co-authors of an 1880s volume on trials for murder by poisoning took up the topic of arsenic, they began by emphasizing that 'notwithstanding the difficulties thrown in the way of the purchase of arsenic' by the Arsenic Act, 'the cases of poisoning by the use of this drug have been so numerous, that it has been difficult to select examples without greatly extending the bulk of this volume.'[40]

*

The bulk of this volume too could be greatly extended by additional accounts of arsenical murder, suicide, and accidental death. But to do so would be to obscure poisoning of a far wider scope, for as much as people had to worry about arsenic in the hands of criminals and the careless, 'distributed broad-cast amongst the population', as *The Lancet* had it, there was a still greater likelihood they would be poisoned by the arsenic cast even more broadly amongst them by brewers, bakers, candlestick makers, and a host of other artisans and manufacturers. To balance the picture of arsenic in Victorian society, it is necessary then, to turn to these other sources of intoxication, beginning with the very food people brought home to their tables.

6

'Sugared Death'

On Monday, 25 October 1858, Joseph Neal, proprietor of a sweet-shop in the Yorkshire city of Bradford, sent an employee to the neighbouring town of Shipley to purchase a quantity of plaster of Paris. What did plaster of Paris, whose usual employment was by artists making moulds or casts, have to do with the making of sweets? Nothing. Nothing, that is, except for being considerably cheaper than sugar. Confectioners in general—not just Neal—had long since determined that by replacing a certain amount of sugar with 'daft', as they had nicknamed the inexpensive plaster, they could enjoy a gratifying increase in their profits.

Nor were sweet-makers the only tradesmen making such cal-culations. Similar manipulations were practised on virtually every dietary item on the market throughout the first half of the nine-teenth century; and though regulatory legislation was enacted in the second half, the law hardly brought an end to such deceits. Adulteration—the secret addition of less costly substitutes for the genuine components of foods and beverages—was rampant through much of the Victorian era. The temptation to replace proper ingredients with cheap, inferior ones, sell the sophisticated item at the price of the real thing, and pocket the savings was sim-ply too strong. Even if a purveyor began his career obedient to con-science, the lower prices charged by morally lax rivals would soon drive him either to join their ranks or to leave the business. As a contributor to a newspaper correspondence column observed, 'one such villain among the bakers or the confectioners of a town may, and indeed, must, thrust honest competition into the bankruptcy list, and constrain those of easier virtue, in self-defence, to adopt the fraudulent practice'.[1]

Neal's assistant applied at the shop of chemist Charles Hodgson, who, bedridden with illness, desired the messenger to come back when he was better disposed. But the messenger had his orders, and he persisted until Hodgson sent a young man who had only recently been taken on as an apprentice to fetch plaster of Paris from a storeroom. The novice apothecary weighed out twelve pounds of the material and the 'daft' was carried back to Bradford and worked into peppermint drops. Only it wasn't daft. What *was* daft was the failure of Hodgson, the ailing druggist, to warn his student that plaster of Paris was not the only white powder stored in the back room, that an unlabelled cask of arsenic was also there (that is not quite true— the cask was labelled, but 'Arsenic' was imprinted on the *bottom* of the barrel). This was another danger of arsenic's colour: it allowed the poison to be mistaken not just for certain foodstuffs and medicines, but for adulterants of foodstuffs and medicines as well. The Sale of Arsenic Act's requirement that the poison be coloured before leaving the shop did nothing, after all, to address the old problem of druggists mistaking the uncoloured arsenic in the storeroom for other white materials. It would soon be suggested that arsenic containers be rigged with bells or some other alarm that would sound on opening, but by that time the apprentice's mistake had killed more than a score of people and grievously sickened ten times that number by means of what *The Times* described as 'little pills of sugared death'.[2]

'The Bradford incident', as the tragedy at once became known, happened to occur just as public dismay over the adulteration of foods and political agitation for some remedy to the problem were building to a head. The first comprehensive law prohibiting adulteration would be passed less than two years later, and a powerful catalyst to that law was outrage over the Bradford poisonings. Nevertheless, arsenic got into Mr Neal's sweets by accident; he thought he was cheating his customers with another substance altogether. Yet for years before the Bradford misfortune, arsenic compounds had been used as adulterants on purpose, and used to such an extent as to make arsenical food and drink yet another significant source of poisoning of the public. We will return to the sad events that unfolded in Bradford, and their aftermath. But first a prelude—arsenic and adulteration before the Bradford incident—is needed.

If not the world's oldest profession, food adulteration cannot have followed too far behind the settlement of the earliest cities. The division of labour that accompanied the transition from agrarian to urban life included a separation of food producers from food consumers that, people being what they are, was promptly turned to profit by unscrupulous producers. Complaints of adulterated bread and wine can be traced back to antiquity, and even though laws were enacted against adulteration from the late Middle Ages on, punishment (fines, imprisonment) was dependent on detection, and detection of adulterants was the most primitive of arts before the nineteenth century. The medieval test for determining an excess of sugar in beer, for example, required an 'ale-connor' clad in leather breeches to pour a pint of the beverage onto a wooden stool, then sit in the puddle until it dried; if on attempting to rise he stuck to the seat, the brewer was guilty.[3]

Adulteration was most prevalent in cities, where people relied more on food products prepared and sold by others, and merchants were less likely to know their customers personally and thus to feel less hesitation about cheating them. Thus as the pace of urbanization quickened in the late eighteenth century, so too did the frequency of adulteration. Yet at the same time, alteration of foods was becoming easier to detect, thanks to advances in the science of analytical chemistry. During the last third of the 1700s, there occurred a veritable revolution in chemistry, a quantum leap forward in both theory and laboratory method that at last made it possible to separate chemical mixtures, including food products, into their component parts. By the beginning of the nineteenth century, the identification of culinary adulterants had become a far easier and more certain procedure than it had been before. It was now possible for two to play at the adulteration game: the adulterator, and the chemist who found him out.

Adulteration 'prevails to an extent so alarming, that we may exclaim, with the sons of the Prophet, "There is death in the pot."' So began the first full-scale exposé of the extent of the abuse in Great Britain, Friedrich Accum's 1820 *Treatise on Adulterations of Foods and Culinary Poisons*. Trained in chemistry in his native Germany, Accum emigrated to London in 1793, at the age of 24, and established a school of chemistry and a chemical supply house in Soho. But it was as an analytical chemist that he made his mark, subjecting foodstuffs sold in the London markets to chemical examination, uncovering contamination for profit everywhere he looked, and at last reporting his findings in the *Treatise*. The white bread that was just then becoming so popular among people of refined taste was commonly made white, he determined, by mixing flour with alum, gypsum, chalk, and/or mashed potatoes (he overlooked the additives resulting from the practice many bakers followed of kneading dough with their feet). The 'tea' that might be taken with that 'bread' very often consisted in part or whole of leaves picked from elder, ash, and other trees and shrubs. The 'cream' that might be added to the 'tea' was frequently milk thickened with arrowroot. If one opted for coffee instead, one might well get a blend of various peas and beans that had been roasted and ground. Ground pepper was almost always made with benefit of matter swept up from the floors of pepper warehouses: 'the sweepings', Accum informed readers, 'are known, and purchased in the market, under the name of P. D. signifying pepper dust'. There was an even more degraded form of the product, the 'vile refuse' called D.P.D., or dust of pepper dust.[4]

But if eating dust—or elder leaves or roasted peas—was an insult, it was not necessarily an injury. Accum's warning that there was death in the pot was provoked by other types of adulteration, by the addition of salts of copper to tinned pickles and green beans to intensify their colour, or by the brightening of sweets with red lead glaze. Merchants were so driven by their 'insatiable thirst' for lucre, he complained, that 'the possible sacrifice of even a fellow creature's life is a secondary consideration'.[5]

The thirst for gain was so powerful that even the revered national beverage, the noble product of the brewer's art, was everywhere sold in debased, and often dangerous, form. By law, only malt, hops, yeast, and water were to be used for the production of beer. But in actuality, Accum revealed, 'the ingredients mixed up in the brewer's enchanting cauldron are placed above all competition, even with the potent charms of Macbeth's witches'. Caramel and molasses were added to impart a dark, rich colour; quassia, a wood extract, was added to simulate the bitterness of hops; peppers and 'grains of paradise' (cardamom pods) and 'Spanish juice' (licorice extract) were added to give sharp flavours; powdered oyster shells were added to remove sourness from carelessly fermented brew; alum and salt were added to enhance the head. In the 1810s, a

Mr Jackson actually developed a business that involved 'teaching his mystery to the brewers for a handsome fee,' his mystery being nothing less than a set of recipes for chemical substitutes for malt and hops. Under his command, a small army of chemists marched about the country carrying samples and price lists for their artificial products and offering instruction in the secrets of their degenerate art.[6]

Yet if drinkers were physically harmed by their beer's adulterants, the blame lay not with caramel or cardamom but with cocculus. *Cocculus indicus*, a bitter-tasting extract of the berries of an East Indian shrub, was widely employed as a substitute for hops. In its native region, cocculus was the lazy man's rod and reel; thrown into water, the berries cause fish to rise to the surface, paralysed by the action of the picrotoxin released from the fruit. Taken by humans, picrotoxin duplicates some of the symptoms of arsenic (burning pain, vomiting, diarrhoea), as well as causing confusion and loss of consciousness (cocculus was also employed as 'knockout drops'); in sufficient dosage it brings about convulsions and death by suppression of respiration. The dosage mixed into beer was lower, of course, but it was nevertheless great enough that when drinkers became addled and passed out they were as likely succumbing to the cocculus as to the alcohol. According to a London physician who admitted to his great fondness for beer—unadulterated beer—cocculus 'knocks you down, so to speak' without producing the initial stage of exhilaration given by alcohol. One was especially likely to be knocked down on Saturday night, when, knowing that sales would be particularly brisk, publicans added more cocculus and other adulterants than usual. It was therefore no surprise, another doctor observed, that 'diarrhoea [is] prevalent on Sunday much more than other days'.[7]

The beer of Accum's day possibly contained arsenic as well, but he did not detect any. Wine was another matter, a product contaminated not only with arsenic but by any number of other adulterants. As early as the 1790s, *The Tatler* had warned readers of London's 'subterraneous philosophers', a 'fraternity of chemical operators, who work underground in holes, caverns, and dark retirements' where, hidden from public view, they transmuted base ingredients into 'the choicest products of the hills and valleys of France. They can squeeze Bordeaux out of the sloe, and draw Champagne from an apple.'[8]

The Tatler offered no specifics as to how the sloe became Bordeaux, but Accum the chemist gave details aplenty to back his assertion that few items 'are adulterated to a greater extent than wine'. Cider was stained crimson with Brazil wood and/or beetroot and sold as red wine. Inferior wines were transformed by addition of alum (to brighten colour), gypsum (to remove cloudiness), filbert shells (to increase acidity), *saccharum saturni*, or sugar of lead (lead acetate, a toxic mineral, to counter acidity), almonds (to add nuttiness), and assorted herbs (to give a floral bouquet). Through the adulterator's art, wines could be tailor-made to any specifications. Did one desire a robust red with undertones of blackcurrant or a suggestion of Italian leather? One that was self-assured without being impertinent? It was child's play for the fraternity of chemical operators. Such were their talents that even before Accum's time they were being celebrated in song:

> One glasse of drink, I got by chance,
> 'Twas Claret when it was in France,
> But now from it moche wider:
> I think a man might make as good
> With green crabbes, boyl'd in brazil wood,
> And half a pinte of Cyder.

'O ye gulled Johnny Bulls', another cynic harangued the public, while you think you are drinking genuine champagne, you actually 'are titillating your exquisite gullets with merely plain home made English gooseberry wine'.[9]

Even corks were falsified, Accum determined, the lower ends stained with red dye to give the appearance of having been in long contact with the supposedly well-aged wine. Finally, used bottles were cleaned of tartrate residue clinging to the sides and bottom by rolling lead shot around inside before refilling them. The shot, which were in fact a mix of lead and arsenic (the addition of a bit of arsenic results in rounder shot), were not always completely removed, resulting in cases such as the one reported by Accum, of a man nearly killed by his bottle of Madeira. There was, moreover, another hazard from wine bottles that escaped Accum's attention. Arsenic was often packaged in wine-sized bottles which, once the poison had been used, were collected by peddlers who sold them to wine merchants. Presumably the merchants would rinse the bottles before filling them with wine, but since residual arsenic adhered to the sides of the bottle as a hard crust, it did not quickly dissolve, and could remain in quantity after washing. There was a particular problem with opaque stone bottles preferred for ginger beer, as arsenic deposits could not be seen. Cases of illness, and even death, from this source were not unusual.[10]

Accum also failed to take note of a more common adulteration of wine with arsenic, one which had been in use for a century or more. 'Wine-coopers', men employed by wine merchants to manage their cellars from the time the beverage arrived in the barrel until it was put into the bottle, were responsible for 'fining' the wine, or clarifying it. The desired method of fining was to add isinglass, a form of gelatin prepared from the air bladder of the sturgeon. Wine-coopers, however, had found that for white wine, at least, arsenic did the job quite as well, and at considerably lower cost. Indeed, although red wines had their colour dulled by arsenic, white ones actually acquired an oil-like gloss: in the argot of wine-coopers, arsenic 'put a face upon it'. An inquiry by the House of Commons in the late 1700s had revealed that as much as 500 pounds of arsenic were used annually in London alone for the fining of white wines.[11]

Arsenic-fined wine was claiming victims as early as the 1720s, when two gentlemen who frequented The Red Lion in Henley died within hours of taking their evening tipple. A companion in their session was one Francis Blandy, who took sick but survived, escaping a poetic demise from wine only to meet a quarter-century later the most prosaic of ends, death by gruel. In an instance in the 1760s, several other gentlemen were killed by wine taken with dinner at an inn, but not before hearing the innkeeper berate their waiter, as soon as they began to vomit, for having 'tilted the cask too high' and drawing off wine from the bottom, where the arsenic finings had settled. And only five years before Accum's book was published, a similar incident occurred in London, newspaper accounts of which caused the public to 'start with amazement and horror' at 'the incalculable mischief' being perpetrated by 'wine doctors'. One writer attempted to calculate the mischief nevertheless, estimating that the quantity of arsenic being put into white wine was sufficient to kill three and a half million people yearly. That such devastation was not actually occurring was owing merely, he proposed, to 'the largely diluted state in which it is swallowed; and it does not follow that it occasions no bad consequences by its slower and more insidious operation'. The insidiousness of so many wines was captured nicely in a bit of doggerel of the day about a country lad who comes to London and has his upright conscience shocked to learn how his cousin, a wine seller, adulterates his beverages. Sent up to the city with

> ... my father's kind blessing,
> To our cousin, the wine merchant, where I soon learn'd
> About mixing, and brewing, and pressing;
> But the sloe juice and rat's bane, and all that fine joke
> Was soon in my stomach arising,
> Why, dang it! cried I, would you kill the poor folk?
> I thought you sold wine, and not poison.[12]

Adulterations were reported in an array of other foods, as well as common drugs, and Accum even published the names of merchants he had found guilty of the abuses. But adulteration was not always so simple a matter as a wine-cooper putting arsenic into his bottles. Dangerous food and drink could come to market through far more complicated mechanisms, through serial adulterations in which no one anticipated that physical injury might result. Accum traced the labyrinthine route, for example, by which a London man was made ill by the Gloucester cheese he often took with dinner. After several episodes of poisoning, the man had the cheese tested chemically and learned it contained red lead. But when he complained to his cheesemonger, the merchant assured him he had added nothing to the product. Undeterred, the man sought out the farmer from whom the monger had purchased the cheese and wrung from him an admission that he had mixed annatto with the cheese, but nothing else (annatto, a yellow-red dye made from the seeds of a tropical tree, was commonly used to give cheese a more intense colour). Further investigation determined that the man who had sold the annatto to the farmer had been dissatisfied with the colour of that particular batch, so had mixed vermilion, a red pigment, with it. Vermilion is a compound of mercury, and not a particularly wholesome substance to consume in quantity—but it is not red lead. Going yet one more step, the London gentleman learned from the druggist from whom the annatto merchant had purchased the vermilion that he commonly added the inexpensive red lead to his vermilion to increase his profit, and did not worry about poisoning anyone because he assumed the vermilion would be used only in house paint. What Accum called 'the circuitous...operations of commerce' worked in wondrous and poisonous ways indeed.[13]

If poison intended for house paint could end up in cheese, almost anything could happen, so Accum's *Treatise* was bound to stir public passions. As one of the book's multitude of reviewers commented, 'bread turns out to be a crutch to help us onward to the grave, instead of the staff of life; in porter there is no support, in cordials no consolation; in almost every thing poison and in scarcely any medicine cure'. The reviewer professed (only half in jest) to be 'almost angry with Mr Accum' for opening people's eyes 'at the risk of shutting our mouths forever'.[14]

But the public never loses its appetite for scandal, and other exposés of adulteration soon followed to satisfy the taste. Among the more popular were *Wine and Spirit Adulterators Unmasked*, authored by One of the Old School; an anonymous *The Domestic Chemist*, which actually attempted to train every man to be his own chemist so as to detect adulterants in his purchases; and An Enemy of Fraud and Villainy's long-winded dissertation on *Deadly Adulteration and Slow Poisoning: or, Disease and Death in the Pot and the Bottle; in Which the Blood-empoisoning and Life-destroying Adulterations of Wines, Spirits, Beer, Bread, Flour, Tea, Sugar, Spices, Cheesemongery, Pastry, Confectionary, Medicines, etc. etc. etc. are Laid Open to the Public, with Tests or Methods for Ascertaining and Detecting the Fraudulent and Deleterious Adulterations and the Good and Bad Qualities of those Articles: with an Expose of Medi-*

cal Empiricism and Imposture, Quacks and Quackery, Regular and Irregular, Legitimate and Illegitimate: and the Frauds and Mal-practices of Pawnbrokers and Madhouse Keepers.[15]

Such works only modestly extended Accum's lengthy list of abuses, but they kept his 'death in the pot' fears at the simmer by maintaining that adulteration was responsible for 'the loss of tens of thousands of human lives every year' in London alone. As the Enemy of Fraud and Villainy put it, how could a person expect any life but a short one 'where every meal ought to have its counteracting medicine'. The only solace to be found in such a situation was that the adulterators were as busy cheating one another as they were the general public: 'The baker abuses the butcher for selling diseased meat; the butcher sneers at the druggist for not knowing the names of his own medicines; the druggist taunts the grocer with selling birch leaves for tea; and the grocer is furiously indignant with the baker for giving short weight.... A plague upon you all.'[16]

Just as amusing was the fact that, doctored food products being the norm, many people seemed to have forgotten the taste of genuine articles and acquired a preference for the flavours of the fake. The lesson was learned by the Lancashire brewer who began his career making ale properly, from malt and hops only, but found his unadulterated product didn't sell. After a period of barely scraping by, he asked a friend for advice. 'Send for an old man from Wigan,' the friend advised, to get someone who could brew 'to the taste of working men'. The secret of the old man from nearby Wigan was to throw a pound of tobacco into each batch of ale; soon the brewer's business was booming. Likewise the business of the retailer of 'gunpowder tea', a brew made explosive by the admixture of large proportions of silkworm dung. 'Its flavour was very peculiar,' a master of understatement commented, 'yet it found a large market.' Or, finally, consider the experience of a grocer who set up shop in Bradford itself, 'foolishly commencing with a determination to vend genuine goods'. His working-class customers complained from the outset. One, for example, 'brought back my genuine Jamaica [coffee], declaring that it was not near so good as—'s'. After repeated instances of this sort, the grocer purchased some of—'s exceptional coffee and found it to be only 30 per cent coffee, the rest being comprised of chicory and other impurities. 'After a contest between conscience and interest, the former gave way,' the grocer confessed. He obtained his own lot of chicory, began mixing it into his Jamaica, and was soon being told 'that my coffee was superior to—'s'. Clearly, consumers cannot be exonerated from complicity in the adulteration follies. As an eighteenth-century compiler of *Wise Sentences and Witty Sayings* recognized, 'If fools went not to market, bad wares would not be sold.' Too many people were too little discerning to even notice the inferiority of their food and drink.[17]

*

Overall, the reaction of the public to Accum and the volumes that followed was one of indignation. Although some found the death-in-the-pot publications excessive, 'indiscreet and mischievous efforts [by] overzealous or designing alarmists...to terrify the public mind', their very sensationalism generated a furore over falsified foods and drugs that was sustained for two decades. The fire was then stoked even higher by the publications of Arthur Hill Hassall, 'the Apostle of Anti-adulteration'. Hassall was a London medical practitioner who was drawn to the adulteration question in the late 1840s. A lecture on counterfeit coffee that he delivered in 1850 brought him to the attention of the editor of *The Lancet*. Subsequently, Hassall was invited to direct an Analytical Sanitary Commission for the journal, a body that would carry out a systematic scientific study of adulteration and publish its findings (in the usage of the time, 'sanitary' meant healthful, being derived from the Latin *sanitas*, health; thus the Analytical Sanitary Commission was charged with using chemical analysis to determine the healthfulness, rather than the cleanliness, of foods). In a series of reports presented from 1851 to 1854, Hassall provided the most thoroughgoing survey yet of the reach of adulteration, reinforcing the traditional chemical procedures with examination of food products under the microscope, a method of analysis in which he was the pioneer.[18]

When 'the urchin who filches a bun is liable to punishment and even imprisonment,' Hassall began his series, the fact that 'the cunning and systematic adulterator' should be allowed 'to go at large unscathed, is an insult to common sense'. Thus at the outset, the chemist/microscopist signalled his intent not merely to detect specific adulterants, but more importantly to bring specific adulterators to justice. Ultimately, he hoped to see legislation enacted to punish food sophistication, but in the short term he relied on the tried-and-true deterrent of shame, measures that would 'entail personal discredit and probable loss', that is, publication of the identity of offenders. Accum had named names too, but to nothing like the extent to which Hassall exposed wrongdoers. He eventually cited nearly 3,000 vendors, complete with the addresses of their shops, and perhaps the surest measure of the reliability of his analyses was that only a handful undertook legal action against *The Lancet* for false statements, and of those few not one was successful.[19]

Hassall's revelations began, naturally enough, with coffee, the beverage that had first brought him to *The Lancet*'s notice. He presented much the same line-up of additives as Accum had found, but now reinforced with drawings of the microscopic structure of coffee beans, and of chicory root, the most common adulterant. In that same initial report, he also dealt with sugar, and in subsequent issues the adulterations of pepper, mustard, bread, tea, milk, vinegar, potted meats, bottled fruits and vegetables, and assorted other comestibles were identified. Through all that, no mention was made of arsenic. But in the spring of 1854, Hassall finally arrived at the category of 'coloured confectionery', and the poison was now brought into the spotlight.[20]

To be sure, the fact that arsenic was often present in sweets was not exactly news. As far back as 1830, a *Lancet* contributor had mentioned the practice among Parisian confectioners of imparting eye-catching colours to their creations by coating them with several different minerals, including the arsenic compound Schweinfurt green. 'Millions of children are thus daily dosed' with poisons, he declared, and not just French *enfants* but English girls and boys too. Indeed, his chemical analyses uncovered the presence of all the same toxic minerals in British-made sweets—except for arsenic, which he was unable to find.[21]

He simply didn't examine enough sweets. Only three years after that paper was published, another *Lancet* article reported finding both Schweinfurt green and a second arsenical pigment, Scheele's green, among the numerous minerals employed to colour 'the showy, but poisoned, baits which are exhibited in every confectioner's shop in London.' Actual cases of poisoning from arsenical confections also appeared in medical literature in the years preceding Hassall's study. In 1849, for example, several children in Marlborough were made dreadfully ill by eating the green leaves of imitation fuchsias used to decorate the cake served at a party. They all survived their encounter with Scheele's green, but others were not so fortunate. In 1853, two brothers died after eating green and yellow decorations on a cake purchased to celebrate Twelfth Night (the green pigment was copper arsenate, the yellow orpiment), and by then Alfred Taylor had already recorded at least ten fatalities among children who had consumed cake ornaments. The fear of green confections such incidents generated persisted well into the twentieth century in some areas. A toxicology text published in the 1950s quoted a Glasgow baker's complaint that any sort of green decoration on a cake 'can reduce the possibilities of sale in many parts of Scotland'. The baker grumbled that he had often had to eat a green-adorned cake himself because he couldn't sell it; 'my customers preferred to go without rather than touch the arsenical-looking things.'[22]

In his 1854 reports on confectionery, Hassall listed more than a dozen toxic minerals regularly used to colour sweets. Yellow came most often from lead chromate (though also from gamboge, a botanical with drastic purgative properties), and red most commonly from lead oxide (red lead); in a sample of lozenges purchased from a Mr Carr of 14 Pilgrim Street, both compounds were present in 'quite poisonous amount'. But yellow was sometimes produced by orpiment and red by realgar, both arsenic compounds, and any green was likely to be copper arsenite (Scheele's green, named for Carl Wilhelm Scheele, the Swedish chemist who discovered it in the 1770s). A merchant in Brick Lane sold candy pheasants standing on grass coloured with Scheele's green in amounts 'highly poisonous', and one in Shepherd's Market offered sugar dogs reclining on grass tinted with an amount of arsenic 'so considerable as to be absolutely poisonous'. Among the cases of absolute poisoning he presented to back up his warnings were the thirty to forty children sickened by candies purchased 'from a Jew, in Petticoat-lane'. To the seller's credit, he seems not to have been aware of the dangers of his merchandise, having purchased it from a 'very respectable' London firm. So very respectable was the company, in fact, the vomit of the stricken children was found to contain copper, lead, and iron in addition to arsenic.[23]

None of those children died, fortunately, but others did. In addition to victims already listed, there were the two children who were killed in 1853 after eating a green pastry ornament they found lying in the street. And there was the 4-year-old whose father brought home a confectionery decoration from a fête honouring Irish soldiers returned from the Crimean War, a decoration tinged with Ireland's national colour. More than a dozen of the soldiers were also sickened by the dessert, nor was this the only instance of a deadly banquet. In 1848, two Northampton caterers were convicted of manslaughter for serving arsenic for dessert at an ordination celebration held in the city's Temperance Hall. They had used Schweinfurt green to colour the fake leaves and cucumber placed atop a blancmange, a practice they had followed for years, but this time 'had used a somewhat larger portion than usual to give a more beautiful colour'. One of the celebrants at the mid-afternoon meal consumed half a pound of the blancmange, 'went to bed at 8, and was a corpse at 5 in the morning'. Criminal charges were an unusual reaction to an adulteration incident, but in this case there was evidence that the chemist from whom they purchased the green had warned them of its toxicity and told them not to use it in food; they had done so nonetheless. Each was sentenced to three months.[24]

Hassall's articles were frequently reprinted in the popular press, and sparked considerable turmoil, especially among the tradesmen whose deceptions he exposed. As one reviewer described the effect, 'a gun suddenly fired into a rookery could not cause a greater commotion' than his publication of the names of dishonest dealers had done. 'Nor does the daylight, when you lift a stone, startle ugly and loathsome things more quickly than the pencil of light' that streamed through Hassall's microscope. Grocers had been thrown into 'a state of great perturbation', the *Family Herald* reported, and many and loud were the howls of protest they lodged with *The Lancet* in defence of their honour as tradesmen and gentlemen. But in reading their complaints, one is struck that they do protest too much, that their overwrought objections prove nothing more clearly than the effectiveness of Hassall's policy of advertising adulterators' names.[25]

Consumers were as upset as the counterfeiters, being stirred to anger and anxiety by the extensive publicity given Hassall's studies. Even humour magazines turned serious at his disclosures, *Punch*, for example, praising *The Lancet's* 'Scientific Detective Force' for discovering such 'an immense quantity of villainous stuff', and for exposing the 'rascality...of the rogues at whose swindling establishments the samples of rubbish were purchased'. In a separate piece, *Punch* turned preacher, calling sweetmakers to atonement: 'Come forth, you trembling Confectioner! [and] with sinking knees and perpendicular locks, confess,' confess and repent of your sin of tempting 'unsuspecting little worshippers' of sweets to 'taste death'. The ubiquity and danger of adulteration were now topics of everyday discourse, and public opinion so vigorously aroused that consideration of protective legislation became imperative.[26]

Historically, legislation has been one of two major strategies employed to address chemical threats in food and the environment; the other has been education. These approaches can be illustrated by their use in the recent battle in the United States against one of the most dreaded poisons of the early twenty-first century: trans fats. Trans fats are a category of unsaturated fats that have been chemically altered to raise their melting point, rendering them useful additions to shortening, margarine, water biscuits, and snack foods. When used for deep-frying trans fats impart appealing flavour and texture characteristics. They also extend a product's shelf life. Unfortunately, the fats also raise serum cholesterol levels and have been linked to increased risk of heart disease and diabetes. Much attention has been given to instructing the public on the problem, consumers being urged to avoid all processed foods whose labels reveal them to contain the fats—just as Hassall warned his contemporaries against purchasing green confectionery. This education strategy can, in effect, mobilize a consumer boycott that pressures producers to change their ways: during 2006, fast food firms across the socio-economic spectrum from Kentucky Fried Chicken to Starbuck's announced they were phasing out their use of trans fats, and early in 2007 the same pledge was made for a cherished American institution, Girl Scout cookies.[27]

Persuading the public voluntarily to shun certain products, however, can be expected to go only so far. Opponents of trans fats recognize that not all consumers will get the message (or heed it if they do), and that not all restaurants can be trusted to end their use of offensive oils. Complete protection requires that trans fats be eliminated by legislation. This second strategy, prohibition, was put into play in December 2006, when the New York City Health Department adopted a statutory ban; since then, several other American cities have followed the example, and one entire state (California, of course). At the same time, there is solid resistance from those who deplore governmental interference with private enterprise and with the freedom of individuals to choose how to live. Consider but three of the comments posted on gothamist.com in response to New York City's ban: 'The people's socialist republic of NY never changes. I can't believe that there are people dumb enough to support such an intrusion into personal choice'; 'A dangerous line is being crossed with laws like this. One that moves us closer to an authoritarian society, where government controls small decisions about how we live and what we consume'; 'FREE COUNTRY? Ha ha ha ha ha ha ha ha ha ... my ass!' Efforts at persuasion, attempts at prohibition, and resistance on laissez-faire and libertarian principles similarly ran through efforts to address all categories of arsenic threats in the nineteenth century.[28]

With respect to food adulteration, the transition from persuasion to prohibition began with the formation of a Parliamentary investigative body, The Select Committee on the Adulteration of Food, in the summer of 1855. Hassall was called as the Committee's first witness. He in essence reviewed his Analytical Sanitary Commission's findings for the full range of food products, but for the purpose of dramatizing the physical harmfulness of adulterated articles he singled out a particular category of edibles: coloured confectionery. Holding out samples of the bright and shiny sweetmeats for Committee members to inspect, he outlined for them how a person enjoying a typical dinner might 'run the chance of a dose of red lead' with his cayenne-spiced curry, and 'be nearly sure to have copper administered to him' from the accompanying pickles; yet while the main course was dangerous enough, 'if he partook of *bon-bons* at dessert, there is no telling what number of poisonous pigments he might consume'. There was an 'enormous consumption' of such candies, so that 'scarcely a year passes' without fatalities. Other witnesses reiterated his emphasis, toxicologist Henry Letheby, for one, identifying the use of mineral pigments in candy as 'the most common and the most serious' of the adulterations practised for the sake of improving a product's appearance: 'There is not an article of confectionery in this country which is not so coloured.'[29]

The Select Committee's first meeting prompted a reaction from *Punch*, in the form of an article advising the public 'What to eat, drink and avoid.' Listing a number of common adulterations, including that of bakers substituting chalk for flour, the author worried that 'if we mix up our crust with our slice of Cheshire, we may be literally unable to tell the chalk from the cheese'. On leafing over, readers met with a full-page cartoon that suggested adulteration could nevertheless be turned to worthwhile ends. Over the legend 'The Use of Adulteration', a young girl is shown standing at a grocer's counter, conveying her mother's request for 'a quarter pound of your best tea to kill the rats with, and a ounce of chocolate to get rid of the black beadles'. Beneath the counter can be seen containers of red lead, nux vomica (a botanic source of strychnine), and... plaster of Paris.[30]

The Select Committee met for nearly two years, gathering evidence from a small army of expert witnesses and considering published critiques such as *The Tricks of Trade in the Adulteration of Food*, an 1856 volume that revealed how confectionery-makers lured buyers with shapes as well as colours. In the sweetmeat shops of Tottenham Court Road, for example, where thousands daily passed along one of London's great thoroughfares, display windows were packed with sugary creations sculpted not just as flowers and animal figures, as one would expect, but also as shoulders of mutton and rashers of bacon and other mouth-watering recreations of the dinner table. Parliament as a whole, however, was at first deaf to the Committee's call for legislative action, reluctant to meddle with the free working of the marketplace. 'The people must take care of themselves,' one critic characterized MPs' attitude; consumers should mind what they're at, and even adulterators' robbery and assault through fraud 'is to be preferred to any interference with the sacred principle of *laissez faire*'.[31]

Protests and poisonings nevertheless did at last provoke the introduction of an anti-adulteration bill into the House of Commons in 1857. The measure failed to pass, and the subject was dropped until a similar bill was set before the House two years later. The 1859 version was voted down too, the oratory that denounced

adulteration as 'a national disgrace' being countered by a battery
of objections to legislative interference, most notably that people
could determine for themselves if the food they bought was to their
liking or if it harmed them: 'It was not an advantageous proceeding,' one opponent thundered, 'to treat the people of this country
like children.' Soon government would have such power as even 'to
lay down what proportion of water a man might put in his grog.'
('FREE COUNTRY? Ha, ha, ha, ha, ha ...').[32]

But, came the rejoinder, did not the people already have enough
to do to earn their daily bread 'without spending time in analysing
it'. Thus did the people's representatives chase one another round
and round. In the end, however, there was a pro-legislation argument that could not be laughed off. As it was put by the speaker
who challenged a colleague for exhibiting such 'vigour in favour
of Free Trade': Had 'his hon. Friend forgotten the Bradford poisoning case?'[33] The Bradford poisonings could not be forgotten,
having occurred only a few months before, and the memory of the
horrifying events caused by carelessness in the pursuit of adulteration would be a potent influence in converting Parliament to support of an anti-adulteration law.

*

The particular adulteration pursued by Bradford confectioner
Joseph Neal, that of substituting plaster of Paris for a quantity of
sugar, was a deceit widely practised (typically 25–35 per cent of
the sugar was replaced). Hassall had pointed it out in his publications, and others had branded it unwholesome as well as fraudulent: 'The effect of plaster of Paris upon the stomach', a London
chemistry professor had informed Parliament's Select Committee,
'is that of a quantity of rubbish'.[34] But when the plaster is instead
arsenic, the effect goes far beyond any quantity of rubbish, as the
citizenry of Bradford learned the hard way.

When Neal placed his order for plaster of Paris under the name 'daft', he was honouring a practice long dear to adulterators of employing obscure nicknames for the fraudulent articles they employed (Accum revealed a number of the slang terms in his treatise: 'multum' for the quassia and liquorice blend added to beer, for example, and 'flash' for the sugared capsicum extract used in brandy and rum. There was even 'stuff', an epitome of opaqueness, which was applied to the alum and salt mixture kneaded into bread.) When the daft arrived, Neal ordered one of his workers to use it to prepare a batch of peppermint lozenges. The employee had performed the task any number of times before, without event, but on this occasion he began to feel ill soon after starting the job, experiencing vomiting and tingling pains in his face and arms; at one point, he had such an attack of sneezing that Neal jokingly asked if he was putting Cayenne pepper into the mixture. Nevertheless, he drew no connection between his sickness and the daft. He apparently completely overlooked the denser, coarser nature of that day's powder compared to the plaster of Paris he was accustomed to working with. Here was the second instance of negligence in what was a rapidly building tragedy of errors.[35]

The third was Neal's observation that the candies took an unusually long time to dry and were darker in colour than usual; they seemingly were not his normal fake confections, yet he put them out for sale anyway. Indeed, he sold a full 40 lb of lozenges to William Hardaker, a vendor in Bradford's Saturday market, marking them down a half penny per pound because of their discoloration. The discounted price and odd hue of the product failed to arouse Hardaker's suspicions either, even when on market day, 30 October, he sampled one of the sweets and became so ill he had to beg a friend to take over his stall. The friend worked into the evening, dispensing an estimated thousand peppermints before closing down.

The mints worked quickly: in the words of a London journalist, 'presently in the streets and in the houses lamentations arose'. By Sunday morning, two young boys had died, and over the course of the day—Hallowe'en—several more fatalities as well as numerous cases of illness resulted from the treats that were in actuality a deadly trick. By the evening, it had been determined that all the victims had partaken of the peppermints, and police fanned out to public houses and other gathering spots to inform the citizenry of the tainted sweets. With the light of the next day, warning placards were affixed to walls throughout the city, urging people to bring any lozenges they had purchased to the police. But for many the warnings came too late. By midday Monday, a dozen had died, and seventy-eight were known to be seriously ill—and that was only in Bradford. Additional victims were succumbing in neighbouring communities. There was, for example, the housewife of East Ardsley whose husband brought home sweets from the Bradford market. After dinner, husband was off to the White Swan for what, one suspects, was his usual Saturday night. When he returned home between one and two, he found his wife vomiting and purging uncontrollably; she died the next morning. In the meantime, the young son of a neighbour had chanced upon one of the lozenges that had somehow fallen onto the ground. He ate it, naturally, and died the next evening. There were so many other cases it was 'impossible to keep a catalogue', reporters declared; the episode was nothing less than a 'horrible story of whole slaughter' that had transformed 'many cheerful homes into scenes of sudden and inconsolable sorrow'.[36]

Meanwhile, police had moved quickly to confiscate Hardaker's remaining lozenges, then descended upon Neal (who 'took to his heels, and ran away from the officers', but was soon apprehended). From the confectioner another 35 lb of mints were seized. These had been added to an assortment of other sweets to form 'Scotch mixture', which, fortunately, had not yet been put out for sale; the policeman assigned to fish the lozenges out of the mixture was twice required to take a break due to itching and stinging in his eyes and hands.[37]

Neal was taken into custody, along with Hodgson the chemist and his hapless apprentice, for an inquest at the Pack Horse Inn. There chemists testified that the lozenges contained as much as 15 gr of arsenic apiece! The wonder, then, is not that twenty-one people died, but that so few perished, particularly since many children were recipients of the sweets. The inquest jury, not surprisingly, remanded the prisoners for trial for manslaughter.

One would hardly have bet on their chances of acquittal, for the entire nation was up in arms over the poisonings, including *Punch*, which did its best to find humour in the situation. In 'Lozenges for Lunatics', it was suggested that henceforth 'a demand to be served with a cheap sweetmeat must imply a fitness for immediate strait-waistcoating', and in 'The Advantage of Adulteration' that dramatists might want to try out a new plot device: 'why not take a leaf from the Lucrezia Borgia *Cookery-Book*' and have the play's characters sit down to dinner, 'and there polish them all off with adulterated sweetmeats'. *Punch* also produced a song to mark the tragedy, 'The Plague of Adulteration' ('For nothing but ill-health can come | From the Plague of Adulteration!'), and the formation of a new lollipop company that would guarantee poison-free sweets was announced. The most striking portrayal of the hazard, though, was a cartoon depicting 'The Great Lozenge-maker', Death, working at his mortar and pestle, a barrel of arsenic to the left and a crate of plaster of Paris to the right (Fig. 4). On a shelf to the rear rests a box

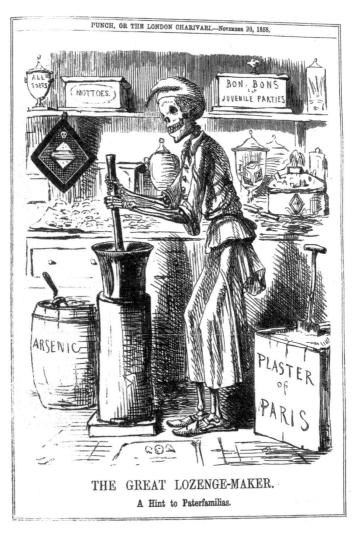

THE GREAT LOZENGE-MAKER.

A Hint to Paterfamilias.

4. 'The Great Lozenge-maker', *Punch* cartoon, 1858

of 'Bon-bons for juvenile parties'. The drawing's subtitle, 'A Hint to Paterfamilias', alerts parents to be watchful.[38]

Yet when the trial of the three men was held, three days before Christmas, the jury could find no violation of a law. The episode was simply a highly regrettable accident, leaving *The Times* to wonder how the druggist who had sent an inexperienced apprentice 'into a garret where were the two tubs of life and death' could be found free of blame. 'There has been a sufficient expenditure of life to insure a very considerable military success,' the paper objected, 'and nothing is gained.'[39]

But something was gained, for 'the Bradford incident' proved to be the last straw in the accumulation of abuses by food and drug tradesmen. Even though the arsenic was an accidental rather than intentional contaminant, it had found its way into the lozenges precisely because of the intent to adulterate, and both the press and the public erupted in outrage that there was no law to inhibit such practices. A letter to the *Manchester Guardian* conveyed the depth of anger that affected ordinary citizens:

I feel, after reading of this horrible catastrophe at Bradford, that it is high time for a new agitation to take place—for us, who are 'the people,' to claim from our Legislature laws to protect us from that foul abortion, born of selfishness and avarice, adulteration. . . . Will anyone tell me what right that lozenge maker had to sell us plaster of Paris for sugar? Why should our stomachs be disordered, our children's health destroyed; nay, all of our very lives shortened, to put money into that lozenge maker's pocket? It is part of a vile system that needs the strong hand of power to abolish it. . . . Until we have laws which make a penal crime of this most dishonest adulteration, we shall not strike at the root of the evil.

The letter was signed 'One of the people', and enough other people vented similar feelings, in letters, in public meetings, and in petitions presented to Parliament, that the legislative body had no choice but to act.[40]

But it did not act immediately. While most members agreed in principle with the need to outlaw adulteration and penalize adulterators so as to prevent future Bradfords, there was the usual haggling over just what wording and precisely what provisions would best accomplish the purpose. Not until the 1860 session was the Adulteration of Food or Drink bill made law, its enactment comprising an early version of an oft-told tale, that of the failure of legislators seriously to address a public health threat until scandal or calamity force a response. America's first significant anti-adulteration law, the 1906 Food and Drugs Act, was debated in Congress for years, but not adopted until *The Jungle*, Upton Sinclair's novel exposing Chicago's meat-packing industry, induced a national attack of nausea. That Act was largely ineffective, yet while its weakness was soon apparent and demands for a statute with sharper teeth quickly followed, nothing was done to amend it until a drug product using a toxic solvent killed more than 100 people in 1937. The 1938 Food, Drug, and Cosmetics Act, still the basic law empowering America's Food and Drug Administration, was adopted by Congress only after what was essentially a repeat of the Bradford incident.[41]

Despite all the legislative fine-tuning, the Act for Preventing Adulteration in Food and Drink was next to useless as an impediment to adulteration. Its provisions were too vague and lenient, its punishments (a maximum fine of £5) too lax to deter violators. To cite but one instance of continued adulteration after its passage, in 1862 three children were killed and two more sickened by arsenical sweets eaten on Christmas Day. The Act's impotence was ridiculed even in children's literature. Kingsley's *The Water-Babies*, published after the Act had been in force three years, details the adventures of a young chimney sweep named Tom in the imaginary land of Other-end-of-Nowhere. There he encounters 'foolish and wicked

people [who] invent poisons for little children, and sell them at
wakes and fairs' (read Bradford market). These villains are breaking
the law, but 'Dr. Hassall cannot catch them', even though 'setting
traps for them all day long', because the law is too weak; so weak,
in fact, as to require supernatural assistance. Hence 'the Fairy with
the birch-rod' is brought in to save the day. She 'will catch them
all in time, and make them begin at one corner of their shops, and
eat their way out at the other: by which time they will have got
such stomachaches as will cure them of poisoning little children'.
When Dr Hassall issued an updated survey of adulteration in 1876,
he reported that arsenical pigments were still being freely used to
colour confectionery. Attempts to strengthen the 1860 law were
enacted in 1862 and 1872, but they too were inadequate. Not until
the Sale of Food and Drugs Act of 1875 was there legislation forceful enough to bring adulteration under some measure of control
and discourage any repetition of Bradford.[42]

The Bradford poisonings, it should be added, also figured in the
adoption of the Pharmacy Act of 1868, mentioned in the previous
chapter. Where confectioner Neal demonstrated the greed of food
adulterators, chemist Hodgson exemplified the carelessness of those
who sold drugs and poisons and the too common ignorance of their
apprentices. Less than five months prior to the Bradford outbreak,
a member of the House of Commons had argued for restrictions
on who should be allowed to sell poisons, by reminding his fellows
of 'those lamentable accidents' periodically caused by negligent or
unqualified druggists. And when that highly lamentable accident
did soon occur in Bradford, it became the battle-cry of proponents
of regulation. 'This fearful tragedy', the *Medical Times and Gazette*
editorialized, 'will, we cannot doubt, force upon government the
necessity of their passing some legislative act to remedy this defect
in our laws.' Those sentiments were echoed in the popular press,

but while legislation was debated in Parliament from 1859 onward, it was not until the 1868 Act that the sale of poisons was finally restricted to qualified chemists and druggists. An influential event in moving along passage of the law, incidentally, was the mid-1860s poisoning of a number of people by arsenic accidentally mixed with cream of tartar by a careless druggist. And where did those poisonings take place? Bradford, of course.[43]

7

'The Hue of Death, the Tint of the Grave'

On a June evening in 1837, a Mr Everitt, professor of chemistry, London, prepared to retire. He blew out a candle—a newly purchased one—and at once the air was filled by the scent of garlic. It will be remembered from Chapter 3 that 'an abominable stinking Smell like Garlic' had long been recognized as an indication of arsenic being heated. It was not, as explained, the most reliable test. But it was a suggestive enough hint that a chemistry professor could hardly ignore it. Next day, Everitt took the candle to the laboratory and determined that arsenic—in the form of arsenious acid, white arsenic—was indeed present in the fumes released from the wick. As noted earlier, the garlic aroma results from the heating of elemental arsenic, not arsenious acid. Everitt the chemist knew that. Thus, he reasoned, when the candle was extinguished, the incandescent wick must provide the right temperature for reducing some of the white arsenic to the elemental state, generating the 'alliaceous odour' he detected. Yet while the candle was burning, there was no odour at all to warn of poison being released.[1]

The candle in question was of a variety new on the market, 'composition candles', as they were being called. Everitt purchased more of the tapers, from several different sources, and determined that white arsenic was present in every one, and in amounts that he believed might well be dangerous. He announced his findings in a public lecture, and there quickly followed confirmations by other scientists, alarming notices in the popular press, a 'Death in the Candle' warning in *The Lancet*, and objections from medical men to the exposure of the public to products that 'may with propriety be called—CORPSE-CANDLES'. Thus did there come to light the presence of arsenic in the wider environment beyond food and drink, the harbinger, moreover, of a host of arsenic-containing manufactures to follow.[2]

If there was any satisfaction to be had in the appearance of poisonous candles on the British market, it was that the threatening items were the handiwork of Frenchmen. Prior to the 1830s, candles were made either from wax, spermaceti (a waxy substance from sperm whales), or, most inexpensively, tallow (beef or mutton fat). In the 1810s, Michel Chevreul, the French scientist who led the way in clarifying the chemistry of fats, found that tallow could be separated into two components, one solid, one liquid. To the solid compound, he gave the name 'stearine', and determined that it had a higher melting point than crude tallow, making it a more desirable material for candles. By the early 1830s, Parisian manufacturers had turned his discoveries to account and were producing stearine candles in quantity. Marketed under a variety of alluring brand names, the candles were received warmly by the public. They were as aesthetically pleasing as expensive wax candles, while being nearly as cheap as the ordinary tallow ones.[3]

But the candles came with a catch. To keep them from being brittle and to give them the smoothness and sheen of the wax product, a certain chemical had to be added to the molten stearine when it was poured into the moulds to cool: white arsenic. The process was at first a tightly guarded trade secret, shared among manufacturers but kept from the public. Early in 1834, however, the secret got out. Authorities confiscated all the candles on the market, prohibited their future manufacture, and, just like that, they boasted, 'every trace of arsenicated candles was obliterated from the capital of France'.[4]

In the meantime, though, the secret had been sold to a London candlemaker, who in turn made the rounds of other manufacturers to share his method—for a consideration, naturally. It must have been a reasonable enough consideration, for from 1835 into 1836 the production of arsenic-stearine candles spread throughout the country. Yet for two years the public remained in the dark about the composition of the prized new candles, kept unaware until Professor Everitt smelled garlic.[5]

Did composition candles truly deserve to be called corpse candles? Common sense agreed with Everitt that they must be dangerous, and a few individuals did report being made ill by them. One man complained of being sickened by the fumes of candles in his hotel room. Another related how the air in a room he lit with the candles one evening 'became exceedingly oppressive', leaving him convinced that the new product was 'a deadly and insidious destroyer'. A handful of anecdotal accounts does not, however, constitute proof of injuriousness, so with that in mind, the Westminster Medical Society, a professional association of London practitioners, in the fall of 1837 appointed a committee to evaluate the danger.[6]

The committee members first applied themselves to analysing numerous composition candles purchased from suppliers throughout London: arsenic was found in every one, in concentrations of ten to eighteen grains per pound, with the cheapest candles containing the highest amounts of the poison. It was additionally determined that the arsenic was mechanically mixed with the stearine rather than dissolved in it, so when the hot stearine was poured into the vertical moulds, arsenic tended to settle towards the candle's top, at the lower end of the mould. Consequently, there was nearly a third more poison near the section of the candle that was sure to be burned than at the base.[7]

But to determine if the arsenic released by combustion constituted a significant health threat, it was necessary to expose animals to the fumes. The committee procured several birds—greenfinches and linnets—and placed them in boxes constructed with small openings top and bottom for ventilation and a glass window through which they could be observed. In half the boxes, composition candles were lit and left to burn for ten hours, in the other half, spermaceti candles were burned for the same period. At the end of each day, the candles were extinguished and the cages moved to an adjoining room free of candle smoke; the next morning the process was repeated.[8]

Pity the poor birds confined to the stearine candle boxes. After just four hours, one of the linnets became 'visibly affected'. It recovered during the night, but next day died after only two hours of exposure to the candles; a second linnet succumbed half an hour later. The following day, additional birds died, while those kept in the boxes with sperm candles showed not the first indication of distress. The stearine-candle animals drank four times as much water as the others, lost their appetites almost entirely, and were attacked with green-coloured diarrhoea. All gave signs of laboured respiration, along with 'a convulsive action of the whole body, backwards and forwards . . . with the head drawn on one side, the eyes closed, and the beaks open and pointed upwards'. One of the birds fell from its perch to the bottom of the box, 'where it made various struggles to fly upwards and regain its station, without success. It, at last, after various crawling attempts, reached the edge of the water-cup, on which it balanced itself in a state of evident convulsion, breathing with difficulty, its beak wide open, and the eyes closed.' It remained in that state for three hours before dying. The finches, being larger, survived longer, but they too slowly succumbed with the same symptoms. When the committee presented its report to the Society, one of the boxes was exhibited so that members could appreciate the degree of thirst experienced by the animals: one bird's 'last struggle' had been to get to its water cup, and 'the Society may see how the little creature, having reached the cup, and by stretching its neck over the edge of it, succeeded in dipping its beak into the fluid and expired in that very position'. The same experiment was done with guinea pigs and rabbits, all of which suffered from the arsenical candles, though none died, while those kept in boxes with spermaceti candles remained unaffected throughout. Finally, the committee member who spent the most time tending the boxes experienced painful irritation of his eyes, a condition that did not alleviate until the tests were concluded.[9]

The committee's written report put forward a question for Westminster Medical Society members to ponder: 'Let us suppose', it was suggested, that London's Theatre Royal Drury Lane, whose chandeliers held 152 tapers, 'were to be lighted with Stearine candles for cheapness sake ... In that case 608 grains of arsenious acid would be vaporized and floating in the air during the time of the performance. Is anyone prepared to assert, that not one of the individuals present ... would receive the slightest injury?'[10]

Perhaps not. But by the same token, was anyone prepared to assert that people in the audience would undoubtedly be harmed? And could he prove it? Any birds in attendance would probably die, that seemed clear enough, and larger animals such as rabbits might sicken. But much larger animals—people—might conceivably come through the entire performance unscathed. After all, those

608 grains of arsenious acid would probably not all be inhaled, and whatever quantity was taken in would be distributed among a large number of playgoers. Each member of the audience might inspire less than a grain, possibly much less, and in three hours or so be freed from the tainted auditorium, not to attend another play for weeks or months.

As would subsequently occur with many another consumer product, the discovery of arsenic in candles raised challenging questions. How small an amount of arsenic was enough to cause injury? How frequently and for how long did people have to be exposed to that amount to be injured? What physical signs or symptoms provided evidence of injury? How severe did the injury have to be, and how great a fraction of the population had to be affected, to justify interfering with the manufacture and marketing of an otherwise useful product? Composition candles did not kill people outright the way rat poison or sheep dip did. Any injury was not sudden, violent, and lethal, but chronic, appearing only after weeks or more of exposure, worsening only gradually, and perhaps so general as to be mistaken for the upsets and aches and fatigue that were periodically experienced by everyone for no assignable reason. Developing an understanding of chronic arsenic poisoning, as distinct from the acute form that had occupied physicians for centuries, would take years of experience with a variety of arsenical hazards. At the time of the candle committee's report, no one could have given a certain answer to another of their questions: 'is it too much to assume, that, whenever a large number of candles of arsenicated Stearine are lighted in a room, a club-house, an assembly, a theatre, or a church...mischief to the health of some, at least, of the parties, may be expected?'[11] Maybe it was not too much to assume such a thing. Maybe it was. Not until much later in the century could an answer be given with confidence.

In the event, it seemed prudent for people to make the assumption and to stop buying stearine candles (that was not quite such a straightforward business as it sounds, since some manufacturers were marketing stearine products as pure wax candles—and at wax prices). Any stearine candles already in the home should be discarded, the committee urged, offering advice for identifying undesirable candles that included the garlic-smell test when the wick was snuffed, and rubbing every candle with the edge of an ivory knife: if made of wax or spermaceti, the candle's sheen was heightened; if made of stearine, it was dulled.[12]

Warnings in the press were also building public resistance to poisonous candles, which in turn pressured manufacturers to desist from marketing arsenical tapers. By the end of 1837, advertisements for arsenic-free brands were common in newspapers, the marketers of Pearl Wax Lights not only declaring 'solemnly and unequivocally' that their product contained no arsenic, but even promising a reward to any chemist who could detect in their product even 'an atom of arsenic' (the switch to non-arsenicated candles was made easier, it might be noted, by the discovery that simple chalk worked on stearine just as well as arsenic did). To be sure, not all candle-makers made the change, and complaints about the sale of arsenical candles would continue for several years more. But complaints were infrequent, and by and large the corpse-candle scare had passed by the end of 1837. Popular demand for an arsenic-free product had altered manufacturing practice for the first, but not the last, time in the century.[13]

Early in 1859, another London chemist reported the smell of garlic when a different type of candle was put out. In this instance, the culprit was not stearine, but *green*. The candles were made of wax, wax given a bold green colour by the addition of copper arsenite, the Scheele's green that was so popular for enhancing the appeal of confectionery. By then, in fact, Scheele's and other green arsenic compounds were being used to pigment an astonishing range of products. 'Indeed,' a pharmacist marvelled in 1879, Britain had for some time been possessed by a 'rage for green colour', a rage 'so general that it is a rare thing to find a shop window where arsenical green is not present on the paper of the shelves or walls, the labels and tickets on the articles, and the wrappers or boxes containing the wares'. The rage for green had transformed the domestic environment as well, everything from the paint people put on their walls to the clothing they put on their bodies being coloured with arsenic. A manufacturer of wallpaper informed Alfred Taylor that public demand for the 'cheerful' colour had become so great he was now using up two tons of Scheele's green per week! Yet at the same time, the public was beset on all sides by warnings of the dangers of green objects taken into the home. Consumers were being educated to recognize arsenical green as two-faced: granted, it was the height of fashion, but it was also—in *Punch*'s unsettling phrase—'the hue of death, the tint of the grave'.[14]

*

Prior to the late 1700s, any rage for green the public might feel had to be satisfied by the mineral substances malachite and verdigris, both compounds of copper that had been known since antiquity. Neither gave much intensity of colour, however, and so both were quickly replaced by the much brighter copper arsenite when that substance was introduced by Scheele in 1778. Scheele's green, also known as mineral green, filled the green niche unchallenged until the 1814 discovery of the even more brilliant copper acetoarsenite. First produced in Schweinfurt, it was referred to as Schweinfurt green, but as methods evolved to vary the depth of colour over a wide range (as many as fifty different shades), a bewildering number of names was adopted to identify the various tones: in addition to

Schweinfurt green, there were Paris green (Parisians referred to it as *vert Anglais*), Vienna green, Munich green, Leipzig, Wurzburg, Basel, Kassel, and Swedish greens, emperor and emerald greens, parrot green, and even, as more imaginative possibilities were used up, 'beautiful green' (to make things properly confusing, it was common for emerald green to be used also as a synonym for Scheele's green). By 1860, these many varieties of Schweinfurt green were being produced to the extent of 700 tons per year in Britain alone, and still more was imported from the Continent. Finally, there was copper arsenate, 'a peculiarly vivid green' that was in wide use by mid-century. All these materials, furthermore, provided a profitable application for the mountains of arsenic being generated as a by-product of the growing mining industry—it couldn't all be used for rat poison. Inexpensive green colouring agents agreed with the economic interests of both ore refiners and a host of manufacturers of domestic goods, as well as with the desires of a rapidly expanding urban middle class intent on enjoying more than the necessities of life and eager to display their disposable income through conspicuous consumption of fashionable goods.[15]

The green arsenicals were employed, in the first instance, as paints—for walls, shelves, and any other wooden item that wanted sprucing up (and for canvases too, being favoured by many of the most celebrated artists of the century). When applied to walls, the compounds inevitably flaked off and injured children who put the dust into their mouths (just as lead paints would continue to do during the twentieth century); in at least one instance, such a paint was found covering the walls of a children's ward in a hospital. But one did not have to eat the paint wittingly, for dust could be removed from the wall by friction and then inhaled. In a German incident that received much attention, clerks at a Königsberg courthouse were poisoned by the fine powder rubbed off a storage room's walls by stacks of documents placed against them. 'A thick layer of green-coloured dust' was spread throughout the building by transport of the documents. The same erosive process worked on Venetian blinds, particles of pigment being thrown off each time the blinds were opened and closed. Paint also came loose from shelves, Alfred Taylor discovered in 1854. Preparing to cut into some bread at breakfast, his eye was caught by patches of green on the loaf's lower crust. He scraped off the patches and found they were composed of Scheele's green, the paint, his baker acknowledged, that had recently been used to cover the shelves on which he cooled his breads. The painter who had done the shelves was aware the pigment was toxic, but 'without arsenic', he protested, 'it was impossible to get a good green'.[16]

Toy manufacturers felt the same way, freely applying arsenical paints to building blocks, dolls, balls, hobby-horses, and the rest. Often the colours were only loosely applied and were easily removed by one of a young child's favourite activities, sucking. There are severe illnesses and even deaths recorded from the sucking or licking of various wooden toys, as well as crayons, chalk, and water colours. Paper and cardboard coloured with arsenical pigments claimed a fair share of victims as well, being employed, as they were, in so great a variety of ways. They were commonly used, for example, to wrap cakes and sweets; a number of cases of poisoning resulted from contamination of the confection by its wrapper, while many others, doctors believed, were overlooked, parents blaming their child's vomiting and diarrhoea on too many sweets. The paper chosen by a prestigious London firm to wrap its chocolates was highly arsenical, yet the confections were promoted with a testimonial from Arthur Hill Hassall himself, that scourge of adulterators; 'the least crease or crumple' of the paper would detach arsenic onto the chocolate, according to the physician who sent a sample wrapper to *The Lancet*, Hassall's own journal. Many of the papers supplied to kindergarten children for art projects were arsenical, a twelve-inch-square sheet of one being found to contain 'double the fatal dose of arsenic for an adult'. Teachers eventually became aware of the toxicity of such papers and began to warn pupils not to put the material into their mouths, but even those children who obeyed might well take the completed project home where a younger sibling knew no better. Children's books were frequently bound with arsenical paper, as were volumes for adults. A young boy who used the back of a green tome from his parents' bookcase as a palette for watercolours nearly died from arsenic ingested by sharpening the tip of his brush between his lips. The book, with fine irony, had been published by a society for the prevention of cruelty to children.[17]

In truth, there was virtually no use to which paper might be applied that did not become arsenical to some degree. Price cards and product labels in shops were often green (a woman was badly poisoned by prunes contaminated by pigment from the price card propped on top of them). Labels on tinned meats and other packaged foods were green, as were advertising handbills and posters, concert tickets, envelopes (including the flap that had to be licked for sealing), paper for lining shelves in cupboards and drawers, and wrapping paper. Shop owners from grocers to milliners covered their packages with arsenical papers. The wrapping on 'an ordinary sized cracker-box', it was found, contained nearly 50 grains of arsenic, while that on just one 'small sized band-box' from a hatter contained 100 grains. A Birmingham infant died after eating paper torn from such a box, a London child was killed by playing with toys kept on a shelf lined with arsenical paper, and so on, down to the man who suffered anal ulcerations after choosing the wrong item to use as toilet paper. In short, as one exasperated chemist objected, 'you can scarcely purchase a bottle of any liquid or solid article of food, delicacy or stimulant, at the present time, without running the risk of getting at least one poisonous dose of arsenic' from its label or wrapping paper.[18]

Playing-cards could have been included in his list, as was learned by the London lady who enjoyed whist and possessed 'a decided preference for green-backed cards'. After just a few rubbers with a new deck, her fingertips became so sore she was unable to deal the cards (the combination of friction from shuffling and warmth and moisture from hands dislodged arsenic not only onto fingers, but into the air as well). The physician who saw her, one of the capital's leading practitioners, Jabez Hogg, suspected arsenic. He advised her to cultivate a preference for different-coloured cards, and once she did, her fingers recovered (playing-cards analysed by a Glasgow chemist were found to hold more than a grain and a half of arsenic per card, or eighty-three grains to the deck). Hogg then made the horrifying discovery that his own children had for some time been playing the game of Forfeits with arsenical cards. They too were made to cultivate a new preference.[19]

At least the children were too young to smoke, else they might have been affected by the Schweinfurt green used to decorate cigar holders or to ornament clay pipes (the latter were responsible for an outbreak of sore throat among medical students in the 1860s). One hopes the oil or gas lamps illuminating their card games were not shielded by green shades, though that's unlikely, since an 1870s survey found arsenical shades to be 'universally employed'. Headaches and eye irritation were blamed on arsenic volatilized from shades by the lamp's heat, and one man whose weak vision forced him to sit close by his gas light, had his lips break out in small ulcers ('eczema arsenicale', physicians called it) that caused 'intolerable' discomfort, especially at night, 'when the lips swelled and became so painful that eating, or even speaking, could scarcely be indulged in'. One hopes also for another unlikelihood, that none of the dresses or trousers or stockings the Hogg children wore were dyed with arsenic compounds.[20]

When condemning 'the excessive desire for rich and beautiful colours' that brought so much arsenic into the home, physicians were especially exercised by society's predilection for rich green fabrics for dresses and other apparel. Muslins in particular were often 'loaded' with arsenic, as one doctor disparaged, harbouring the poison in amounts that were, in another's words, 'enough to startle anyone'. Certainly London practitioner George Rees was startled when he analyzed a sample of green muslin intended for a ball gown and found it to contain more than sixty grains of Scheele's green per square yard—and so loosely incorporated into the fabric 'that it could be dusted out with great facility'. Since twenty yards of fabric—or more—were required for dresses 'under crinoline regime', the ladies to be met at the best parties were concealing in excess of 1,000 grains of arsenic on their persons. 'Our fair charmers in green whirl through the giddy waltz', a physician exclaimed, 'actually in a cloud of arsenical dust....Well may the fascinating wearer of [such a gown] be called a killing creature': she was literally drop-dead gorgeous, as she 'carries in her skirts poison enough to slay the whole of the admirers she may meet with in half a dozen ball-rooms'. (The theatre was no safer, apparently, the performers in a certain ballet being 'nearly all...more or less poisoned' by the green costumes they wore in their portrayal of water nymphs). One could now understand the true source of 'the pallor and languor so commonly observed in those who pass through the labours of a London season'. It was not to be attributed to 'ill-ventilated crowded rooms and bad champagne' after all, but to the inhalation of arsenic 'shaken from the clothing of a number of poisoners, who, though blameless, are not the less pestilential'.[21]

One did not have to be a belle of the ball to poison and be poisoned, however, for the less costly fabrics used to make dresses for women of lower station were equally arsenical. The threat was so broad in its scope that Henry Letheby developed a simple test for women to use when shopping to determine if a dress was dangerous. Given general circulation by *The Times*, his test consisted of applying a drop of ammonia to the fabric; if the spot turned blue, copper must be present, and copper was almost never found in textiles unless combined with arsenic (as in Scheele's green and Schweinfurt green). Thus if ladies would just carry about a phial of ammonia, 'instead of the usual scent bottle', his easy method 'would betray the arsenical poison and settle the business immediately'.[22]

It's unclear how many women actually employed the Letheby test, but those who did were well advised to take along their ammonia when shopping for any item of clothing, not just dresses (the fabric for ladies' hats, for example, was sometimes cut from the same material used for gowns: in the film version of *Gone With the Wind*, the stylish bonnet that Rhett presents to Scarlett on his return from Paris has precisely the tint and sheen of Scheele's green). Numerous poisonings and several deaths were linked to exposure to arsenical shirts, pants, and stockings, 'the evil effects of the socks' being 'especially well-known to the public'. People (including at least one MP) were disabled from walking or even standing after wearing arsenic-dyed stockings, leaving an editorialist to ask 'if socks may be dangerous' (socks!), could there be any manufactured article at all 'in these days of high-pressure civilization [that] can possibly be trusted'. The list of apparel that could not be trusted stretched on, to gloves, boot-linings (which killed several California miners), the paper collars and cuffs that enjoyed a period of vogue in the 1870s, and even men's hatbands, which could produce unsightly and uncomfortable eruptions on the forehead (head sores could result as well from the several brands of hair pomade that included arsenic in their composition). Not even dolls' clothes could be trusted, children being poisoned by sucking or chewing on their playthings' dresses.[23]

The fabrics from which dresses and socks and hatbands were made, furthermore, were also given a variety of non-sartorial applications. Nurses at a mental asylum, for example, tried to cheer the place up by hanging green curtains in their quarters: 'within a few months, nearly every nurse on the staff had been, or was, under medical treatment', complaining of headache, gastric upset, irritated eyes, anaemia, and neuralgia. Eventually the curtains were examined and found to contain arsenic to 'an astonishing extent'. When the curtains were removed, the nurses improved. Students at an engineering college were bothered by digestive and other problems for more than a year before it was determined the muslin wall drapes hanging in their rooms were highly arsenical. A wife and husband endured illness for months until their green calico bed curtains were incriminated and disposed of. A woman experienced poor appetite, constipation, and shooting pains in her legs for a year and a half before her physician realized she was being poisoned by the green muslin she made into curtains, cushion covers, and other decorative articles as gifts for friends. A woman suffered skin eruptions from carrying her brightly coloured purse, and children were sickened by the cloth linings of their bassinettes and perambulators. The lament voiced by *The Times* was an all-too-accurate summation of the situation: 'there are so many possible forms of accidental poisoning... lying in ambush on all sides of us.'[24]

And on top of us. In the late 1850s, a new fashion accessory became de rigueur for ladies of elevated taste, that of hats and caps adorned with elaborate constructions of feathers and artificial flowers, leaves, and fruits. The botanical components of fancy headdress almost always included components of a green tint; the leaves attached to a garland of artificial grapes, one analysis determined, held a grain and a half of arsenic apiece. This 'arseniferous verdure' might seem appealing to male admirers, but 'to the eye of science' it was simply 'an indication of death'. In confirmation, a London girl died in 1862 from sucking on headdress grapes tinted with Scheele's green. Never was the axiom *il faut souffrir pour être belle* (it is necessary to suffer in order to be beautiful) more apt.[25]

The event that brought headdresses into the headlines, though, was the death of another London girl the year previous. Matilda Scheurer was employed at age 18 as an 'artificial florist', that is, a producer of fake flowers. There were more than 10,000 such workers in Britain, most of them in London and more than half under the age of 20, some as young as 8. Their work involved cutting leaves from muslin that they had coloured green by dipping the fabric in wax and then dusting it with Scheele's green, or by kneading a solution of the green powder into the material. With either process, their hands and other areas of skin were exposed to the direct irritating effects of the pigment, while the poison was also diffused through the air of the workroom ('dusty beyond belief' is how one visitor to a facility described the atmosphere; 'devil's dust' is what another called the floating powder) and inhaled countless times over the course of the fourteen- to sixteen-hour work days that marked the busy season. The green material also lodged under the fingernails and from there easily became mixed with food. Workers typically began to feel ill within days of taking the job, and Matilda Scheurer was soon plagued with stomach pain and vomiting, the dejections of her stomach being 'very greenish'. In November 1861, she had a vomiting attack so violent her mother took her to a physician, who diagnosed poisoning by some irritant mineral. The diagnosis was of little use, unfortunately, for the girl remained 'in the greatest pain' and at last endured 'a death of great agony' (her last hours were troubled with convulsions 'every few minutes' and foaming at the mouth; she complained that 'everything she looked at was green'). An inquest was held, and the autopsy disclosed arsenic was broadcast through her body; the jury returned a verdict of accidental death from copper arsenite.[26]

By the time of that 'accident', the dangers of employment in artificial flower workshops were known to at least some physicians. More than a year before, Arthur Hassall had redirected his concern for Scheele's green to its use by flower-makers and described their situation as 'wretched in the extreme', every one showing signs of arsenic poisoning. Contact of Scheele's green with their skin produced 'ugly-looking sores' on the face, hands, and 'other parts of the body'. Other parts included the scrotum (nearly 90 per cent of the flower-makers were young women, but men were employed in the trade too), where the roughly folded skin trapped the powder and extended the time of exposure, resulting in 'greenish pimples' that oozed a yellowish discharge and made walking difficult. The injuries were so disabling that nearly all workers had to leave the job periodically. When they did, symptoms went away, but once recovered, flower-makers usually returned to the only employment at which they were skilled, and a new round of poisoning began.[27]

The poisonous nature of the trade had been pointed out to the men who ran it, and some employers had responded by encouraging their workers to wear gauze masks. The flower-makers found the masks uncomfortably warm, though. Some women worked with no facial covering, others made makeshift masks by lifting their aprons up and tying them around their heads below the eyes, still others placed a layer of muslin over their mouths. If the apron or muslin were green, it would only have exacerbated the problem, but even if of an innocuous colour, a loosely tied sheet of fabric was an imperfect precaution against tiny particles of poison floating in the air.[28]

And still the list of products exposing people to arsenic is not ended. It runs on through wine and cookware to copper coins and coal. Wine bottles were sometimes sealed with green (i.e. arsenical) wax that could contaminate the liquid it covered. The copper from which pots and bowls were made usually contained arsenical impurities, which could be released into food when acid or salt were present, and the same problem existed with the tin used to can foods. Coal released arsenic into the atmosphere when it was burned: a Manchester physician found appreciable amounts of the poison on the leaves of evergreens during the winter months, and worried that 'a material amount' of poison must be inhaled by city residents. Glycerine, the base material for manufacturing nitroglycerine for dynamite, was generally tainted with arsenic. Fake animals intended as toys for children were often dusted with an arsenic powder to preserve their fur from insect depredations, with serious cases of poisoning resulting. In 1848, *The Lancet* reported the cases of two children nearly killed from playing with a stuffed bunny given them by their mother.[29]

Arsenic could protect more than stuffed animals from insects. There were a number of brands of moth killers that were sold to safeguard carpets, furs, and clothing; the advertising materials and packaging for these preparations might acknowledge they were poisonous, but made no mention of arsenic. Nor did the advertisements for the many formulations of rat poison, brands such as Scatter Rats, Raticide, Rat Dynamite, and Baker's Cooling Physic (Fig. 5). Then there was Shoo Fly, fly papers being yet another category of arsenical product. The papers were made from strips

ESTABLISHED 1820.

KILLING NO MURDER!

BAKER'S

COOLING PHYSIC,

FOR DISTROYING WITHOUT TROUBLE

BUGS, FLIES, BLACK BEETLES, WASPS, RATS, MICE & COCKROACHES.

DIRECTIONS.—For Flies or Wasps. Pour a little into Oyster Shells or saucers, and place them in different parts.

For Bugs.—Do not take the Bedstead down, but wash the joints, by introducing a feather, and the same way, if the Bugs are in the walls.

Black Beetles, Cockroaches, Rats and Mice. Soak crumbs of Bread in it, & scatter them about, the vermin will eat it greedily & die instantly.

Sold by Oilmen, Grocers, Toymen, &c., in Bottles. at 3*d*., 6*d*., and 1*s*. each, and in Family Bottles, (glass) at 2*s*. 6*d*. **It is POISON.**

MANUFACTORY: HEN AND CHICKEN LANE, WALWORTH.

5. Advertisement for Baker's Cooling Physic

soaked in a solution of arsenic and sugar, then dried for sale. In the home, the strips would be placed in bowls of water to which flies would be drawn by the sugar that dissolved. The papers were widely disseminated—'there is scarcely a house without them'— and were advertised as 'perfectly harmless to animal life of a higher order than of our insect pests'. In fact, they generally contained five or more grains of arsenic per sheet, more than enough to kill any child who might be drawn to sugar water as irresistibly as a fly. Such fatalities did occur, and one person was sickened by drinking beer in which poisoned flies were floating. To sum up, a multitude of items attracted consumers by their colour, then poisoned them when taken into the home. Yet there is at least one nice thing to be said for green arsenicals: they would never be mistaken for flour or sugar, and their colour likewise inhibited employment for homicide. The possibility of murder was not eliminated altogether, though. One enterprising villain cut open green figs, lined them with Paris green, and mailed them as a present to his victim.[30]

*

Throughout the chapter to this point, arsenic in domestic products has been repeatedly blamed by physicians as the source of death and sickness. In some cases, there could have been no serious questioning of the diagnosis. Matilda Scheurer, the girl who sucked the artificial grapes, the child who ate paper from a hatbox: all were exposed to significant levels of the poison and it was found present in their bodies. In other instances, the connection was demonstrated by the fact that symptoms went away when an arsenic-containing item—curtains, bed drapes, lightshades—was removed from the sick person's environment. But in many other situations, the degree of damage done by arsenic, if any, was difficult to demonstrate. Arsenical candles killed birds, but did they seriously harm people? The Westminster Medical Society's investigative committee supposed so, but their 'evidence' was largely hypothetical. 'Is anyone prepared to assert' that no one 'would receive the slightest injury?' and 'is it too much to assume, that...mischief to the health of some, at least...may be expected?' are not unequivocal statements. They are of the 'it stands to reason' brand of argument, drawing on common sense and intuition rather than demonstration. Likewise the 'cloud of arsenical dust' discharged from the dresses of the whirling 'fair charmers in green': the dust could hardly be a salubrious addition to the air of a ballroom, but was it demonstrably dangerous? Belles weren't falling to the floor vomiting, beaus weren't complaining their legs were too weak to dance. Mounting a conclusive case against some sources of arsenic was a trickier proposition than with others, and many physicians were initially sceptical that domestic arsenic poisoning was a widespread problem.

Overcoming that scepticism took time, the evidence against it piling up steadily but slowly in the form of clinical histories—many published in professional journals, many more simply related at medical society meetings or in hospital corridor conversations—of patients who had been exposed to low levels of arsenic and were exhibiting certain signs and symptoms of illness. Gradually, patterns began to emerge, aggregations of different symptoms coming to be recognized as showing up consistently among such patients. At first, physicians were reluctant to attribute the patterns to arsenic because they frequently administered the substance in comparable amounts as medication. Indeed, for most of the nineteenth century medical practitioners prescribed arsenic preparations as cures for a host of maladies, and with an enthusiasm that knew only the broadest bounds. The popularity of arsenical therapy, and the health problems it caused, will be explored in Chapter 9. For now, the point is that doctors who believed that small quantities of arsenic were a potent agent for restoring the sick to health were not readily persuaded that those same quantities could make the healthy sick. It was only as case after case of poisoning was reported that resistance was worn down to the point of collapse and the profession convinced of the extensive occurrence of chronic arsenicism.

Not until the 1880s was there a professional consensus on the clinical picture of chronic arsenic intoxication. Early signs of poisoning included loss of appetite, nausea, periodic vomiting, and weakness. The mucus membranes of eyes, nose, and throat were affected. 'Irritation and smarting of eyes and nostrils is often the most marked symptom,' the irritation sometimes lasting for months (at least one man lost his sight from arsenic inflammation), and frequently accompanied by ulceration of the mouth and tongue, sore throat, a persistent dry cough, and hoarse voice. Skin eruptions of different types usually appeared, along with patches of brown pigmentation on eyelids, on the neck, in armpits, and in advanced cases on just about any area of the skin. A physician's perception of the artificial flowers and leaves used to adorn the female head was thus somewhat different from that of the ladies: 'The brilliant ball-room wreaths—green with an unearthly verdure—which contrast so bewitchingly with the complexions of the fair wearers, never fail to remind us', a London practitioner commented, 'of the reddened conjunctivae, the eczematous eruptions, the burning fauces, and short, hacking coughs we have met with in our morning *clientele*' in the city's hospitals. He might have been reminded as well of the nervous system injuries that eventually followed, the tingling and numbness of hands and feet, with actual paralysis of the appendages occurring in extreme cases.[31]

That was the 'average' patient history. But as with all forms of illness, individual cases could differ widely from the norm: 'symptoms are notoriously varied in character,' one physician wrote; they 'present many apparent anomalies [and] follow little regularity of manifestation'. One victim's miseries were concentrated on her skin, another's in his nerves. Some patients suffered severely, even unto death, while others got off with nothing worse than 'a low and miserable state of health' or a 'general impairment of health'. At that lower level of impairment, of course, diagnosis was sometimes iffy: it was not unusual, doctors knew, for chronic arsenicism to imitate other complaints so closely 'that those who are not alive to the real cause of the mischief are liable to be misled'. The early symptoms were often 'shrouded in mystery, and, consequently, for every case of chronic poisoning made known, hundreds possibly pass unnoticed or unrecognized'. An 1896 court case illustrates the uncertainty that could exist even down to the end of the century. A Croydon woman who believed her health had been damaged by green drapes brought suit against the shop where she had purchased them. One of the two medical experts called to testify at the trial supported her claim, but the other denied she was a victim of arsenic poisoning and the judge ruled in favour of the merchant. Yet even if individual victims of arsenical products did sometimes go undetected, the products themselves were firmly incriminated by the last quarter of the century: there simply were too many victims who had been correctly diagnosed.[32]

An important aid to diagnosis came into play during the second half of the century: urinalysis. Arsenic taken into the body is slowly excreted in the urine, elimination continuing for one to several weeks after ingestion; its presence can be easily demonstrated by the Marsh or Reinsch tests. When linked with the constellation of symptoms known to be characteristic of arsenic, a finding of the poison in the urine tightened the diagnosis. Urinalysis also gave a measure of the magnitude of the public's exposure to arsenic. Several studies were done on sizeable patient populations during the later years of the century, both on patients suspected of being poisoned and patients taken at random. The most extensive analyses, performed at Harvard in the 1880s, found arsenic in urine samples from more than 30 per cent of the patients tested. Some of the patients had been taking arsenical medication, so the state of their urine was no surprise. But many had not been on medication, and when arsenic-containing materials in their domestic environment were removed, the arsenic in their urine soon disappeared. Here was a graphic demonstration of the difficulty of living an arsenic-free life in the Victorian world.[33]

Exposure to arsenic did not inevitably lead to sickness or death. There were many people who had arsenical products in their homes

and arsenic in their urine who exhibited no evidence at all of compromised health. Individual resistance to the poison seemed to vary
widely, and doctors granted that 'in by far the greater number of
cases of domestic exposure no ill result follows'. Yet if the number
of cases was modest as a fraction of the overall population, in the
aggregate it was considerable. The absolute number of victims was
much too great to be tolerated, doctors argued; it represented a
public health problem of formidable proportions. So pervasive was
arsenic in the domestic environment, it was easy for physicians to
succumb to hyperbole in addressing the threat. Even as staid an
institution as the *British Medical Journal* got carried away, accusing
arsenic of opening the way to 'the invasion of every conceivable ill
to which flesh is heir', including moral depravity:

According to the purity or impurity of the air we breathe, so are human
beings influenced both physically and morally; crime itself lurks in
poisoned dens; and if we surround man, woman, or child with a poisonous atmosphere, from whatever source, we hinder healthy development...and sow the seeds of physical and mental incapacity for every
avocation of life.[34]

That exaggerated the threat, but there still was a problem that
had to be addressed. The question was how to address it. Lawsuits
were one way of discouraging producers from marketing arsenical
goods, though as the woman from Croydon learned, it was not the
most reliable measure; nor could it be afforded by the many. Publicity that frightened consumers away from poisonous products and
forced manufacturers to switch to safer procedures was another
way, and, as seen earlier with candles, the tactic could be effective.
But the surest bet for elimination of the hazard was prohibitory
legislation.

To many physicians, the arsenic question seemed just that clear-
cut. After all, there were already laws in force protecting the public

from arsenic in other contexts. The Act to Regulate the Sale of Arsenic placed restrictions on the purchase of the poison. Yet while 'a pennyworth of arsenic must not be sold unconditionally, "over the counter"', it was pointed out, 'a ton might be sold, without a question being asked as to what is to become of it, to a manufacturer of paper-hangings!' Similarly, a druggist noted, anyone could 'without making any direct purchase at all...obtain from an old meat can, a bottle label, a grocer's wrapper, a child's picture book, a worn-out artificial flower...as much arsenic as will enable him to inflict deadly injury'. There was also an Act for Preventing Adulteration in Food and Drink, which prohibited the addition of arsenicals and other toxic or fraudulent ingredients to comestibles. Certainly it was an anomaly 'that a grocer who adds chicory to our coffee should be fined, while a paper-stainer who lays a family prostrate by arsenical poisoning...is allowed to go free.' To many, a regulation to outlaw the employment of arsenic for any domestic purposes whatever seemed an obvious and unobjectionable extension of laws that were already on the books. It was time, surely, for Parliament to intervene to stop practices that were 'worse than many crimes'.[35]

But for members of Parliament, the matter was not so simple. Health was a social good, without question, but so was wealth; arsenic was to be found in such a great range of manufactures that eliminating it would have significant economic repercussions. An ever-present theme in the history of public health legislation throughout the world has been this tension between private interests and public welfare: 'It too often happens', one arsenic antagonist complained, 'that vested interests...carry the day against...those precautions for the public good which a wise humanity and the most evident responsibilities earnestly and plainly recommend.' It still happens too often, but in nineteenth-century Britain it happened even more frequently, for in that self-consciously free and democratic nation (as well as in America, which at the time had no arsenic legislation whatever), the political environment was, in a physician's agitated summation, one in which 'liberty runs mad' and 'the rights of individuals and of industrial pursuits are deemed too sacred' to permit legislative interference.[36]

Certainly a determination to support British arsenical manufactures ran through opposition to poison legislation, virtually to the point of equating injury to industry with injury to consumers. Even Hassall paired his reminder that it was a 'duty' for doctors 'to guard with jealous eye the public health' with the admonition that in doing so they should be careful not to 'unnecessarily interfere with trade and manufactures'. Even those who most strongly supported legislative intervention worried that while a law restricting British manufacturers would do no damage to intramural commerce, since all companies would be playing by the same rules, it might damage the nation's competitiveness against countries that did not have such laws.[37]

As was evidenced in the debate over the food adulteration bill, laissez-faire was a 'sacred principle' in British political life. It could be overcome, but never without a battle, so even the most zealous of those striving to eliminate arsenic from manufactures were resigned to an arduous uphill struggle. Reactions to the death of Matilda Scheurer, for example, took repeated note of the fact that France and Germany had prohibited arsenical flowers, but 'our free-trade governmental spirit does not admit of that free and easy way of redressing evils and nuisances'. From the 1837 report of the Westminster Medical Society on stearine candles (Britain was 'the only country in Europe where the public health is so little regarded by the governing powers') to an 1884 exposition on arsenical fabrics (Britain 'is behind most other civilized countries' in protecting citizens from poison), medical reformers repeatedly voiced frustration over legislators' reverence for the sanctity of unrestrained commerce. Parliament's passivity toward the marketing of arsenical products 'sufficient to poison whole armies of people' was, *The Lancet* insisted, the most profound demonstration of 'the extent to which our Government carries the principle of respecting freedom in trade'. England was such a 'gloriously free country' that anything was allowed, 'even to the slow poisoning of our little ones'.[38]

More than a few members of the public shared that respect for freedom in trade, if judging only from the attitudes exhibited at inquests on arsenical deaths. Those impanelled at Matilda Scheurer's inquest, remember, ruled that while her death was caused by the arsenic she was unavoidably exposed to in her employment, it was nevertheless 'accidental'. A like interpretation was made by jurors at the inquest on a child killed by green paper. When 'after a brief consultation' they returned a judgment of 'Natural Death', the coroner 'expressed his entire dissent from the verdict'. The reply of one juror was, 'Oh, we are willing to admit that the use of green paper is objectionable'—but death was still natural.[39]

Such deaths were natural because parents were adults who had freely chosen to purchase the goods that poisoned them and their children. Yet while it was a fine notion to think of consumers as free agents who should be permitted to decide for themselves what products they would or would not buy, how could they decide whether or not they wanted to risk being poisoned if they did not know which products contained poison? If manufacturers genuinely respected the ideal of consumers as consenting adults free to purchase whatever appealed to them, a physician submitted, they should be only too happy to label their goods 'highly impregnated with arsenic' and let buyers make their choice. Freedom in business was all well and good, it was granted, but should freedom be so freely interpreted as to allow 'manufacturers to saturate our walls, furniture, or clothing, with subtle poisons?' Further, what of the conscientious manufacturers who no longer impregnated their goods with arsenic (there were some, in fact)? Were they not entitled to protection against 'such unprincipled competition' as came from those businesses that used arsenic without admitting it? There was more than one way in which laissez-faire was unfair.[40]

Respect for commercial interests had a hold even on some physicians, as was demonstrated clearly in the aftermath to the Matilda Scheurer tragedy. People needed protection from arsenic, a leading medical journal editorialized, but protection was best provided by education, 'so that persons knowing a trade to be dangerous, may protect themselves by refusing to embark in it'. It was no business of 'the *State* [to] hinder...young women [artificial florists] from destroying themselves for a beggarly livelihood'. Nevertheless, the majority medical reaction to the stories of Scheurer's death was an outcry for legislative action, an outcry that came with most practical effect from the public health official for the parish in which Scheurer had died (Medical Officer of Health was the formal title of the position). Demanding that 'something ought to be done', he called the attention of the Home Secretary to the dangers of arsenical manufactures, who passed the matter on to the Privy Council, who in turn requested that their own Medical Officer of Health investigate 'the use of the poison in the arts, and its effect on health and life'. Thus were the wheels of government set in motion towards the consideration of protections against arsenical hazards in the workplace and home. They were not to roll far.[41]

Investigation of health effects associated with artificial flower production was assigned to London physician and professor of forensic medicine William Guy. Visiting a number of workrooms and interviewing workers and their bosses, Guy determined that flower-makers suffered serious effects indeed. Most of the workers were young, half of them 20 and under, and many complained of symptoms that could be related to arsenic. Nearly all experienced the onset of what felt like a common cold within an hour of taking up the day's work, developing headache, runny eyes and nose, and sneezing. Other symptoms were not universal, but occurred in some combination in virtually everyone. Constipation; diarrhoea; green nasal mucus; green vomit; green urine; pimple-like eruptions breaking out on the face, sometimes covering other areas of the body, growing in size till they resembled smallpox, and leaving scars when they abated; sloughing off of patches of skin and formation of ulcers in the denuded areas; sores on the fingers; shedding of hair; darkening of the complexion to dusky or olive; disruption of menstruation; ulceration of the genital organs, leaving them so tender that 'in several cases the lower part of the body has been so severely affected that the young women were unable to sit down' (workers thus afflicted were reassigned to sweeping the floor, which did not require sitting). Flower-makers were not infrequently made invalid for weeks at a time, Guy learned, but he was able to substantiate only one case of death from the employment: that of Matilda Scheurer.[42]

To Guy's mind, only one death was not enough. If his inquiries had turned up 'several' fatalities, he stated in the summation of his 1863 report to the Privy Council, 'I should have thought it right to suggest the absolute prohibition of such branches of manufacture'. A single death out of thousands of workers, however, could not justify such a 'measure of extreme precaution' as prohibition. Extreme measures might play well with the French and Germans, who had indeed submitted to arsenical legislation of that sort. But for Britons, Guy reminded, there was an 'obvious objection... to all restrictions on the liberty of manufacture, and to every interference of the

Government in the affairs of individuals'. He entertained the idea that government might require firms involved in the manufacture of arsenical products to provide more spacious workrooms so as to decrease the concentration of dust in the air. But he questioned the practicability of enforcing the requirement given the number of businesses involved, and worried that the expense of improvements in the workroom environment would lower the competitiveness of British businesses against firms from countries lacking such laws. And would legislated improvements even work, he wondered, given the sad truth that 'the majority of the working classes of both sexes are very uncleanly in their habits, and very reckless in their proceedings'. Even if working conditions were bettered, workers would still fall ill, and when that happened, the solution was that they should 'abandon their employment...suspend it for a time'. The effects of arsenical pigments, after all, while 'disagreeable and even painful', did 'soon subside and pass away' when workers removed themselves from exposure (this conveniently overlooked the fact that, as another who investigated the flower-making industry pointed out, 'the workers generally dread the occupation, but dread still more the alternative of being without work'). Children, Guy conceded, were a special case and might be prohibited from working with arsenic until the age of 18. In that way, the handling of arsenic would be placed exclusively in the hands of people 'of an age to judge and to act for themselves, and who might be fairly held responsible' for any injuries they incurred. As for protecting the public, it should be enough to require that all arsenic-containing paper products be stamped with the words 'arsenical paper' and that producers of items for children (confectioners, toymakers) be disallowed from purchasing arsenic compounds.[43]

One could hardly ask for a more succinct primer on the laissez-faire approach to social policy, nor, apparently, a more persuasive one, for after Guy's report Government lost interest in arsenical manufactures for more than a decade. Attention would be rekindled in the late 1870s, but that development is best reserved for the next chapter. In the meantime, there would occur a decline in the distribution of arsenical domestic items despite the lack of legislative interference.

*

Guy had argued in his report to the Privy Council that 'enlightened public opinion' was much to be preferred to prohibitory legislation. People awakened to the presence of arsenic in ordinary household products, he reasoned, would surely stop purchasing them, which would compel manufacturers to stop making them, which would free workers from exposure to the poison.[44]

Guy's argument was a strictly pragmatic one, but the same conclusion could be drawn from a moral analysis. Was it not a safe assumption, the *British Medical Journal* asked, 'that the very leaves which are at this moment giving an artificial verdant splendour to the locks of some of our countrywomen are just the very leaves whose production effected the death of this poor girl', Matilda Scheurer? Yet if publicity could just 'bring home to the hearts of our *grandes et belles dames* the fatal cruelties' that their passion for artificial flowers inflicted on members of their own sex, would not *les dames* change their style? The deadly trade could be ended if only women would be content to wear 'the sere and yellow leaf' instead of the green one.[45]

Laudable as were the intentions of the *Journal*, the argument from morality was given its most compelling expression—just as the Victorian ethos would have it—by women, in particular by the women of a fledgling health organization called the Ladies' Sanitary Association. Using 'sanitary' in the traditional sense of all things related to health, the Association was founded in 1857 for the dual purposes of educating women on how to protect their families' health, and inspiring them to work for the remediation of social and economic conditions that generated illness. The lady sanitarians composed and distributed health tracts by the thousands ('Woman's Work in Sanitary Reform', 'How to Manage a Baby', 'Why do Women not Swim?'), and sponsored lectures throughout the country ('On the Blessing of Clean Homes').[46]

Being for the most part female, flower-makers were solidly in the purview of the Ladies' Sanitary Association. Shortly after Scheurer's death, two members of the Association submitted a letter to *The Times* in which they informed the public that the unfortunate girl was just an extreme illustration of the misery endured by hundreds; surely now that women were being made aware of the situation, they would abandon green adornments for some 'more becoming colour'. Who needed Parliamentary intervention when the weapon of sisterly love was at hand?[47]

Such an appeal had worked before. In the 1790s, the world's first organized consumer boycott was mounted in England against sugar from the West Indies. Through lecture and pamphlet, the Anti-Saccharine Society directed attention to the miserable existence of slaves exploited on the sugar plantations. It became politically incorrect, we might say, to eat sugar, and consumption of the product dropped significantly. The Ladies' Sanitary Association saw itself as a worthy successor to the Anti-Saccharine Society. The letter to *The Times* had, in fact, been preceded by a tear-provoking story in *The English Woman's Journal* written by another member of the Association. The author, who had visited many of the flower-making workshops, presented a fictionalized account of 'silent, seething depths of suffering yet unfathomed'. Katy, a young girl paid a pittance to make artificial flowers for the firm of Leech and Vampire, had been kept 'on green' for days, 'till her face was one mass of sores, and she was threatened with blindness'. The other girls in the garret workshop were deadly ill too; by the morrow, they would 'be on the floor like poisoned rats'. Katy's torture is drawn out over several pages, yet though she is still alive at the end of the story, it seems certain she will soon be in heaven with another who 'lies dead through her temerity' in making flowers: Matilda Scheurer. Lest the moral somehow be missed, the author observed that in the workrooms in which other trades were carried on, 'a considerable proportion of elderly females are found', but among artificial florists, old women did not exist.[48]

Katy's story ended with a prayer that women would henceforth shun green accessories, and more than a few readers vowed they would. 'I did not know, and multitudes beside me do not know,' one woman wrote the *Woman's Journal*, that the wreaths 'were procured at such a fearful price'. Now that women did know, they most certainly would not prove 'deaf to the voice of humanity'. Others were not so sure, suspecting that the voice of shame was all that most women would hear. They would respond only when publicity given to the sufferings of those who made artificial flowers had caused the wearing of them to be 'looked upon as of *mauvais goût*', in bad taste. Then, like their fur-coat-wearing counterparts of a century later, women would turn to inoffensive alternatives. In the end, it was probably neither fashion nor compassion that led to a decline in the purchase of arsenical clothing, but simply people's anxiety for their own skins. By the 1860s, the dangers of most items coloured green had been made well known and consumers were beginning to shy away from them: in 1863, a medical observer of the scene declared that the demand for products known to contain arsenic 'has visibly diminished'. The degree of that diminution will be explored further in the next chapter.[49]

But even supposing every woman, man, and child in the kingdom joined the ranks shunning green clothing, paper, and paints, arsenical sickness would not be ended, for the poison came concealed by other disguises. The green pigments were often combined with non-arsenical colours to create shades quite distinct from green, so it was not sufficient, *The Lancet* stressed, for consumers 'to be chary only of the more gaudy hues'. Reds, blues, and even blacks could be arsenical. The occurrence of certain symptoms together should raise a red flag for physicians whether any green materials were in the patient's environment or not; indeed, towards the end of the century a 4-year-old boy was poisoned by playing with ... a red flag. Around that same time, an American baby nearly died before arsenic was discovered to be in the blue satin lining of his bassinette, and both nurses and charges at a Massachusetts orphanage were sickened by arsenic in the blue dresses worn by the nurses; two infants died.[50]

This uncertainty was compounded even further by the introduction of a new category of colouring materials in the 1850s, the aniline dyes, organic substances synthesized from the colourless coal tar derivative aniline. In just a few years, aniline dyes became available in an assortment of brilliant colours, including green, and were eagerly welcomed as replacements for arsenical colours. The most economical procedures for synthesizing aniline dyes, though, incorporated arsenic in several stages of production, and the poison was often retained in the finished colour. These new pigments did not produce the extent of injury wholly arsenical ones had, but a number of instances of arsenic poisoning from aniline-dyed clothing, gloves, handkerchiefs, and other items did occur. There was even a case of a woman killed by colouring artificial flowers with an arsenical aniline compound.[51]

Aniline dyes aside, however, there remained yet one more common household item bearing the tint of the grave.

8

Walls of Death

Diphtheria was a devastating disease of childhood in former centuries, outbreaks of the infection being positively dreaded by parents down to the very close of the 1800s (an anti-toxin protective against the infection was introduced in the 1890s). There was thus good reason for neighbourhood alarm when in 1862 a child in London's working-class Limehouse district died with a diagnosis of diphtheria. As was usual following the report of a potentially epidemic disease, the Medical Officer of Health for the parish made a visit to the home. The duties of a Medical Officer of Health included monitoring levels and causes of morbidity and mortality in his district, examining foods for evidence of adulteration, overseeing offensive workplaces such as slaughterhouses and chemical plants, and inspecting sites of disease outbreaks. In the days predating the germ theory, infectious diseases such as diphtheria were attributed to poisons inhaled from a malodorous, 'miasmatic' atmosphere supposed to be generated from garbage, sewage, and other decomposing organic material. Thus Dr Thomas Orton's visit to the Limehouse quarters was for the purpose of examining the building's drainage, ventilation, and general sanitary situation. His finding, surprisingly, was that everything was 'in capital condition', indicating diphtheria had not been present. Soon, however, another of the children came down with a sore throat and died,

and again the surgeon in attendance, Mr Horton, diagnosed diphtheria. Over the next weeks, the family's two remaining children
passed away with similar symptoms, and their deaths too were
blamed on that same disease. Panic began to spread through the
tenements, even though another inspection of the home concluded
there was no malignant atmosphere. Surgeon Horton and Doctor Orton were at odds—but only until the physician took note
at last of the green wallpaper in the children's bedroom. It then
became clear that the painful, constricted throat the children had
complained of had not been due to diphtheria at all; the culprit
was Scheele's green.[1]

Here was the final type of application of arsenical pigments
to paper that caused widespread poisoning: the manufacture of
green wallpapers. The 'rage for green colour' responsible for so
many of the hazards cited in the last chapter not surprisingly
extended to the decoration of the walls of rooms. As a letter to
the *British Medical Journal* asserted in 1871, such papers were 'to be
seen in the majority of dwelling-houses, from the palace down to
the navvy's hut' (though it seems unlikely the typical navvy would
possess either the funds or the inclination to paper his hut). The
papers were in the majority of hotels, too, as the writer had discovered on a trip the previous summer, when he had had to turn
down 'upwards of seventy lodging-houses' because none could
provide him a room without green wallpaper.[2]

The paper on the walls of the Limehouse children's room was
determined (by Henry Letheby) to hold three grains of arsenic to
the square foot, a lethal amount, but unusual only for being so
small; one authority quoted twenty grains per square foot as 'an
average proportion', and another claimed the number reached seventy in the most heavily coloured papers. It is easy to understand,
then, that of all the domestic products that were dyed or painted

to satisfy the rage for green, none stirred up so agitated a medical reaction as wallpaper. 'When the atmosphere of dwellings all over the kingdom...is thus more or less poisoned with arsenic,' Alfred Taylor stated, it is 'a question of great national importance.'[3]

The question emerged as one of national import only towards the end of the 1850s. By that time, wallpapers had been manufactured for three centuries, though production was limited until the late eighteenth century, when the Industrial Revolution and increasing urbanization greatly expanded the ranks of homeowners who could afford such luxuries. The bourgeois taste for domesticity and for costly furnishings and decor as a material demonstration of social rank and personal merit opened the market to increased manufacture of many household goods, wallpapers not least. At first, green papers were coloured with the traditional mineral pigment verdigris or by mixing blues and yellows of plant origin. But once Scheele's green began to be produced in quantity, it was adopted as an improvement over the old colours and became a common constituent in wallpaper by 1800. Further, technological innovations such as production of papers in continuous rolls instead of large sheets (1797) and machine printing of patterns in place of labour-intensive hand application (1841) brought prices down to levels generally affordable.[4]

During the same period, candles were being replaced by oil and gas as the chief sources of illumination. Producing more light than candles, the new lamps did not require pale-coloured reflective walls, so wallpapers in dark shades—such as Scheele's and Schweinfurt greens—were now suitable. By 1858, a manufacturer could venture an estimate that as many as 100 million square miles of arsenic-coloured paper were to be found on the walls of homes in Great Britain; or, as Taylor so trenchantly observed, wallpaper now 'furnishes arsenic to the million'.[5]

For the manufacturer, such extensive coverage was a matter for boasting. For the medical profession, it was a matter for concern. Just the year before, the first substantive warnings of danger from green wallpapers had been sounded. In 1857, Birmingham physician William Hinds published an article relating his personal experience with the papers. Several years before, he recounted, he had decorated his study with 'bright and elegant' wallpaper. Within two hours of his first evening reading in the room, however, he was overcome by 'an inclination to vomit' accompanied by abdominal pain and light-headedness. Hinds retired for the night, but on returning the next evening, the nausea, pain, and light-headedness were repeated. Still, he laboured on—one wonders how—until after some days the coincidence between the onset of his miseries and the papering of the room finally struck him. Scraping away some of the green pigment from the paper, he analysed it, found it full of arsenic, and promptly had the paper removed. His symptoms never returned.[6]

Hinds nevertheless allowed eight years to elapse before putting his experience into print, supposing his had been an idiosyncratic reaction, 'unique and unparalleled', and that other people, less sensitive, would not be affected. That notion was exploded in the winter of 1856, when he was consulted by a Birmingham businessman and his wife, both suffering from weakness, inflamed eyes, headache, and sore throat. Even their parrot was sick, refusing to eat, drinking water almost continuously, and being 'constantly drooping' (behaving, that is, exactly like the birds enclosed in the stearine candle boxes in the 1830s). The man soon became so ill he travelled to the seaside in a last-ditch attempt at regaining health— and succeeded, in just a week. Then, alas, he returned home and in two days was back to abnormal. When it was suggested that the bright green wallpapers that had recently been applied to two rooms of the house might be at fault, the man had the papers taken down and within the week he, his wife, and the parrot were hale as ever.[7]

'A vast deal of slow poisoning is going on in Great Britain,' Hinds now believed, but the source—arsenic dust dislodged from wallpaper—was not understood by the profession. In some papers, he reported, pigment was very loosely attached, so that a napkin 'just rubbed lightly' over the surface picked up considerable quantities of the colour. How could a vast deal of poisoning not occur, then, when 'a puff of wind or an ordinary current of air floats off myriads of particles' of arsenic?[8]

Hinds's incrimination of green walls brought other critics out of the woodwork. Early in 1858, Alfred Taylor, called as a witness before a parliamentary committee considering a bill to regulate the sale of all poisons, not just arsenic, introduced into evidence a piece of wallpaper on which 'the colour is put on very loosely indeed' and therefore, he maintained, must be harmful. Only days later, a London physician submitted a letter to *The Times* detailing how within three weeks of papering his study in the autumn of 1856 he became 'completely prostrated'. When he moved his work to other rooms, his condition improved; when he returned to the study, prostration came on again. Unaware that wallpapers contained arsenic, he drew no connection between his illness and the paper in his study until reading Hinds's article a year and a half later. He had his paper immediately subjected to 'chymical scrutiny' and copper arsenate was found; with that, the paper, 'though a costly, new, and handsome one, was speedily stripped off the walls' and his health as speedily returned. He had regularly used the room since then without injury. Dr Halley's letter was followed by that of 'A Sufferer', who told *The Times* much the same story about himself, adding the postscript that when he informed

his decorator he was distributing poison, the man 'denied the possibility of ill resulting, and offered to eat a pound of the paper' to
prove the point.[9]

Yet while still more medical men weighed in with the opinion
that there must be many cases of wallpaper poisoning going undi-
agnosed, serious doubts about the risk were expressed by other
figures. Foremost, of course, were the paper manufacturers themselves, who spoke as if they too would be willing to eat their product by the pound (his rooms were covered with green paper, one
announced; 'look, I can rub it hard, I can lick it a dozen times
with my tongue and nothing comes off'). Manufacturers generally
embraced the strategy that would prove so effective in the twentieth
century for the tobacco industry, the fossil fuels industry, and other
producers of materials damaging to human health or the environment. A cigarette company executive in 1969 urged colleagues to
always bear in mind that 'doubt is our product': by raising doubts
about scientific consensus, by questioning the absolute certainty of
the case against tars and nicotine—or arsenic—an industry can
delay, or forestall altogether, the forming of public agreement that
a product is harmful and in need of regulation.[10]

The opinions of manufacturers clearly had to be taken with a
good pinch of salt. They were hardly medical experts, and their
judgement was necessarily influenced by their economic interests.
But it was also the case that, at first, there was no consensus among
medical scientists that wallpapers were a threat to health. Arthur
Hassall, for one, doubted that wallpapers were harmful. In as vivid
a revelation of the intensity of the rage for green as can be found,
Hassall informed a scientific journal in 1859 that he was writing his
article in a room decorated with 'a green Turkey carpet, a green
velvet sofa, several green morocco chairs, and three green table covers'. If the arsenical Cassandras were right in their views, then 'in

the first place, I ought to be very ill...and secondly, I ought (which would be a serious sacrifice) to get rid forthwith of the greater part of the furniture contained in the room which I habitually occupy'. The furniture would not be sold, though, for he was not the least bit ill, and was confident that neither his carpet, nor his sofa, nor any wallpaper were releasing arsenic into the atmosphere. His own examinations of papers had persuaded him that except for a few cheaply made products, green pigments were too tightly bound to the paper to come loose; the chance of being poisoned by wallpaper, therefore, 'is not very great'. Such nonchalance about wallpaper might seem to be in conflict with Hassall's denunciation of the dangers attending artificial flower-making, discussed in the last chapter. But the wallpaper evaluation preceded his investigation of flower-making by some months, and arsenical dust was visibly present in the air of flower workshops.[11]

Hassall was hardly the only medical man initially sceptical of wallpaper as a source of illness. There was, after all, room for doubt. First, as with exposure to stearine candles or green playing cards, the symptoms produced by proximity to arsenical wallpaper could be so mundane as to be dismissed as inconsequential or else assigned to other causes. It was perfectly reasonable for a London professor who 'could not account for what was amiss with me' to draw the conclusion he must be suffering from overwork. His discomfort was always at its worst after he had spent long periods at reading and writing in his study (a green-papered room), and he always felt better after taking a break from work to attend a dinner party or other extramural function. In some situations, unfortunately, supposing another illness was involved could significantly worsen the problem. When a wallpaper victim lost weight and developed a sore throat and coughing, for instance, the diagnosis might be consumption— pulmonary tuberculosis. For that, the standard treatment was bed rest and avoidance of cold air. Confined to a bedroom papered in green, its windows tightly sealed to keep out draughts, the supposedly consumptive patient 'breathes constantly an air loaded with the breath of death'. When death at last arrived, it was indeed due to consumption—consumption of arsenic. Further, doctors could not escape noticing that many, if not most, of the people who lived with green wallpaper displayed no symptoms at all; being, in Taylor's words, 'most fortunately constituted', they could 'breathe arsenical dust with impunity'. As a consequence, if only one member of a family was *un*fortunately constituted, he alone would suffer and the wallpaper would escape incrimination because the rest of the household had also been exposed to it.[12]

The question of wallpaper poisoning was complicated as well by uncertainty over the mechanism involved. Many physicians initially agreed with Hassall that only the most shoddily made papers shed dust into the air. Some also took it upon themselves to disprove the only other possible mechanism, the generation of arsenical gases from the paper. That seemed an unlikely occurrence on the face of it, as the pigments did not evaporate at ordinary temperature. But to put the possibility beyond question, several investigators carried out experiments. In one trial, a wallpapered room was tightly sealed for thirty-six hours, then much of its air drawn through a respirator: 'not a trace of arsenic was detected'. The test was then repeated seven times over increasingly lengthy periods, up to nine days in the last, and still not a trace turned up. Therefore, the investigator decided, it could be 'very safely concluded' that poisoning from wallpaper pigments 'has been disproved' and that the symptoms experienced by Hinds and others were only 'accidentally' connected to wallpaper exposure, and in actuality were 'ascribable to other causes'. Hinds begged to differ, offering to furnish any doubter with arsenical paper to cover a room in which he must then spend a few days: 'let the experimenter undergo the same experience as we who have suffered, and I shall have little doubt that he will come out of the trial fully convinced'.[13]

Several decades later, it would be discovered that a poisonous vapour actually was released from arsenical wallpapers, but in the meantime, from the late 1850s to the 1890s, solid arsenic, in the form of very fine dust, would receive all the blame. Hassall's doubts notwithstanding, dust would be demonstrated to be detached from all types of green papers, not just the cheap ones with no sizing (adhesive) or coating of varnish to hold the pigment fast. In response, medical opinion moved steadily towards agreement that any arsenical papers could cause harm. The conversion of T. Lauder Brunton, one of the Brahmins of London medicine, is reflective of the shift. When Brunton first read accusations that wallpaper was poisonous, he threw the articles 'into the wastepaper basket' as nonsense. Soon after, however, he had his consulting room papered in green and shortly began to experience symptoms 'of such a serious character as to endanger life'. He spent the rest of his career arguing for the prohibition of arsenical pigments in domestic products.[14]

The key in shifting medical opinion was the demonstration of something more than that pigments could be rubbed off intentionally, as Hinds had done. That represented a threat, to be sure: in the early 1850s, a 3-year-old nearly died from chewing slips of green wallpaper, and in the 1870s two children were badly poisoned by an art project that involved green paint they made by rubbing their wallpaper with saliva-moistened fingers. But people did not, as a rule, chew their paper or rub it with wet fingers. For wallpapers to be taken seriously as a wide-scale menace to health, it had to be shown that pigment came loose on its own.[15]

Alfred Taylor provided evidence in 1858, collecting sizeable quantities of arsenic dust from the tops of instrument cases in a London optician's shop. The shop staff had not noticed any deleterious effects from their paper, but two years later *The Lancet* reported the death of a 3-year-old boy who had expired with symptoms of arsenic poisoning, whose evacuations and organs were found to contain the poison—and whose play area was found to be coated with arsenic dust. The paper that lined the room—'this horrible paper'—was one-third Scheele's green by weight: to inhale the air of the playroom was to court 'violent and horrible death'. Letheby, who analysed the paper, was left shaking his head: 'When our artificers and manufacturers will learn caution in respect of the use of such poisonous pigments I know not.' Not soon.[16]

Reports of the detection of toxic dust on shelves and furnishings of wallpapered rooms became commonplace in the early 1860s, but sediments of arsenic were not, by themselves, taken as conclusive proof that wallpapers poisoned people. It was uncertain just how much arsenic might be in the air at any time, and how much inhabitants were taking in. The presence of arsenic in the room was a theoretical explanation of an inhabitant's illness, but the empirical demonstration, physicians believed, was that illness disappeared when either the person or the paper was removed from the room. The many cases reported in medical literature through the 1860s and 1870s have that as their common line of argument: people became sick when surrounded by arsenical papers and recovered when separated from the papers (and became sick again if they returned to the papered rooms).

To select just a few examples from a lengthy list, the professor who supposed himself to be a victim of overwork at last came to suspect his wallpaper after fainting one night in his study. Making a point of avoiding the room for several weeks, he regained his health fully and then, 'by way of a test', returned to his study for an evening of work. By bedtime, he was ill again; but once he had the paper removed he was able to work every day in the room with no bad effects. A family who periodically went on holiday to a second home on the Isle of Wight had a similar experience. Whenever there, they would get sick; on leaving, they would improve. The wallpapers at last coming under suspicion, they were tested and every room in the house determined to be layered with arsenic. The papers were stripped and discarded, and on subsequent holidays the family were free of symptoms. A Yorkshire physician treated his ailing children for months, 'dosing and doubly dosing' with no benefit until he came to wonder about their wallpaper. He took the paper down, 'and from that day they have never required a single dose of medicine, and now, instead of pale faces, they have rosy cheeks'. A London woman sickened soon after moving into a new house, and her Persian cat lost its fur and broke out with 'a peculiar skin eruption'. A friend suggested the green paper in her bedroom might be at fault, so the woman traded rooms with her maid. She recovered—and the maid became ill. The room's paper was removed and the maid got better; whether the cat did as well was not recorded. Finally, there was the Cambridgeshire farmer whose family's health improved once he took down the wallpaper, but at the expense of his livestock. He threw the paper into the yard, planning to dispose of it once his bare walls were refinished. Before he could accomplish that, however, three farm animals got at it, ate it, and died.[17]

There was the possibility, of course, that all those people improved in health for psychosomatic reasons—they had read about poisonous wallpaper, become convinced they were being poisoned by it, so when the paper was taken away, they felt better. But then how did one explain the young man whose wallpaper was taken down 'much against his will, as he was an utter unbeliever in the possibility of arsenic in that shape hurting him'? He, too, was soon feeling much better. 'We have here,' Taylor declared of the large aggregate of such cases, 'as close a connexion of cause and effect as we can reasonably expect to find.' (It wasn't necessary to be a scientist to notice the connection. In one house, the servants referred to the green bedroom as the 'haunted chamber', and advised newcomers to the household, 'Oh! you needn't try to sleep in that room; I never could take any breakfast when I slept there.' The woman issuing the warning didn't blame the wallpaper, though; she simply believed 'there was something not "canny" about the room'.)[18]

*

The public were alerted to the uncanny properties of green wallpaper not only by the press, which regularly reprinted medical journal articles on the subject, but also by fictional explorations of the problem. As early as 1862, a widely read weekly, *Chambers's Journal of Popular Literature, Science, and Arts*, discomposed readers with a short story about young Sir Frederick Staunton, the orphaned ward of an uncle who wishes him out of the way in order to inherit his estate. The scheming uncle sends him to live with a kindly vicar, the latter being instructed to give Frederick the best bedroom in the parsonage, a room with wallpaper of 'a rich deep emerald hue', with curtains and carpet to match. Shortly before the nephew's arrival, Vicar Harper learns that local folk believe the house to be cursed by a monk from the days of Henry VIII: 'Several deaths had occurred in the green chamber in particular, for the most part blooming girls who had faded and pined under "the curse" until their dim eyes had looked their last at the emerald-tinted walls.' Still, instructions are instructions, so the unsuspecting vicar houses Frederick in the accursed room, the young man soon falls ill, and

despite the efforts of a local surgeon continues to decline until tee-
tering on the very edge of his grave. At that juncture, a renowned
physician is summoned, who immediately upon stepping into the
green room recognizes it for what it is, an 'envenomed den' swathed
in 'arsenic enough to poison a regiment'. Frederick is moved to a
safe chamber and quickly recovers his health, his uncle loses his
anticipated wealth, and the vicar is rewarded by Frederick with an
assignment to a much more lucrative parish.[19]

Seven years later, short story gave way to novel with the publication of *The Green of the Period*, an anonymously authored volume
with a subtitle that promises suspense (*The Unsuspected Foe in the
Englishman's Home*) and phrases that warn of hidden peril ('the verdant assassin' was 'slaying its unsuspecting thousands' with 'green
paper fever'; wallpapers 'were now coiling me . . . in their grasp, day
and night'). The promise goes unrealized, sadly, as in the end the
plot, if such it can be called, is little more than a series of eye-glaz-
ing lectures delivered by protagonist Sir Robert Chichester (he who
had been brought 'nearly to the grave' in 'an arsenical den') to com-
panions Lord Henry Douglas and Mr Fortescue as they tour the
Continent. For Chichester, it is not enough for the friends peacefully
to contemplate the majesty of the falls of the Rhine; they must also
be informed of the miserable fate of the four Limehouse children.
Standing in Chamonix, gazing raptly at Mont Blanc, Douglas and
Fortescue are brought crashing to earth by the recitation of medical
reports of people sickened by wallpaper. Crossing into Switzerland,
they are not allowed to marvel quietly at the grandeur of the Alps,
they must also listen to a recounting of the suffering of Matilda
Scheurer. Yet the friends keep coming back for more, repeatedly
begging Sir Robert to read them still another medical article or to
tell them once again about the time his physician diagnosed him as
a case of 'arsenical heart'. When at long last (page 178), Chichester

takes leave of his fawning entourage, it is only so he can rush back to London to begin his crusade 'to rid England of "THE GREEN OF THE PERIOD"'. In this, he enjoyed some degree of success. Two years later, a lay correspondent of the *British Medical Journal* related that he, his family, and their servants had all been poisoned by wallpaper without suspecting a thing until his doctor placed a copy of *The Green of the Period* in his hands.[20]

Plodding plot and vapid prose were not failings of a second wallpaper novel, *Minsterborough*, the 1876 creation of London physician Humphry Sandwith. Blending medical expertise with modest literary talents, he concocted a lively three-volume potboiler employing all the clichés of Victorian melodrama. The villain of the piece, Lord Buckton, is ruler of Hillborough Hall, in the hitherto sleepy town of Minsterborough, Yorkshire. When Buckton's wife suddenly takes ill, then dies, the town's older physician declares her to be a victim of English cholera. A more astute young practitioner, however, suspects arsenic, and indeed detects a small amount in the lady's vomit. Her viscera are therefore removed and 'sent in sealed jars to Mr Herapath, of Bristol, the first analyst in England' (Alfred Taylor was still alive and if he read the novel no doubt took offence; the author's selection of Herapath as number one perhaps reflects the loss of prestige Taylor suffered in the Smethurst case).[21]

When the great man of Bristol finds arsenic in the organs, an inquest is called and events take a familiar turn, familiar, that is, to any who had followed the Smethurst trial. Lady Buckton, it is soon revealed, had been married twenty years ago in Scotland to a Mr Fraser, who was subsequently persuaded somehow by Lord Buckton's father that the marriage was invalid. Heartbroken, Fraser enlisted in the army and shipped out to India, where a year later he received a letter from Buckton informing him that his sweetheart had died. The woman is alive, of course, and has even given birth to a daughter sired by Fraser. She also is in line for a significant inheritance, an inspiration for the wily Buckton to woo and wed her, and to take in her child. Recently, though, the clergyman who performed the first marriage has learned of the false death report of two decades gone by and has written to Fraser, now a major, that the lady is alive though ill, and that the marriage had in fact been perfectly legitimate. The major hurries to Minsterborough, arriving too late to reclaim his bride, alas, but just in time to tell the inquest jury how Buckton has robbed him of his 'wife and her fortune'.[22]

It is now all quite obvious what has transpired. Buckton, a 'haughty-looking man', a 'brawling kind of ruffian', a 'brute' who has ever treated his wife badly, has seen his designs on her wealth shaken by Fraser's return so has hastened the frail woman's death with arsenic. When it is shown that he has recently purchased the poison (to destroy crows and magpies, he laughably claims), the jury pronounces the Lord guilty.[23]

Yet during the trial, Lady Buckton's daughter Helen, now grown into a young woman as lovely as her namesake of antiquity ('her face and figure...were simply a poet's dream'), mentions in testimony that her mother's last days were spent in the green bed-room. On hearing this, the town's young chemist rushes off 'in hot haste' to Hillborough Hall, returning just as the judge accepts the jury's verdict and sentences Buckton to death. As the prisoner turns 'pale as a corpse', loud scuffling is heard at the back of the court. A man pushes forward 'by might and main, to the witness-box; men swore, as he tore through the crowd; women screamed, for the man looked crazed; his coat was torn, his cravat hanging loose, his hair dishevelled, and he carried in his hand a mass of what looked like coloured paper'. Somehow, the chemist has found time to analyse Lady Buckton's wallpaper, has determined it to be

arsenical, and 'is prepared to prove that anyone living in that room
would inevitably...absorb sufficient [arsenic] to cause death'. His
evidence comes too late to alter the verdict, the judge informs him,
but it will be sent to the Home Office and the Secretary may well
advise a pardon. Just like Smethurst, Buckton does get his pardon,
but Lady Buckton's marriage to Fraser is declared fully legal and
the Lord is denied his hoped-for inheritance. Otherwise, all ends
happily. The courageous chemist soon wins the hand of a lady he
has yearned for from afar, while her brother conquers the heart of
the sublimely beautiful Helen.[24]

*

This trilogy of wallpaper sagas built upon the extensive publicity
given the menace in the popular press, leading the public to view
any green-papered room in the terms used by Alfred Taylor in the
late 1850s, as 'a complete chamber of death to all who entered it'.
But in truth, wallpaper did not have to be dyed in the green of the
period to be deadly. The physician treating a woman who developed headaches and lethargy soon after her house was redecorated
had the green wallpaper in her sitting room analysed and was surprised to learn it held only traces of arsenic. The blue and white
paper in her bedroom, however, was heavily arsenical, and when it
was removed her symptoms subsided. As with the domestic items
that formed the subject of the last chapter, colour was an uncertain signifier of chemical composition. Arsenic compounds were to
be found in blues, reds, pinks, yellows, browns, grays, even white.
'Papers of any colour and of any shade may be arsenical,' doctors
explained, 'so that there is absolutely nothing in the appearance of
a paper by which we can form any opinion as to its arsenical or non-
arsenical nature.' In America, the Michigan State Board of Health
in the 1870s put together a book of arsenical wallpaper samples in
all colours, titled *Shadows From the Walls of Death*, and placed copies in

every library in the state. Harvard's Countway Library of Medicine holds a booklet containing a number of wallpaper samples, most of them green, but with many other colours represented as well; a strip of light blue paper adorned with silvery flowers has the words 'much arsenic' pencilled on it. The collection also contains a bright red arsenical ticket to a Bible lecture by nineteenth-century evangelical preacher Dwight Moody. Yet the public in both countries were frustratingly slow to absorb the message that arsenic was not necessarily green. As late as the mid-1880s, an English expert on arsenic in the home complained that people's minds were still 'so strongly prepossessed with the term "arsenical green," that it seems almost impossible to root out the erroneous impression so prevalent, namely, that green is the *only colour* to be avoided'.[25]

One of the last to absorb the message was the queen. In 1879, Victoria reprimanded a gentleman for being late for his audience. When, however, he begged her pardon by explaining he had been ill during the night because of his green wallpaper, 'Her Majesty was greatly startled,' apparently ignorant of the fact such things were going on in her realm. Offering an 'expression of deep concern', she had an attendant remove a strip from the wallpaper in the room, and, when it tested arsenical, acted with the 'considerateness for the comfort of those about her person so proverbial of Her Majesty'. An immediate order was issued that every bit of wallpaper in the whole of Buckingham Palace be removed right away, thereby ensuring the future safety of the palace's residents while simultaneously providing her subjects with a lesson 'to suppress decorations calculated to insure a torturing death'.[26]

Her subjects were quite ahead of her on that matter, as by 1879 heated efforts to suppress poisonous wall decorations were well underway. Only the previous year, the violet powder tragedy had left the country shocked by the ease with which arsenic could invade innocent people's lives. In the wake of that catastrophe, a public-spirited writer named Henry Carr had sent enquiries to a number of physicians and chemists soliciting information on arsenic in common household articles, the responses from which he used to put together a pamphlet to educate the public about *Our Domestic Poisons*. Wallpapers, dresses, and sundry other products contaminated with arsenic were dealt with in the body of the pamphlet, but Carr opened his presentation with the assertion (or threat, as some would see it) that 'Parliamentary action and legal restraint are evidently demanded for the protection of the public' from arsenical manufactures. That was not just his opinion. He had asked the doctors and chemists he consulted for their ideas about how to address the arsenic problem, and a single theme dominated their replies: 'I wonder much that... Parliament does not take the matter up'; 'I do hope the disgraceful use of poison in fabrics may be prohibited by a stringent Act of Parliament'; 'I suppose... that the evil will continue, and will probably increase, unless those uses of arsenic are prohibited by Act of Parliament' (this last from John Simon, Medical Officer of Health of the Privy Council and the foremost figure in the field of public health at the time). Alfred Taylor had something to say too, of course, expressing full support for an Act of Parliament to prohibit arsenical goods 'except under condition that products carry a skull and crossbones emblem with underneath the motto *Memento mori*'.[27]

'Remember you must die' if arsenic continues in free distribution was a warning being issued from other circles as well. Shortly after Carr's pamphlet came out, one of his correspondents, Jabez Hogg (he whose children had once amused themselves with arsenical playing cards), delivered a lecture to the Medical Society of London on skin and eye diseases caused by arsenic, in which he stated it was 'imperatively necessary' for the sale of arsenical papers to be outlawed. So impressed was the society by his talk, officers appointed a committee to explore the question further, and this committee too called for statutory restrictions on arsenic manufactures. Likewise did a committee formed in 1883 by the National Health Society, an organization dedicated to spreading knowledge of health matters among the populace. Among other actions, this committee solicited information from more than twenty European governments relative to arsenic legislation in their countries; a number banned arsenic from wallpapers, fabrics, and just about everything else, and several others had prohibitions against specific uses such as candles or confectionery. Add to these measures the voices of individual physicians speaking out against arsenic, and it can be appreciated that by the early 1880s there was no little pressure being directed towards government to act against arsenical products. Yet while the National Health Society's committee drew up a bill and placed it in the hands of a physician MP for introduction into Parliament, the effort went no farther. There would be no law to prohibit the manufacture or sale of wallpaper or any other domestic product containing arsenic.[28]

The danger from arsenical manufactures nevertheless subsided steadily over the last two decades of the century, for in the process of making the case for a law, critics had so thoroughly worried the public that consumers took a vote against the poison on their own. Afraid of being sickened or killed, they voted with their feet, taking their business to manufacturers who guaranteed non-arsenical products. It might be true that Schweinfurt green was a colour 'which for brilliancy is not to be surpassed', but by the second half of the century there were other pigments being synthesized that were appealing enough—and did not contain arsenic. Thus, just as women had moved away from green gowns and headdresses, so did the public turn against wallpapers once they were perceived to be destructive. Manufacturers had little choice but to honour the new consumer demand. To be fair, a few paper producers seem to have stopped using arsenical pigments soon after the first cases of poisoning were reported, before there was significant public pressure to do so. London's Woolams and Co. ceased the production of arsenical papers as early as 1859, and in the aftermath of the Limehouse deaths in 1862, another manufacturer exhibited his non-arsenical green papers before a medical association meeting in London (they were deemed 'beautiful' by the doctors in attendance).[29]

Most producers of wallpaper, however, were of a mind with the men who offered to lick their products or eat them: the papers were completely safe. Such was the opinion of one of the most successful manufacturers in Britain, William Morris, the leader of the arts and crafts movement and prolific designer of domestic ornamentation across a spectrum from furniture to tapestry to stained glass. Morris began designing wallpaper in 1862, making liberal use of arsenical pigments in his creations. Eventually he would eliminate the arsenic in response to public demand, but he seems never to have accepted that the papers truly were harmful. As late as 1885, he declared that it was 'hardly possible to imagine' a 'greater folly' than 'the arsenic scare'. Doctors had been 'bitten' by a kind of 'witch fever', he laughed, blaming wallpaper when they were unable to come up with any other cause for their patients' problems (it was his own belief that 'the source of all illness' was the water closet, an expression of the widespread fear in the 1880s of 'sewer gas', foul-smelling, supposedly noxious vapours that leaked from sewers into houses through toilet drains). Colleagues in the industry shared Morris's contempt for the poisoning theory, touting their workmen—men 'who have been daily employed for many years in manufacturing large quantities of these colours'—as being 'in the regular enjoyment of perfect health', or, even better, 'lusty specimens of manhood'.[30]

It was, of course, easy for manufacturers genuinely to believe that their employees were unaffected by working with arsenic. They were hardly objective evaluators of the situation, and in any event the symptoms produced by exposure were, to non-medical observers, readily attributable to other complaints. By contrast, physicians, once their awareness of the problem was raised, discovered all the same injuries among men engaged in wallpaper production as were common among artificial flower-makers—the hazards of this and other arsenical occupations will be considered in detail in Chapter 11.

What most sharply concentrated manufacturers' minds, however, was not medical evidence but the public's growing fear of arsenical paper. How could it turn a profit if people were afraid to buy it? By the early 1870s, it was being reported that the publicity given the dangers of arsenical papers had rendered them 'much less fashionable', and manufacturers were responding with safe products (it helped that new, improved non-arsenical pigments were being developed in quantity by then). An inquiry into wallpapers conducted by a parliamentary commission in 1876 found the same trend. A spokesman for the firm of Carlisle and Clegg testified to the commission that consumers 'very often compel us to use non-arsenical green', with the result that production of such papers was 'very materially diminishing'. Manufacturers had reached agreement that, 'it now answers our purpose better to make goods free from arsenic'. Arsenic-free paper had become good business: products were being marketed under the description Patent Hygienic Wallpapers, and advertisements proudly announced products as 'FREE FROM ARSENIC'.[31]

Consumers had only the manufacturer's word that products were pure, however, and some guarantees were not worth the paper they were written on. One writer protested that a paper sold 'by one of the first firms in London—printed on the back "non-arsenical," proved to be highly arsenical'; another determined that every sample of eight papers certified to be non-arsenical did in fact contain the poison in significant amounts. When a Boston dealer complained that the free-from-arsenic papers he had imported from an English firm had been found by American chemists to be heavily contaminated, the manufacturer responded with an analysis from his own chemist that baldly charged the Yankee scientists had made a mistake. After a second set of analyses performed in America again demonstrated the papers to be poisonous, the manufacturer washed his hands of the matter, refusing to take the papers back or make reimbursement, and leaving the conscientious Boston dealer no choice but to try to sell the product with an open acknowledgement that it was arsenical: 'so much for the value of a "manufacturer's guarantee"', an American physician huffed. In 1880, Woolams and Co., the originators of arsenic-free papers and recipients of a gold medal for contributions to public welfare awarded at a major London health exhibition, discovered that a batch of pigment purchased from a manufacturer who guaranteed it to be non-arsenical in fact contained the poison. By the time the discovery was made, however, the pigment had been used to produce a large quantity of wallpaper. Refusing to market the paper, Woolams sued the pigment producer for £370 for the loss incurred; the jury rejected the suit on a legal technicality.[32]

At the other end from Woolams were the dealers who treated customer enquiries about safety 'with withering contempt, descant[ed] upon cranks and other offensive persons' who drummed up unnecessary alarm, and bullied clients 'who may not wish to be considered imbeciles into buying without a guarantee of any sort'. Perhaps the *British Medical Journal* was right in objecting that 'there is no safety now-a-days from being poisoned against one's will, except for having every paper in your house analysed by a reliable analytical chemist'. Reliable chemists cost money, unfortunately: 'the public desire to know whether their papers are arsenical or not, but they are unwilling to pay for the information'. Consequently, some consumer champions urged the public to test their papers for themselves: tear off a strip of paper, people were told, light it, blow it out, 'then smell the smoke which issues from the still ignited, but not blazing, paper. If it contain arsenic, the smell will be that of garlic.' Alternatively, one could extrapolate from the old canary in the coal mine test, as there were in fact cases of canaries dying when their cages were put into arsenic-papered rooms (and also, as has been seen, of parrots sickening and cats losing their fur; there were instances of ferns withering too).[33]

Nevertheless, chemical analyses of wallpapers were demonstrating a sharp drop in the use of arsenic. In 1874, a survey of the wallpaper problem had concluded that notwithstanding all the publicity given to the danger, arsenical papers 'are still made and used to an enormous extent'. Only a quarter of a century later, in 1900, a report issued by the Home Office announced that British wallpapers were now 'practically arsenic-free', containing at most 'infinitesimal amounts'. A similar drop occurred in the United States over that period, likewise from consumer insistence on non-arsenical paper.[34]

Even so, it took some time for wallpaper poisoning to disappear. New arsenical papers were not being put up, perhaps, but old papers remained on walls, and even if they had been layered over with safe papers, preventing pigment from being detached, a hazard remained. In 1891, the Italian chemist Bartolomeo Gosio discovered that several fungi (most notably *Scopulariopsis brevicaulis*) could grow in the paste used to apply wallpapers and act upon arsenic in the paper to release a toxic vapour. Arsenical fumes had been suggested as the cause of wallpaper poisoning as early as the 1850s, but the idea had been dismissed with the observation that arsenic could not be volatilized at ordinary household temperatures. The incriminated fungus, on the other hand, growing as a mould, operated at regular temperatures and set free arsenic even from underlying layers of paper. The chemical nature of the gas was a mystery at first—'Gosio's gas', it was called, and wallpaper poisoning referred to as 'Gosio's disease'; the gas was finally identified in the 1930s as trimethyl arsine. In the meantime, cases of arsenic poisoning of people living in rooms with non-arsenical papers on top of arsenical ones were regularly reported (a medical journal article in the 1870s described a room with thirteen layers of paper on its walls, most of the layers containing arsenic).[35]

Despite the deaf ear Parliament turned to calls for the prohibition of arsenical wallpapers, artificial flowers, ball gowns, and all the rest, the tide of arsenic-tainted consumer products that had once threatened to swamp British society had been turned back by the end of the century. Where legislators had baulked, consumers had rallied, spurred by the alarms sounded by the medical community and publicized in the popular press. Exercising choice, shunning arsenical manufactures, the public had applied sufficient economic pressure to force industry to comply with the new preferences. People could have helped themselves still more, though, by shunning their doctors' prescriptions for arsenical medications.[36]

*

But before proceeding to arsenic as medicine, it's necessary briefly to address the question: was Napoleon killed by wallpaper? After his defeat at Waterloo, the emperor was exiled to Longwood House, on St Helena, in the South Atlantic, where he lived another six years. When he died in 1821, several people close to him removed clippings of hair from his head, and these were passed down for generations as keepsakes. First in 1960, then more extensively in the 1990s, the hair samples were subjected to chemical analysis, and all were found to contain abnormal levels of arsenic. The news was welcomed by some Napoleonic scholars as verification of their theories that he had been poisoned by English and/or French conspirators determined to prevent a repetition of the escape from Elba (death by arsenic poisoning was also suggested by the fact that when his body was exhumed twenty years after death for removal to Paris, it was found to be remarkably well preserved). By others, it was interpreted as evidence he had succumbed to wallpaper poisoning. There was green paper in the room in which he died, and a fragment of the paper in the possession of an English woman tested positive for Scheele's green in 1992. The damp maritime climate of St Helena, furthermore, was ideal for the generation of Gosio's gas from the wallpaper.[37]

But could Napoleon's arsenic have come from other sources? He may well have been treated by his physicians with one or more of the arsenical medications to be discussed in the next chapter. In addition, at least according to stories bandied about during the nineteenth century, he was so fearful of being poisoned in his later years he gave himself small amounts of arsenic on a regular basis in the belief he could thereby establish immunity to the substance.[38]

The matter was cleared up, after a fashion, in 2008, when analyses of hair taken from Napoleon at various times well before his death (1805, 1814, 1816, 1817) showed quantities of arsenic in all samples similar to those in the post-mortem locks. There were no significant increases in arsenic intake in his last days, merely a long-term exposure comparable to that of other people of the time; indeed, hair from Josephine and from his son had levels of arsenic similar to his. So much for the assassination theory, and though it appears the Longwood House wallpaper did not kill him either, some of the arsenic in his hair quite possibly derived from that as well as from earlier wallpapers he had been exposed to. So while Napoleon may not have been killed by wallpaper, he possibly was to some degree poisoned by it.[39]

9

Physician-Assisted Poisoning

It has never been more unpleasant to be sick, or more dangerous, than during the nineteenth century. The ailments that people
suffered were very often infections with highly disagreeable symptoms and serious risk of mortality. The remedies employed against
tuberculosis, smallpox, cholera, typhus, and the rest were, furthermore, generally useless. There was an effective treatment for
malaria in the form of quinine, but for it to accomplish a cure dosage had to be rigorously managed and physicians were frequently
not up to the challenge. Until the 1820s, moreover, quinine was
not available as a pure compound, but only as a component of the
South American tree bark called cinchona, whose dosage was even
more difficult to regulate. There were also a few drugs that relieved
certain symptoms: opium acted against pain and sleeplessness, for
example, and a host of laxatives were at hand to relieve torpid
bowels. But for the most part, a person's chances rested chiefly
with a strong constitution and good luck. The strong constitution
was needed not just to ward off the illness; it was essential also
for resisting the medications, for even the good remedies had deleterious effects. If not carefully monitored, opium could replace
insomnia with sleep eternal (and was addictive as well); cinchona
could damage both eyes and ears, and even cause death in the
hypersensitive; and the laxatives then used were so violent as to

result in severe dehydration (most have long since been abandoned as dangerous). The most popular of these cathartics, calomel, was a mercury compound that also caused ulceration of the mouth, loss of teeth, and even destruction of the jawbone. Another favoured drug, the vomitive tartar emetic, contained antimony, a mineral that could inflict much the same damage as arsenic in addition to causing forceful ('cyclonic' was one doctor's word) evacuations by mouth. Physicians recognized the toxic nature of their drugs, but used them nonetheless because they believed them to work, and reasoned (as do oncologists today) that temporary poisoning was a small price to pay for staying alive.[1]

That a single substance could act either to heal or to kill was not a new idea: 'within the infant rind of this weak flower', Friar Laurence reveals in *Romeo and Juliet*, 'poison hath residence and medicine power'. Still, it was one thing to suppose that a delicate flower might possess such properties, and quite another to think of arsenic, the deadliest of minerals, as also an agent of health. 'Had it been announced to the World, a century or two ago,' Staffordshire physician Thomas Fowler wrote in 1786, that 'the most violent mineral Poison...had been found experimentally to be a Medicine of most surprising activity and efficacy, yet safe in its Administration; the Account would hardly have been believed.' It was still not easy to believe, Fowler recognized, but experience had convinced him it was true, and the book he published detailing that experience— *Medical Reports of the Effects of Arsenic*—would convince so many fellow practitioners as to raise arsenic nearly to the level of supposed cure-all for most of the nineteenth century. Arsenical medication would also serve as a prolific source of chronic poisoning.[2]

Fowler overstated his point in asserting that preceding centuries would have been amazed at hearing of arsenic being used as medicine, for arsenical compounds had been prescribed in limited ways since the time of Hippocrates, the fourth-century BC physician revered as the 'father of medicine'. Hippocrates used both orpiment and realgar as escharotics, caustic materials to destroy tumours and ulcers on the skin. The celebrated herbalist of Nero's day, Dioscorides, found orpiment to be effective also as a depilatory, or agent for removing unwanted hair from the body. By the eighteenth century, such preparations as Lanfranc's collyrium, Hellmund's ointment, and Frère Côme's paste counted among the considerable number of arsenic combinations then in use against any form of skin eruption or external growth.[3]

External application was not without danger, for the poison could be absorbed through the raw surface created by its caustic action. But internal administration, the traditional method for murder, seemed riskier, and it was that which Fowler had in mind in presenting his discovery as unexpected and hard to believe. Nevertheless, arsenical compounds had, in fact, been given internally as medicine before Fowler; it was just that they had been taken primarily in the form of so-called patent medicines, secret recipe pills or potions peddled by laymen whom the medical profession regarded as quacks. Although therapeutically useless, they commonly contained substances that caused physiological effects such as vomiting, diarrhoea, or urination so as to impress purchasers that the drugs were operating upon the system; arsenic appealed because it produced both vomiting and diarrhoea. Since the composition of these nostrums was a closely guarded secret, patients rarely knew that they were swallowing arsenic. But those that did know, or suspected, considered the medications dangerous and loudly warned the public against them as 'detestable Wickedness' sure to lead to a 'most fatal Consequence'. Thus, even though arsenicals had been used medicinally for centuries, Fowler was justified in supposing that the profession would find it hard to credit his discovery that they could be both effective and safe when taken internally.[4]

The full title of Fowler's book specified that his *Reports* related primarily to the *Effects of Arsenic, in the Cure of Agues*. Ague, derived from a Latin term for fever, was a common synonym for malaria. Today, malaria is thought of as a tropical disease, the great affliction of non-industrialized countries. But prior to the twentieth century the infection was rife throughout Europe and America, and as Physician to the General Infirmary of the County of Stafford, Fowler had frequent opportunity to treat the victims of ague. In his time, of course, no one knew yet of the protozoan parasites that cause malaria's alternating bouts of chills and fever, or of the role of mosquitoes in the transmission of the disease from person to person. But physicians did have available a somewhat effective therapy for ague in the form of cinchona.

Cinchona did not, however, work for everyone, quinine being more active against some species of malarial parasites than others. The percentage of quinine in the bark varied, furthermore, from one sample to another, making dosing something of a matter of guesswork. Finally, the drug was often administered in cases in which it was inappropriate, for since it suppressed the fever of malaria, doctors were given to thinking of it as a general febrifuge, a drug that would lower fever in any disease. It would not. Many cases diagnosed as ague or some closely similar condition resisted cinchona, so many as to render it necessary to find, in Fowler's words, 'a powerful vicarious Remedy' for the ailment.[5]

As it happened, a vicarious remedy for ague was at hand. The Tasteless Ague and Fever Drops, a patent medicine, had won favour with the public in the malaria-ridden fens of East Anglia during the 1770s ('tasteless' was an important attribute, for cinchona bark was quite bitter on the tongue). It was not, in truth, effective, but inertness never stood in the way of a patent medicine gaining acceptance. Advertised with extravagant claims that stimulated the buyer's hope and thereby the placebo response, recommended against ailments that in many cases would clear up sooner or later whether medicine was taken or not, patent nostrums were time and again given false credit for cure when recovery occurred. To be sure, there were rare instances in which patent remedies, as well as folk medicines, yielded valuable drugs: digitalis is a particularly famous example of an active pharmaceutical discovered in a non-official medication. But Tasteless Ague and Fever Drops were an example of nothing more than the capacity of patients for self-delusion.

As a rule, physicians did not deign to experiment with concoctions peddled by the medically unschooled ('empirics', doctors called such pretenders, because, ignorant of medical science and theory, they relied purely on trial and error bumbling). But in exceptional circumstances, if a product enjoyed particular éclat and/or the condition it purported to cure was especially troublesome, curiosity could overcome professional dignity and motivate a doctor to give the nostrum a try. 'When the patent Ague Drops began to acquire some Reputation in the Country,' Fowler wrote, 'they were occasionally adopted in the Hospital Practice of this Place,' the Staffordshire Infirmary; and, he added, the Drops 'were found efficacious'.[6]

In the autumn of 1783, some two years after the occasional employment of the Ague Drops began, Fowler was told by the apothecary to the Infirmary that there were chemical reasons to suspect the remedy contained arsenic. The physician then made up a preparation of white arsenic in solution with a potassium salt, compared its action to that of the Drops, and found it to be very similar, but stronger. After diluting it to roughly the same strength as the patent medicine, Fowler started using his solution in earnest to treat ague cases, though without telling patients they were being given arsenic. Eager to avoid the 'disagreeable Association of Ideas' of arsenic with poison, he decided to call the medicine simply 'the Mineral Solution' (later *Solutio Mineralis*). The results obtained with the euphemistic remedy were startling: of 247 patients diagnosed with ague, 242 he pronounced cured by his treatment. Many of these patients, moreover, were people whose illness had been plaguing them for weeks and who had taken cinchona and other medicines to no avail. It was difficult to resist Fowler's conclusion that he had found a wondrous new therapy for ague.[7]

On closer reading, however, the case reports raise doubts. Fowler acknowledged, for example, that some patients responded indifferently to his solution, but then rapidly improved when given cinchona. These were counted among the cures, as it seemed to him the solution must have paved the way for the bark to act more efficiently. This reasoning also failed to take account of the fact that attacks of malaria generally subside after two to four weeks, and while relapse is common, it may not occur for some time, leading the doctor to suppose he has accomplished a cure no matter what medication might have been given. Even more troubling are the low-key references interspersed among the records to patients who, experiencing no improvement, stopped coming to the Infirmary. In Fowler's eyes, their lack of response was due not to any inadequacy in the medication, but to their inability to stay the course of treatment to the end; he saw no need to include those feckless invalids in his statistics. The preconception that when patients failed to improve it must be their fault, not the medicine's, is seen again in his accounts of using the solution to treat 'Headachs': 'it is probable had she continued her Attendance', he wrote of a woman who ceased her visits to the Infirmary, 'the Treatment would have proved successful'. Would it? In Fowler's defence, he is far from alone in showing a bias toward the assumption that a medicament *hoped* to be effective must in fact be so; it is a failing common to physicians throughout history.[8]

Then there was the question of safety. Patients may not have known in their minds that the *Solutio Mineralis* was actually arsenic solution, but their bodies soon figured it out. On 14-year-old Dorothy Perkins, 'it operated from the Time she had taken the second Dose, as a violent Emetic, attended with Nausea, and painful Griping and Purging, for the Space of ten Hours'. With another patient, 'her Face and Eyes became so swelled every Morning, she could scarce see till towards Noon'. Some combination of these reactions occurred in most patients, but generally the responses were no worse than those produced by other drugs, so there seemed no reason to withhold the solution on account of side effects. To Fowler, the closing sentence of his book was fully justified: 'I flatter myself its Reputation will soon be established on so firm a Basis, as to render it highly useful, not only to the present, but future Generations.'[9]

*

Highly harmful to future generations was nearer the mark, yet its reputation was soon established nonetheless. Though some practitioners counselled caution, other doctors tried the solution and agreed with Fowler. Even the timid now fell into line, and the preparation quickly became a therapeutic mainstay: as early as 1809 it was praised as 'almost as *certain* a medicine as we possess throughout the whole range of our materia medica'. That same year, it was accepted into the *London Pharmacopoeia*, the official register of professionally approved remedies. The mineral solution also began to be identified more honestly, as *liquor arsenicalis* (it was a solution of potassium arsenite, with a touch of lavender added to give a distinctive flavour and prevent it being mistaken for water and swallowed accidentally).[10]

Before long, however, everyone was referring to the remedy by the simple name of Fowler's solution, and employing it against numerous complaints besides ague. As with many pre-twentieth-century drugs, once it was recognized to be useful in one ailment, it was tried against others and soon determined to be effective against them as well. Fowler's solution steadily acquired the reputation of 'the multipotent drug', a drug that operated (by an American doctor's metaphor) as one of medicine's 'therapeutic mules': it performed 'the hardest kind of work under the most adverse conditions, with the least amount of exertion'.[11]

One field in which the mule worked its hardest was asthma. 'Her breathing is easy, not even wheezy,' an English practitioner recorded of an asthma patient after he had treated her with Fowler's solution. Different though it was from malaria, asthma was regarded as one of the diseases most responsive to arsenic. Asthma patients were in fact subjected to a barrage of arsenical therapies, being dosed with Fowler's solution, given inhalations of a mist containing white arsenic, and directed to smoke pipes in which arsenic was sandwiched between layers of tobacco in the bowl. Soothing vapours could also be delivered by cigarettes, with sometimes arsenic alone mixed with the tobacco (typically one and a half grains per cigarette), more often the plant product stramonium added too. The second form of smoke worked particularly well, since stramonium contains atropine, an alkaloid that dilates bronchial vessels and assists breathing. A typical cure was that of the woman who had suffered with asthma for more than twenty years, 'taken every species and form of medicine' as well as being regularly bled, but with no benefit. In desperation, she turned to arsenic/stramonium cigarettes, and 'from being in a state of constant breathlessness', incapable of 'the slightest exertion', she became able to move about normally. Asthmatic attacks still occasionally occurred, but were at once ended by a cigarette (she rolled her own, incidentally, adding upwards of three grains of arsenic; surprisingly, swollen eyelids were the only untoward effect she experienced). Another asthmatic, so short of breath she laboured to climb the one flight of stairs in her home, was, after six weeks of treatment with Fowler's solution, 'able to go from the bottom of the steps in the Crystal palace "right off" up to the top, without the slightest embarrassment, and greatly to her own astonishment'.[12]

No less astonishing were the results reported for chorea, a condition of involuntary jerky or spasmodic movements of the facial muscles or limbs. In the 1850s, arsenic was used to treat a 16-year-old boy who for ten days had been afflicted with 'writhings and agitations of the body so strong, as to render it necessary to impose the whole weight of a grown-up person in order to retain him in bed'. When food was offered, his jaws clamped around whatever utensil or vessel was placed to his lips; on one occasion he bit through a glass, cutting his tongue so deeply as to cause profuse bleeding. Various remedies were tried, none had any effect—until he was given the mineral solution. Within three weeks, 'every symptom of his malady had disappeared'. Seeming miracle cures of chorea were commonplace accounts in medical journals. 'I have never known the remedy to fail,' one doctor stated; for another, it was 'an infallible cure'.[13]

Then there were skin diseases. By the end of the century, the editor of a textbook on therapeutics could summarize that arsenic had been 'the most extensively used internal medicine' for dermatological problems for many years, so much so 'that there are few diseases of the integument in which it has not been employed'. In small quantities, arsenic does indeed improve the appearance of

the skin, for a time at least, creating a milk-and-roses complexion
by dilating capillaries. It can also relieve certain skin conditions:
Fowler's solution would be a trusted remedy against psoriasis, in
fact, on into the middle of the twentieth century. But in the nineteenth century, the solution was entrusted with the cure of all skin
ailments, from simple acne (nothing was more reliable against
'the unwelcome visitor') to eczema, hives, and anything else that
erupted or itched: 'Nor has it failed in any of these diseases in a
single case when fairly and fully tried.' The remedy would even
cure skin problems that were side effects of other drugs. Epileptics
were often treated (ineffectively) with bromides, for instance,
which produced an unsightly 'bromide rash', a rash that resisted
all treatments—except arsenic. Eventually arsenic would be added
directly to bromide medications so as to prevent the rash from
developing in the first place.[14]

The list of additional ailments that one physician or another
decided could be cured with arsenic falls only a little short of an
index of all the ills to which flesh is liable. Diphtheria was treatable,
one practitioner claimed, by removing the membrane that formed
in the patient's throat, then swabbing the raw area with Fowler's
solution to prevent a new membrane from forming and closing off
the airway. Other doctors reported success with Fowler's solution
against worms, anemia, heart palpitations, rheumatism, tuberculosis, typhus, syphilis, disorders of the uterus, menstrual irregularities,
morning sickness in pregnancy (as well as 'the morning vomiting
of drunkards'), diabetes, rickets, rabies, epilepsy, Hodgkins disease,
hallucinations, lymphoma, heart disease ('a valuable adjunct to digitalis'), and snake bite (the famous Tanjore pill, a mix of arsenic and
black pepper, was an anti-venom popular among British forces in
India, and it was rumoured that some fakirs took it as a preventive
measure against cobra strikes). Dr Livingstone himself announced

from the heart of Africa that arsenic seemed to counter the bite of the tsetse fly. Another physician proposed that drops of Fowler's solution might be used actually to *prevent* people from catching scarlet fever, diphtheria, influenza, or just about anything else: 'in arsenic we have ... a perfect prophylactic in most infectious diseases'. That same practitioner—at a date well past Lister's introduction of antiseptic technique into surgery—also expressed certainty that if patients were treated with the drug several days before any major operation, survival rates 'would be even far better than they are now'.[15]

This last opinion drew on a longstanding belief in arsenic as a tonic, a drug that elevated the level of physiological activity in the body (in small doses, it does stimulate circulation and weight gain): as early as 1830, a London physician remarked to a medical society gathering that arsenic patients experienced 'unusual excitement of the system', feeling 'wound up after the manner of a musical instrument overstrung'. The observation was immediately seconded by a colleague who pointed out that the tonic action extended to the reproductive system. It was a sexual stimulant, he explained, a useful fact discovered by accident when he employed the substance to poison flies and 'was struck with the unusual aphrodisiac excitement which it produced amongst them before they died'. At the other emotional extreme, even depression with suicidal tendencies, a *mental* illness, was reported as curable by arsenic. The catalogue of complaints presumed vulnerable to the *Solutio Mineralis* could be continued at some length, but it should already be clear how by the 1880s a doctor could have come to the conclusion that 'if a law were passed compelling physicians to confine themselves to two remedies only in their entire practice, arsenic would be my choice for one, opium for the other'.[16]

Fowler's solution is itself a radical abridgement of the list of medications based on arsenic that was utilized by Victorian physicians.

It was far the most popular item on that list, but practitioners also had recourse to Pearson's solution (potassium arsenate), Donovan's solution (arsenic iodide), Bieto's solution (ammonium arsenate), de Valagin's solution (arsenious acid dissolved in hydrochloric acid), and still other solutions. In the 1840s, arsenic was discovered to be present in the springs at spas such as Bath, where people had long treated multiple ailments by taking the waters. The discovery was not much of a surprise, for many springs built their reputation on being 'chalybeate waters', that is, iron-containing, and arsenic was known to be almost universally present in iron ores. But the discovery of arsenic in the waters did offer a new rationale for the presumed beneficial effects of spa therapy. Nor were arsenic preparations limited to liquids. The oldest dosage form of all—the external application of arsenicals as pastes or salves, favoured by the physicians of antiquity—also continued in use, as a depilatory, and to remove warts and moles. Arsenic was given as pills, inhaled as vapour, taken by enema, and, after the hypodermic syringe was introduced in the 1850s, received by injection. Not even mother's milk was safe from being exploited as a vehicle: a nursing infant affected by eczema, to cite one case, was cured by arsenic given to its healthy mother.[17]

All this respect for the health-promoting powers of arsenic in small doses naturally interfered with physicians' recognition of chronic poisoning from similar levels of exposure in the environment. One practitioner's contribution to the wallpaper debate, for example, was the observation that it was 'quite possible' that people living in green-papered rooms actually profited from the experience: 'the arsenic may act medicinally and be beneficial, and I think I have seen it to be so'. Laymen thought they had seen it be so too. At the height of the investigation into stearine candles in the 1830s, one manufacturer's response to medical criticism was the cheeky remark that he and his fellow entrepreneurs were only following the example of Fowler's solution, their candles being 'a new method of strengthening the stomach by the vapour of that mineral'.[18]

*

The survey of arsenical medications could be continued, but at some point it becomes necessary to stop and ask the question: how could Victorian physicians have been such fools? How could they possibly have believed they were curing epilepsy with drops of Fowler's solution? Or diabetes, which requires insulin? Or rabies, which is invariably fatal in the absence of vaccine injections? Were they mass-hallucinating under the influence of other drugs? Were they all smoking something even stronger than asthma cigarettes?

In truth, they were anything but fools. Yet their evaluations of the effectiveness of arsenic were prejudiced by certain psychological influences, the same influences that led them to suppose bleeding and leeches and calomel and many another useless therapy were valid. These were psychological forces, furthermore, that had distorted the therapeutic judgements of physicians throughout history and which practitioners today have not entirely escaped.

Prior to the establishment of the germ theory in the 1880s, doctors had no understanding of the causes of most of the serious ailments they had to treat. They thus had no sound guide to what they should be trying to accomplish with drugs in order to achieve a cure. Rather than looking for compounds that would kill or inhibit the growth of micro-organisms, they had to fall back on interpretations of illness formulated on the basis of bedside observations of patients and the course of their diseases, with little assistance from laboratory science. Over the centuries up to the 1800s, any number of theories had been set forth as explanations of pathological changes underlying sickness, but while these differed greatly from one another in terms of details, they were fundamentally of a piece. Since the time of Hippocrates, disease had been character-ized as a dynamic process in which the body released evidence of internal alterations in the form of external evacuations. The sick person vomited, had diarrhoea, excreted more urine than normal, generated more phlegm, sweated heavily, and/or exuded pus. The composition of the body changed with illness, causing the balance between individual components to shift away from the normal state. If the equilibrium that existed in health disintegrated, the object of treatment must be to restore the physiological harmony that had been disrupted.

The restoration of integrity rested on what today we would call a holistic interpretation, an analysis of illness on the basis of each person's age, sex, constitution, environment, living habits, life stresses, and 'diathesis' (or innate tendency towards particular types of illness). The ability to thoroughly analyse how a person was affected by the interaction of all those factors was a main constitu-ent of medical wisdom, and one might expect that prescriptions for treatment would therefore have been as varied as the people for whom they were designed. But if the explanation for physi-ological disequilibrium was unique for each patient, the effects of sickness were in great measure the same, the disordered excretions that flowed from the invalid's body and betokened internal disar-ray. Thus treatment ended up being much the same for everyone, the administration of drugs that produced manifest alterations in excretions or other bodily functions and that could be visualized as exerting an impact on the system that might jar it back in the direc-tion of balance. The specific drugs and combinations that might be prescribed would vary from one patient to the next according to the individual physician's preferences and experiences, but in the end just about everyone could count on receiving medication that made him vomit or defecate or sweat or that produced sensations (stimulation, nausea, decrease of pain, drowsiness) that signalled the inner economy was being altered.

It is easy to understand how a frightened and medically unenlightened patient could conclude that the drug producing those effects was doing him good. But how does one account for physicians coming to the same conclusion? Doctors' readiness to credit their treatments as effective is rooted in three Latin phrases: *vis medicatrix naturae, placebo,* and *post hoc, ergo propter hoc.* The concept of *vis medicatrix naturae,* the healing power of nature, had been used since antiquity to explain why most people who got sick eventually got better, whether ministered to by a doctor or not. Even in epidemics of Asiatic cholera, half the people infected recovered. Hippocrates had been the first to call attention to the fact that the body did not passively yield to the assaults of illness, but struggled to restore itself to normalcy. And although they knew none of the details of the functioning of the immune system or other physiological processes involved in recovery before the very end of the century, Victorian physicians recognized that there were innate curative mechanisms in the body and often interpreted their therapies as methods of stimulating and supporting the action of the *vis medicatrix.* 'Boast as doctors often will of *their* cures,' a mid-century American physician remarked, 'this *vis medicatrix naturae* is the chief doctor after all.'[19]

Yet the fact that doctors administered their cures anyway further increased a patient's chances of improvement, for being told by a physician that this pill or that mineral solution was active medicine aroused the placebo response. Derived from the Latin for 'to please', the placebo response is a positive physiological reaction to any item perceived by the patient as medication, no matter how pharmaceutically inert it may in fact be. Victorian physicians were aware that placebo reactions occurred, and even prescribed placebos (bread pills, flavoured water, and similar 'drugs') to 'amuse people who are morbid on the subject of health'. People could be 'cheated into a feeling of health by globules', doctors laughed, and patients given only 'a teaspoon-ful of—nothing—will actually thank you for saving their lives'. Physicians ridiculed such gullibility, yet failed to see that most of the drugs *they* believed to be genuinely active were also simply nothing. Indeed, prior to the twentieth century, the most potent remedy physicians of any era had in their arsenal was the placebo.[20]

Since doctors were familiar with the placebo effect and the power of the *vis medicatrix*, we might think they would have realized that through those two forces many patients who got better did so on their own, with no help from the therapy and often in spite of it. But instead, their thinking was shaped by the third Latin term, *post hoc, ergo propter hoc*: after this, therefore because of this. The phrase is used by logicians to identify a particular fallacy of reasoning, the supposition that because event B occurs soon after event A, B must be caused by A. In most circumstances, the illogic is obvious—not many people believe that 'cock-a-doodle-doo' makes the sun come up. But the interaction between patient and physician is no ordinary circumstance. One desperately wants help, the other strongly desires to provide it, and both hope the prescribed drug or procedure will work. Unlike the situation with the rooster and the sun, there is a plausible connection between treatment and recovery, so if the patient does indeed get better, the drug will surely be given the credit (if not, it will be because the disease was too strong or treatment was started too late, not because the drug was inert).

There are a number of glaring instances of *post hoc* thinking with respect to arsenic in nineteenth-century medical literature.

An old woman confined to her chair by rheumatism had a quarrel with her servant girl...the girl struck back by putting arsenic in the woman's tea...the woman drank only a little before getting sick...after recovering from the poison she found her rheumatism was relieved...the accidental arsenic apparently had cured her. An 'excessively backward [and] very unsociable' 2-year-old, incontinent of urine and faeces, got into some rat poison. He lingered near death for a week, but pulled through, and once over the attack 'his dirty propensities ceased, he easily learned new words, and was ready to make friends with anybody'. 'Beneficial effects following arsenic poisoning' was the title given the report in *The Lancet*.[21]

Today we eliminate *post hoc* reasoning by subjecting new drugs to clinical trials in which large numbers of patients are given either the proposed drug or an inert substitute, with neither patients nor physicians knowing who is receiving which. Only if a significant advantage is found for drug patients over placebo patients will the medication be presumed therapeutic. There was some attempt at such statistical comparisons by the 1830s, but study methods were crude by modern standards, and in any event were applied to only a handful of drugs and procedures. The placebo-controlled, double-blind trial would not become normative until well into the twentieth century. Victorian physicians, for the most part, drew conclusions on the basis of small numbers of patients, the ones that they personally treated. Each doctor formed an impression of the efficacy of a drug from the results he obtained with his own patients, results often biased by the tendency to remember cases with positive outcomes more clearly than those with negative ones: a fourth Latin phrase figures in here, *per enumerationem simplicem*, or counting only the favourable cases. Journal articles reporting successes with a remedy usually presented fewer than ten cases, often only three or four, to substantiate therapeutic claims. If several other physicians came up with similar results, agreement would form that the treatment truly was useful. Critics sometimes reproved colleagues for the error of generalizing from too few cases (had this only been 'duly appreciated by the profession, how much less should we now have to *unlearn!*'), but they were not listened to. It's not surprising, then, that all sorts of pharmaceutically negligible substances—not just arsenic—ended up on the register of potent medications. At a time when there was no effective treatment for epilepsy, for example, a Scottish physician could aver that 'antiepileptics abound'.[22]

To this point, a somewhat one-sided account of the medicinal use of arsenic has been presented. As it turned out, not all physicians became disciples of Fowler. The Stafford physician's observation that some might find it hard to believe so violent a poison was also a medicine was a prescient one. More than a few practitioners did question both the efficacy and the safety of the remedy, Orfila, for one, protesting that even if used with 'extreme precaution', arsenic would produce 'alarming symptoms'. This was in 1820. By 1840, the sentiment had become widely shared, and not just with respect to arsenic, but for medications in general. During the 1830s, there took place a revolt against the traditional therapeutics based on bleeding and harsh evacuative drugs. There was a deep philosophical basis for the reaction that it is unnecessary to delve into here. For present purposes it's enough to know that an attitude of therapeutic scepticism took hold among a portion of the profession, an attitude that combined a suspicion that most drugs were ineffective and many dangerous, with a belief in placing greater reliance on allowing the body to heal itself. 'The nature-trusting heresy', America's Oliver Wendell Holmes dubbed this orientation, and lay observers joked that while old-style physicians were still killing their patients, the new breed were just letting them die. The joke greatly oversimplifies the situation, for therapeutic sceptics hardly abandoned therapy altogether: they were physicians, they were impelled to do something more than hold the patient's hand and spoon chicken soup into his mouth. Rather, they steered a more moderate course, seeking a middle path between the extremes of nihilism implied in the joke and of heroic interventions that had ruled for centuries. Even Holmes, who courted professional censure with his remark that if most of the drugs then in use were to be thrown into the sea, 'it would be all the better for mankind—and all the worse for the fishes', continued to employ most of the traditional therapies. He and other nature-trusting heretics simply cut back on doses and gave relatively more play to the *vis medicatrix naturae*.[23]

Given that environment of scepticism, along with arsenic's reputation for deadliness, it is not surprising to hear from doctors in the 1840s that 'a very large section of the profession repudiate [arsenic] altogether', hurling 'invectives against the temerity and recklessness' of the doctors who did prescribe it; 'no medicine has met with so much prejudice as arsenic', with the result that there was 'a tendency to saddle it with all conceivable consequences'. A physician who confided that he regarded Fowler's solution as invaluable, and 'would sacrifice nine-tenths of the *Materia Medica* for arsenic', quickly added that he stated such convictions '*privately*, for the prejudice against it is very strong'. A colleague backed him up, saying he was acquainted with several practitioners who prescribed arsenic freely 'but who dare not avow it'. Yet while calomel and tartar emetic and other drugs that Holmes proposed dumping into the ocean did steadily decline in popularity during the second half of the century, Fowler's solution somehow held its ground, even rallied. Towards the end of the 1850s, a Scottish physician took note that 'much of the dread and apprehension of its [arsenic's] poisonous effects...have happily been overcome'.[24]

How the dread and apprehension were overcome is not easy to fathom, for arsenic's potency was exhibited chiefly in the production of side effects. Some of these have already been encountered in case records from Fowler's *Medical Reports*, and the catalogue would be extended considerably by others. But as a hardworking therapeutic mule, arsenic could not be dispensed with merely because some disagreeable reactions followed its use. The trick was to manage the dosage so as to minimize the reactions, a task to which Fowler himself devoted a goodly amount of time and thought. With experience, he came to the conclusion that eight to twelve drops of the solution was the effective dose (for adults; for children, three to five drops sufficed). Doses were to be taken twice a day, raised to three times if the illness put up a fight. An average dose of ten drops contained 0.06 grains of arsenic. Thus a person on a thrice-daily schedule would swallow close to a fifth of a grain of the drug each day, not nearly enough to cause acute poisoning, but clearly enough to provoke toxic reactions in many patients over the course of the one- to two-week treatment period Fowler considered necessary. His *Reports* reveals a physician taking great pains to closely monitor each of his patients, lowering or even stopping the doses temporarily when negative signs appeared. Yet even with those precautions, two-thirds of his subjects, he estimated, suffered undesirable effects.[25]

Doctors would wrestle with dosage regulation through the entire nineteenth century. Some were profligate, one practitioner from the Midlands, for example, bombarding children with twenty-five drops of Fowler's solution at a time. The great majority of physicians, however, recognized such doses as excessive, 'a powerful steam-engine without a safety-valve!' as one called it. 'Let us use the medicine,' he argued, 'but use it discreetly,' so as not to bring about 'the destruction of our fellow-creatures!'[26]

In order to use the drug discreetly, it was essential for the doctor to familiarize himself with the early signs of its toxic action. It is no less essential for readers to be familiar with the signs as well, at least if they wish to appreciate fully the discomforts that Fowler's-treated patients were made to undergo. 'I never knew a patient become fond of arsenic,' wrote a London physician. Reflecting on his long experience administering the drug, he recalled that 'many a patient' had begged, 'please don't order me arsenic, for it always makes me feel so ill'. Those who were ordered the drug were 'without exception glad to leave it off, and always experience improvement in general health when they do'.[27]

Who would not be glad to leave off a medicine that produced burning of the eyes, tender, swollen gums, coated tongue, and skin rash? It was nevertheless deemed necessary to continue dosing until these signs of 'its peculiar action on the system' manifested themselves: 'hot-eye' was generally accepted as the signal that the dosage should be cut back or the intervals between doses lengthened. The physician had to constantly juggle to keep benefits greater than injuries: arsenic 'requires nice management, else it will not only fail, but may do mischief'. Keeping the drug in check included never prescribing it for nursing mothers, for their babies could be poisoned by their milk.[28]

The therapeutic juggling act was complicated by the fact that patients varied over a broad range in their individual susceptibility to the medication. The skin rash was often succeeded by a dirty coloration of the complexion that could take the form of 'the colouring one sees among Arabs' in one case, or of 'a boiled lobster appearance' in another. A man given arsenic for a skin condition soon acquired pigmentation so dark as to prompt his physician to diagnose Addison's disease (an endocrine condition that produces bronze pigmentation)—and to prescribe more Fowler's for treating that. Only after six months and repeated bouts of abdominal pain for his patient did the doctor come to realize that his case of Addison's was actually a case of arsenic poisoning. Arsenic was stopped, and the man's skin slowly returned to normal.[29]

A form of individual susceptibility that was especially serious was the tendency of some patients to develop peripheral neuritis, painful inflammation of the nerves of the arms and legs. Cases of neuritis from fabrics and wallpapers have been met with in previous chapters, and they seem to have been just as common an occurrence among people treated with Fowler's solution (odds are, in fact, that more than a few unfortunates were taking arsenical medication while living in houses with green curtains and green wallpaper). The case of a 12-year-old girl who was 'cured' of chorea with Fowler's solution is representative. Within a fortnight of her cure, she began to experience weakness and painful tingling in her legs. Within another week, an even more distressing aspect of peripheral neuritis appeared, paralysis of the muscles below her knees, resulting in 'ankle drop', drooping, unresponsive feet. Other patients had wrist drop, some incurred drop in all four joints. As a rule, months were required for return to normal after quitting the medication.[30]

Physicians ascribed a plethora of other side effects to arsenical medication. Among them were swelling of the legs (one patient's extremities puffed up so badly in the evenings 'as to hang over his shoes'), impotence ('sexual desire greatly diminished, with almost impossible penile erection'), weakened voice ('particularly in singing, with a constant tendency to crack'), and lowered powers of concentration and memory. Karl Marx stopped taking arsenic because it 'dulls my mind too much, and I needed to keep my wits about me'.[31]

Not least among such untoward effects must have been the dyspepsia complained of by so many Victorians. Dyspepsia was just

a fancy way of saying indigestion, but it was interpreted at the
time as a wide-reaching condition that could include such diverse
symptoms as nausea, vomiting, flatulence, diarrhoea, insomnia,
headache, numbness of the extremities, anxiety, and depression.
As vague as any malaise could be, dyspepsia was an almost irresistible label for people to apply to whatever mysterious thing was
ailing them. Those pursuing the life of the mind seem to have
been especially prone to the complaint: Huxley, Spencer, Carlyle,
George Eliot, and Robert Browning were just a few of the intel-
lectuals tortured by dyspeptic attacks. But the symptoms of dyspepsia were such a close match with the effects of arsenic, and
so many sick people were treated with arsenic, that a persuasive
argument can be made that many dyspeptics were in fact the victims of arsenical medication. Possibly the most pre-eminent such
case was Darwin. The naturalist's nearly lifelong poor health has
been variously diagnosed as a physical problem (malaria, ulcer,
gout, even lingering effects from seasickness experienced on the
Beagle voyages) or a psychological one (hypochondria stemming
from resentment of a domineering father). Darwin's symptoms,
however, duplicated many of those connected to Fowler's solution
(right down to the 'brown out-of-doors complexion' described by
his daughter even after he ceased spending time outdoors), and he
began taking arsenic to treat eczema as early as his university days.
Thus, as John Winslow has proposed, *Darwin's Victorian Malady*, his
dyspepsia, may well have been a case of 'Fowler's disease'.[32]

*

It might seem there could be nothing else to add to the index of
Fowler's solution side effects. But there was, in fact, something
much worse than dyspepsia or neuritis: cancer. In the 1820s, a
London practitioner had suggested that cancer of the scrotum was
caused by the arsenic to which smelter workers were exposed, but

his evidence was not conclusive and no strong arsenic–cancer link would be forged until near the end of the century. In 1887, surgeon Jonathan Hutchinson presented several cases at a meeting of the Pathological Society of London that indicated epithelial (skin) cancer could develop in patients who were treated with Fowler's solution over a period of time. One was that of an American physician given arsenic for psoriasis. After fourteen years of treatment, small tumours appeared on his palms and soles, and then a tumour beneath the skin on his left hand, which eventually broke through to form a raw ulcer. All the growths were excised and determined to be cancerous. The man travelled to London and Vienna for treatment, in the end having both hands amputated, but he nevertheless died a year and a half later; nodules of epithelial cancer were found in his ribs, lungs, and other parts of the body. Discussion following Hutchinson's talk was divided over whether the five cases he had presented demonstrated a true connection between arsenic and cancer or not, but soon reports of skin cancer following arsenic therapy began to be published by other physicians and opposition to the idea steadily gave way. By the mid-twentieth century, it would be accepted that arsenical medication often generates wart-like growths on the skin—keratoses—that may eventually, even several decades later, develop into epithelial cancer (cases of skin cancer induced by Fowler's solution would in fact continue to be reported into the 1950s). In subsequent years, it would be recognized that repeated ingestion of arsenic could engender cancer of the lungs, bladder, and other organs.[33]

There is a sad irony in the discovery that medicinal arsenic can cause cancer because arsenic had for centuries been one of the chief measures for *treating* cancer. The disease itself has been around since the days of dinosaurs, whose skeletal remains show evidence of cancerous growths. Tumours have been discovered in the mummies of ancient Egypt, and by the fourth century BC the disease had acquired its name, Hippocrates calling it *karcinos*, or crab (breast cancers sometimes resemble crabs, having a large central mass with outward-stretching tendrils). Our words carcinoma and carcinogen derive from the Greek name, obviously, while cancer itself is the Latin word for crab.[34]

That ancient pedigree notwithstanding, cancer could be detected to only a very limited extent before the middle of the nineteenth century. There was no way of looking deep inside the body of a living person until the discovery of X rays in the 1890s, so only those cancers that were visible, or broke through to the surface, or produced palpable swelling caught physicians' attention (tumours were often found after death, of course, once autopsies became common in the 1700s). Consequently, medical awareness of the disease was dominated by skin and bone tumours, cervical cancer, and breast cancer, in which tumours ulcerated, eating through tissue to the skin and releasing a foul-smelling discharge. Until the emergence of histology in the 1850s, furthermore, there was no ability to distinguish reliably between tumours as malignant or benign on the basis of their cellular make-up, so physicians erred on the side of caution, supposing any unusual growth was probably cancerous. In the 1830s, for example, a London practitioner confidently reported the cure of 'incipient cancer' in both breasts of a middle-aged woman: his treatment consisted of the administration of Donovan's solution (arsenic iodide) and the application of leeches to the breasts.[35]

Whether truly malignant or only presumed so, a tumour was most effectively dealt with by surgical excision. Even breast cancers had been cut away since ancient times, albeit by the somewhat crude method of simply amputating the breast and controlling bleeding by burning vessels shut with a hot iron. By the nineteenth century, both surgical technique and methods of haemorrhage control had been refined considerably, but until the introduction of ether anaesthesia in 1846 mastectomy remained a horrifically painful ordeal (the most harrowing first-person account of pre-anaesthesia surgery of which I'm aware is that of a mastectomy endured by the English belletrist Fanny Burney in 1811. I read her account every year in a course on the history of medicine and to date have had three students faint; her story is made even more upsetting by the fact that her tumour was in all likelihood benign). Surgery also involved a high risk of infection, until the 1870s at least, so any less traumatic way of removing a tumour was welcome.[36]

A few physicians reported success treating cancer with Fowler's or other arsenical solutions. Some attacked tumours of the cervix with vaginal douches comprised of arsenic with other drugs (opium and hemlock were popular additions). But the strongest faith was placed in erosion of cancerous growths. Arsenic is an escharotic, a caustic material that burns flesh away. That action, furthermore, is even more pronounced on quick-growing tissue such as tumours. Consequently, as early as the 1500s arsenic salves of diverse composition were being applied to skin growths and to breast malignancies that had ulcerated. During the 1700s, a Frenchman who adopted the name Frère Côme popularized a mixture of arsenic with several other ingredients that became widely adopted as Frère Côme's paste. The paste was a compound of arsenious acid, cinnabar (red mercuric sulphide), burnt juniper, and dragon's blood (an Oriental plant resin, not quite so difficult to come by as the name would suggest), and was held in esteem by physicians and surgeons throughout Europe.[37]

Although Frère Côme's preparation did often destroy the visible tumour, it had no effect on metastases and must have regularly failed to achieve a permanent cure. Consequently, much tinkering was done with the formula, in terms of both ingredients and proportions, until by the early 1800s there were a number of combinations identified individually by their creators (Hunter's caustic, Rousselot's powder, Dupuytren's caustic powder) and referred to collectively as the *pâte arsenicale*, or arsenical paste. If applied by expert hands, we are told, the *pâte* 'separates the mass from the surrounding parts, in the same manner...as a nut comes out of the shell; or, as if it had been cleanly dissected by the knife'. The many reports of success with arsenic, however, have to be greeted sceptically, for, as explained above, the frequency of misdiagnosis must have led to the 'cure' of many growths that were harmless.[38]

In Britain, the most highly regarded preparation was Marsden's mucilage, developed by William Marsden, surgeon and founder of a cancer hospital in London (now the Royal Marsden Hospital). Made by combining white arsenic and powdered gum arabic with sufficient water to form a paste, the mucilage was painted onto the surface of the tumour to cover roughly a square inch. As tissue was destroyed, it was made to slough off with the aid of a bread-and-water poultice. A new application of the mucilage was then made, and the process repeated, often over the course of several weeks, until the growth was completely erased. 'By this mode of treatment,' Marsden asserted, he could 'arrest and even destroy a cancerous action' so decisively that he had 'not yet seen a single instance of the disease returning in any of the cases thus treated'. Figure 6 is an engraving taken from before and after photographs of a patient treated for cancer of the lip by Marsden. Three and a half years after the treatment, there had been no recurrence of the disease.[39]

Marsden's and other arsenical pastes could not have accomplished cures very often, and physicians sometimes admitted that all arsenic could do was slow the progress of the disease. Even

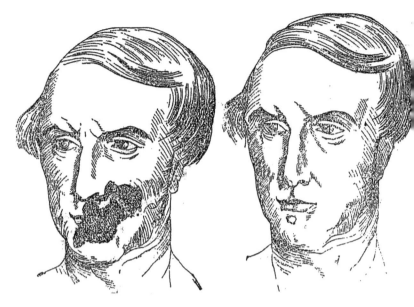

6. Before and after treatment of lip cancer with Marsden's mucilage

then, there was consolation in having a medicine 'that can, when death is inevitable, strew flowers on the borders of the tomb'. But extended quantity of life came at the cost of lowered quality, as arsenical treatment caused sharp, burning pain in the area of the tumour, and it was not uncommon for acute poisoning to ensue. In the 1830s, a supposed breast cancer patient died with 'vomiting and violent colic . . . great suffering' only two days after application of the *pâte arsenicale*. Cancer patients were also subject to all aspects of chronic intoxication, for the disease was just as eagerly treated with Fowler's solution and other forms of internal administration (after the development of the hypodermic syringe, arsenic solutions were sometimes injected directly into the tumour).[40]

To hear doctors tell it, the cancer patients who truly suffered were those who put themselves into the hands of cancer quacks. Of these, there seems to have been no shortage. 'Charlatanism', a Scottish practitioner lamented early in the century, 'still marches through the land, making woeful havoc, and bringing, if not immediate death, inevitable destruction to the health of thousands of deluded victims annually.' To be sure, charlatans promised relief from all manner of ailments, but then as today dread of cancer was particularly likely to drive people to seek help in dubious places. The 'cancer-doctors' relied primarily on arsenical pastes much like those employed by physicians, but, in the eyes of professionals, were criminally negligent in their application. Hertfordshire's Mr Chamberlain, who misleadingly billed himself as a 'herbalist', and Mrs Warren, the Irish 'Cancer Curer', were just two of the more notable lay healers who were tried for manslaughter after their arsenical treatments went amiss (both were convicted, but in the latter's case reluctantly, the jury foreman appending to the verdict the statement that 'but for her a great many people would be in their graves').[41]

There were also a half-hundred or more patent medicines containing arsenic. The Sale of Arsenic Act of 1851 placed no restrictions on medicinal preparations of the poison, so brands such as Arsenauro, Aiken's Tonic Pills, and Gross's Neuralgia Pills were freely marketed for those preferring self-treatment and could make their own woeful havoc (Fowler had warned when announcing his solution that making it directly available to the general public 'is to put a two-edged Sword into the Hands of the Ignorant'). Those stricken by the wrong edge of the sword included the man who was poisoned by using an arsenical hair-restorer on his scalp and the 9-year-old girl who was killed by a patent arsenic powder her stepmother applied to treat the child's ringworm. One man died merely from using a can that had previously held an arsenic patent medicine as a beer mug. Finally, whether Arsenauro or Fowler's solution, patent medicine or professional remedy, arsenical medications should not have been left within the reach of children. But, inevitably, they were, and young ones unwittingly sickened and killed themselves as readily with medicine as with rat poison.[42]

Even foetuses were killed by arsenic preparations, it being common knowledge that the poison was an effective abortifacient. Some women took patent abortion pills containing arsenic, some turned to standard medicinal preparations, many resorted to the plain white arsenic of the shops, administering it orally and/or vaginally. Whichever measure was taken, the result was usually the poisoning, if not the death, of the woman as well as the foetus. People were at risk as well from non-arsenical remedies that had been contaminated with the poison during manufacture, including such common medicinals as sodium bicarbonate, Epsom salt, Glauber's salt, glycerine, and preparations of iron and bismuth. Impurities could get into medicines as well from coloured arsenical paper used to cap remedy bottles.[43]

And then there was dentistry. Even today, with high-speed drills and potent local anaesthetics the norm, the prospect of a visit to the dentist strikes fear into the hearts of millions. In the nineteenth century, a dental appointment truly was an ordeal, and not just because of slow, hand-operated drills and non-existent or unreliable anaesthetics. During the 1840s, it became popular in dental practice to attempt to relieve pain in decayed or abscessed teeth by destroying the dental pulp, the soft material inside the tooth that contains blood vessels and nerves. It made sense that if nerves were cauterized, they should stop hurting; and what better to choose for a cauterizing agent than arsenic? If it could eat away a cancerous tumour, a little bit of tooth pulp should pose no difficulty at all, so by 1850 it was standard practice among dentists to apply to painful pulp a mixture of creosote, morphine, and arsenic. The creosote was the vehicle, used to create a thick paste, while the morphine was intended to dull the pain of the arsenic's attack on the pulp. Once the tooth's nerves were dead, they could be removed and the tooth filled (or 'stopped', in the terminology of the day). In theory, it was a simple yet efficacious way to save a tooth from extraction.[44]

In practice, the procedure worked well for some patients, not so well for others. The morphine was not always adequate to suppress the discomfort of arsenic's action fully. Some of the arsenic could escape into the mouth, be swallowed, and produce the usual poisoning symptoms. Worst of all, the caustic action of the arsenic did not always stop with the pulp, but penetrated down into the alveolus, or socket of the tooth. The resultant inflammation was attended by an 'increase of pain to a frightful and almost unbearable extent' and eventual loss of the tooth as the socket was destroyed. A sample case of pulp destruction gone wrong is that of a woman in whom 'day after day, the pain continued with increasing intensity...the face was much swollen, the alveolus acutely inflamed, and an offensive discharge escaped from the wound'. In the end, after 'two months' intense suffering; and all the necessary medical expenses', the three treated teeth had to be extracted anyway, along with another that had been healthy at the outset. In another case, an officer stationed in India who was given the arsenical paste suffered such pain he had to come home on sick leave. Once there, he lost his upper molars and a sizeable portion of his upper jawbone. As British dentists slowly turned against the practice ('It played me ugly tricks...In fact, I have no hesitation in writing, it is bad'), they sometimes shifted the blame to their American counterparts, who had introduced the method: Yankee practitioners, it was well known, were keen on 'violent remedies', so the profession should give careful scrutiny to any treatments 'said to be American'.[45]

Medical science underwent extraordinary progress in the late nineteenth and early twentieth centuries, fostering a burst of new and more effective remedies that culminated in the sulpha drugs in the 1930s and antibiotics in the 1940s. The onslaught of 'wonder drugs' swept away nearly all the therapeutic standbys of the nineteenth century, Fowler's solution included: the preparation disappeared from Britain's *Pharmacopoeia* after the 1952 edition (and from America's five years earlier). That did not mean an immediate end to the use of the solution. While it had long ceased to be looked upon as a near-panacea, it had continued in use against psoriasis through the first half of the twentieth century. As late as the 1950s, dermatologists had to be scolded for having fallen into a 'habit' of resorting to Fowler's solution whenever 'one is at one's wit's end in a resistant skin case'.[46]

It was also during the 1950s that Fowler's solution made a brief comeback in the treatment of asthma, albeit in disguise as a remedy called Gay's solution. Gay was a Mississippi practitioner who achieved striking results in asthma patients using Fowler's solution combined with other drugs. His solution was warmly adopted at first as preferable to steroid therapy in difficult cases. Before long, however, it came under attack as too great a risk for producing skin cancer and quickly fell from favour (the same objection was being raised against the use of Fowler's solution in psoriasis). The basic component of Fowler's solution, arsenic trioxide, was employed through much of the twentieth century in the treatment of some forms of leukaemia, and other arsenicals are still utilized against trypanosomiasis, or sleeping sickness (so Dr Livingston was correct in asserting that arsenic protected from the bite of the tsetse).

A number of organic arsenic compounds also came into broad use in the 1900s, most notably arsphenamine, a cure for syphilis introduced in 1910 and the first of the century's wonder drugs. But, as an American physician has recently put it, compared to the 'grand therapeutic station' held by arsenic throughout the nineteenth century, 'the magic is gone'. Given its record in the 1800s, one can only add 'good riddance!'[47]

10

'A Very Wholesome Poison'

The 1857 murder trial of Madeleine Smith was reckoned by all to be 'the most exciting and interesting trial which has occurred during this century' in Scotland. Certainly it had all the ingredients of intrigue and scandal anyone could want: an intense but doomed love affair between an attractive young woman of social standing and an older man of foreign ancestry and low station; a slow, undignified, and painful death; a mix of circumstantial evidence that pointed in some instances to the guilt of the accused, in others to her innocence; and a verdict that seemed up for grabs down to the moment it was delivered, and that even then was frustratingly inconclusive. The only thing needed to complete the drama was erotically charged *billets-doux* between the lovers. The trial had that as well, a veritable slew of love letters, in fact, letters bursting with— as one who read them shuddered—'disgusting details'. 'I pray God I may never see such again,' a journalist reporting on the proceedings told readers; 'Ugh!' How could it *not* have been the trial of the century? Yet it was more than that, for the trial also served to publicize still another way by which people might unintentionally poison themselves with arsenic.[1]

The daughter of a prominent Glasgow architect, Madeleine Smith was only 19 when she met Pierre Émile L'Angelier, twelve years her senior. The son of French immigrants to Jersey, Émile, as he liked to be called, had been working as a warehouse clerk in Glasgow for several years when he was smitten at the sight of the lovely Madeleine strolling down Sauchiehall Street, the city's fashionable promenade, one day in the late winter of 1855. A veteran of romantic dalliances, Émile was able to charm his way into her affections by spring. By summer, she was writing letters to 'Dear, Dear Émile' ('I love you with all my heart and soul'), and meeting him for midnight trysts in the woods bordering the family country home. By fall, they were secretly engaged and fantasizing about being wed the next year, and already calling one another 'husband' and 'wife' in their correspondence.[2]

The engagement was secret because Madeleine's father, who had learned of the relationship early on, forbade her to continue seeing a mere clerk: 'he hates you with all his heart', Madeleine confided in one letter to Émile, and, in another, 'Papa would rather see me in my grave than your wife.' Mr Smith wanted to see her the wife of William Minnoch, a Glasgow native and family friend with a solid business position and bright prospects, and eventually the daughter would come around to Papa's way of thinking. But in the interim, for more than a year and a half, she would write to Émile almost daily, gushing out declarations of love and devotion and swearing, prophetically, that 'only death shall break [our] engagement'. She would regularly summon him to wee-hour whisperings through the bars of the street-level window of her Glasgow bedroom, on occasion even sneaking him into the house to partake of 'the pleasure ... of being fondled by you, dear, dear Émile'. At last, on the sixth of June 1856, in the darkened wood by the country home, afire with passion (even though Émile, coughing and sneezing with a cold, could hardly have been irresistible), she surrendered her virtue. Within hours, at five the next morning, Madeleine was back at her writing desk, asking 'were you angry at me for allowing you to do what you did? Was it very bad of me?' Yes, he replied, what she had allowed was very bad indeed: 'Why, Mimi [her pet name], did you give way after your promises' (of saving herself for their marriage)? 'You had no resolution,' he scolded (and on top of that, the experience 'did my cold no good'). He, fortunately, did have resolution: 'I will never again repeat what I did until we are regularly married,' he vowed. The very next month, he repeated what he had done—more than once.

There was something else about Mimi that was as troubling as her feeble willpower. In her post-defloration letter, she had flatteringly told him of 'a good deal of pain during the night', but had confessed as well that 'I did not bleed in the least.' 'My pet,' Émile wrote back, 'I do not understand ... your not bleeding. For every woman having her virginity must bleed.' He tried to salve his wounded ego by telling Madeleine 'you must have done so [bled] some other time'—perhaps she had somehow injured herself bathing. But misgivings about the purity of his 'dearest and beloved wife' were minor compared to the ones he was feeling about William Minnoch. All the while that Madeleine was professing her undying devotion, reports were coming to Émile that Minnoch frequently visited the Smith household, and accompanied Madeleine on walks and to concerts and the opera (the latter, by improbable coincidence, was Donizetti's *Lucretia Borgia*). His Mimi did little to assuage the worry, referring to Minnoch in her letters as 'pleasant' and 'most agreeable ... I like him very much better than I used to do.' She even took to referring to him as Billy. Yet she repeatedly denied the rumours Émile had heard that she was contemplating marriage with Billy, assuring him that she would ever have but one love. After an evening of sweet-talk at her window in late January 1857, Madeleine wrote, 'Émile, what would I not give at this moment to be your fond wife,' then added teasingly that 'my nightdress was on when you saw me. Would to God you had been in the same attire.' Less than a week later she accepted William Minnoch's proposal of marriage. Five days after, she informed her erstwhile 'husband' they must henceforth 'consider ourselves as strangers...my love for you has ceased.' Madeleine had had her youthful fling; now it was time to settle down.

Émile responded exactly as one would expect, letting Madeleine know he had kept all her letters and would hand them over to her father if she persisted in her commitment to Minnoch. 'Will you, for Christ's sake, not denounce me,' she begged in reply. 'I shall be undone. I shall be ruined.' She pleaded with him to return the letters to her, or to destroy them, wailing that if he should 'denounce me to Papa [he] would kill me'. In a postscript, Madeleine asked Émile to come to her window at midnight.

He did come to see her again, but without the letters. Not much more than a week later, Madeleine bought sixpence-worth of arsenic, telling the chemist it was to be used to kill rats. The next morning, Émile suffered an attack of vomiting and abdominal pain that incapacitated him for a week and left him sickly the rest of his abbreviated life. A month later, he received his last letter, an invitation to another evening at the window. He accepted—and before noon the next day he was dead.

An autopsy was performed, revealing an inflamed stomach and a great deal of arsenic in its contents. At the same time, all those letters that Émile had saved had been discovered by the police, and subsequently the poison registers of the city's druggists were examined. When three purchases of arsenic were found associated with the name Madeleine Smith, it seemed obvious that L'Angelier had been murdered by his mistress to stop him from exposing her to her family and fiancé. Madeleine was arrested on 31 March. Her engagement to William Minnoch was broken off, and the two would never speak with one another again.

The trial of Madeleine Hamilton Smith was held in Edinburgh beginning on 30 June 1857 and running until 8 July. Each day, a largely sympathetic crowd gathered to see Madeleine brought to the court and, at the end of proceedings, taken back to her cell. Each day, newspapers throughout Britain reported all the details of testimony and argument. There was, to be sure, much to incriminate her, not least her questionable character. An entire day of the trial was devoted to reading all her letters aloud, and even though the more salacious sections were edited out, the abandon with which she expressed her love to Émile, particularly after she had given her hand to another, could not have made a positive impression on the jury. Nor could the prosecuting attorney's references to the 'improper connection' the unmarried woman had enjoyed with her victim more than once, have helped her situation.[3]

In contrast to the profile of licentiousness drawn by the prosecution, however, there was the observed behaviour of the woman at the trial. As a reporter for *The Times* described it, 'She stepped up the stair into the dock with all the buoyancy with which she might have entered the box of a theatre.' Her perfect self-possession might be a sign of extraordinary self-control, of course. But could it not also be explained, *The Times* asked, by 'a proud conscience of innocence?' Madeleine's composure in the face of the gallows was remarked upon widely (she never once was so discomfited as to require smelling salts, one awestruck observer noticed), and jurors were as susceptible as journalists to the impression that such coolness was evidence of a guiltless mind. More solid matters to take into account were the lack of any witnesses to a meeting between

Émile and Madeleine the night he died; hints in Madeleine's letters that Émile was threatening to kill himself, buttressed by the statement of a friend of L'Angelier's that he had once contemplated suicide over another failed love affair; and, most damning, the discovery of a total of eighty-eight grains of arsenic in the dead man's stomach. Scotland's top toxicologist, Robert Christison, testified that he was not aware of so great a quantity of the poison having ever been found in the stomach of a murder victim. Because of L'Angelier's heavy vomiting, the original dose must have been much greater than eighty-eight grains, and so large an amount, the defence argued, would have been virtually impossible to administer without raising the victim's suspicions. It was, rather, a quantity typical of what suicides usually gave themselves in their determination to ensure the job got done ('it is in cases of suicide that double-shotted pistols are used'). True, no arsenic was found in L'Angelier's possession, nor was there any record in area druggist shops of him buying the poison; but it was, as defence counsel pointed out, not all that difficult to obtain the substance under the table or by pilfering.[4]

There was much for jurors to ponder, and thus a full twenty minutes passed before a verdict was returned. By a vote of thirteen to two (at that time in Scotland, only a majority decision by the fifteen-man jury was required), they had decided that the murder charge was 'not proven', invoking a curious provision in Scottish law that allows an option beyond 'guilty' and 'not guilty'. The so-called 'Scottish verdict' of 'not proven' is a statement by jurors that they find the case for the defendant's guilt short of fully convincing, yet are not entirely persuaded of the prisoner's innocence either (the two dissenters in Madeleine Smith's trial voted 'guilty'). 'Not proven' allows the accused to go free, yet leaves her or him under a cloud of doubt, ever after to be suspected of having been cleared only because not quite enough evidence was turned up. In a Wilkie Collins romance of the 1870s, the union of two newlyweds teeters for more than 300 tedious pages on the husband's shame over a 'not proven' verdict in the arsenic-poisoning death of his first wife; only when wife number two uncovers proof that her predecessor committed suicide is her spouse able to deem himself worthy of her love. As for Madeleine Smith, the room in her Glasgow home where she entertained Émile is today used as solicitors' offices, so there is a chance the stain of 'not proven' may yet be removed from her name.[5]

In Smith's case, the cloud was to be darker than for most. Only months after the jury let her off, in part because of the plausibility of the defence argument that L'Angelier must have committed suicide, Christison reported that he now knew of a case in which even more than eighty-eight grains of arsenic had been found in the stomach of a person who without question had been murdered. In 1842, he had analysed the contents of the stomach of a man killed by arsenic mixed into whisky punch and found thirty grains of the poison, a remarkable enough quantity in itself. But in the aftermath of the Smith trial, the physician who had attended the dead man fifteen years earlier contacted Christison to say he had removed sixty grains of arsenic before handing over the stomach contents to the professor. Thus a total of something more than ninety grains must have been administered without the victim's awareness, a fact that knocked the props out from under the assertion that so much as eighty-eight grains could not have been taken unintentionally. Christison graciously refused to speculate on Smith's guilt or innocence, and indeed the case against her was not proven. Nevertheless...[6]

Another poisoning that came too late to influence the Smith decision was the 1863 murder by Alice Hewitt of her mother. The

Stockport factory worker cleverly secreted the arsenic in pork pies, and no suspicion was aroused until she collected the money on a life insurance policy on her mother that had been activated only the day before the woman died. Mrs Hewitt's body was exhumed, arsenic was detected, and the daughter was tried and sentenced to death. In this instance, the body held no less than 130 grains of the poison—explaining why the corpse was 'found to be undecomposed'.[7]

The Smith verdict was applauded by the crowds in Edinburgh, but in Glasgow the decision was much less popular. To journalists there, she was a 'woman of strong passion and libidinous tendencies' with the power to 'startle and appall us', not a desirable neighbour. To find peace, Madeleine moved to London, where, four years later, she married a man who would rise to the position of business manager for William Morris, the most notable manufacturer of arsenical wallpapers. After her husband died in 1910, she moved to New York City, where she married again. Smith died in 1926, aged 93 and in poverty; a movie biography, *Madeleine*, appeared in 1949.[8]

When the jury had been deliberating in 1857, two final considerations had helped tip the balance towards 'not proven'. In her pre-trial statement to police, Madeleine had confessed that the true purpose of her arsenic purchases was not to poison rats, but rather to improve her complexion. Then during the trial, two of L'Angelier's acquaintances testified that the man had told them he took doses of arsenic 'regularly' for his health. Much was made of these points by defence attorneys, because one provided an innocent excuse for Madeleine to have the poison in her possession, and the other suggested Émile probably had the poison available for suicide. In both instances, however, this personal utilization of arsenic was connected not to medicinal use—Fowler's solution or some related therapeutic agent—but to a distinctly separate source of arsenic employment, a source that added yet another opportunity for people to poison themselves.[9]

*

Only six years before the trial, in 1851, a Vienna medical journal had published an article that set off heated and lengthy debate among scientists over the physiological effects of arsenic. Physician Johann von Tschudi announced there that among the peasantry of the southern Austrian region of Styria it was a common practice habitually to consume quantities of arsenic well above the lethal dose. Further, not only did those who took the poison escape all harm, they positively flourished on it. Users gradually habituated themselves to the substance, beginning with small doses of half a grain or so, taken several times a week, then slowly increased intake until they were swallowing four to eight grains or more with impunity; quantities as high as twenty-three grains would be reported in later studies. Von Tschudi believed that only a minority of the rural population indulged in the custom, but since the practice was generally frowned upon and therefore not freely admitted, it was impossible to know with certainty just how many *Giftesser*, or poison-eaters, there were.[10]

That such a thing could be done was surprising enough. But *why* was it done? Why would anyone risk a deadly dose of the most frightening poison of all? For men, the answer was that it increased energy and endurance. In mountainous Styria, working the soil, herding sheep, and felling trees was more than usually taxing. Yet, the area's residents had discovered, those physical challenges could be easily met simply by taking arsenic: 'the operation is surprising, and they will ascend with facility heights which previously they could climb only with great difficulty in breathing'. Small doses of arsenic are in fact stimulating and accelerate metabolism (in biochemists' terms, the arsenite ion promotes oxidative phosphorylation), so there was a sound empirical basis for the peculiar habit.[11]

Women worked the mountainsides too, of course, and many of them had also adopted the practice. In their case, though, arsenic was taken not so much for stamina as for beauty. A 'spare and pale dairymaid' von Tschudi interviewed had an admirer whom she wished to enchant even more. She took up arsenicophagy, and in just a few months, 'had become stout, rosy-cheeked, and altogether quite to her lover's satisfaction'. Such results for women dovetailed with a second reason men became arsenic-eaters: the habit, they had discovered, produced 'strong sexual desire'. Desire coupled with heightened virility ('the sexual power was increased') and presented with rosy-cheeked maidenhood resulted in an 'inordinate number of illegitimate children' in arsenic-eating regions, as high as 60 per cent of all births, some estimated. A British man who read about the Styrian practice and then adopted it, became '*notorious* for his amorous propensities'—until eventually dying from the poison's effects.[12]

There were yet more attractions to arsenic consumption. It was thought to heighten courage, so poachers, whose line of work involved a good bit of risk, often took it. It was believed to increase resistance to infection, to prevent hangovers, and, not least, to extend life. Most remarkably, physical superiority continued even into the grave. It was the practice in Styria that graveyards, once filled, would be closed for a period of twelve years and then all bodies be removed and taken to a charnel house so the ground could be readied for new tenants. On such occasions, it was easy to tell who had been an arsenic-eater and who had not: the former were so well preserved as to be 'recognizable by their friends'. Their maintenance of human form while lying for years in the coffin was thought by some, in fact, to be the origin of the legend of the vampire. Legend aside, Styrians seemed to demonstrate that, used properly, arsenic could be 'a very wholesome poison'.[13]

The life of an arsenic-eater was not, however, all roses and no risks. The number of victims of too large or too frequent doses, von Tschudi reported, was 'by no means trifling'. The dairymaid who transformed herself from pale and spare to pink and stout, for example, could not leave well enough alone. Hoping to become even more voluptuous, she increased her dose and 'fell a victim to her vanity'. Even survivors were condemned to a sort of living death, for, it was supposed, if a person abandoned the habit, true arsenic poisoning ensued, and he must at once resume the practice or face a grim death. The myth was so compelling as to spawn stories of physicians exploiting the addictive power of arsenic as job insurance, secretly dosing children with it till they had been transformed into 'regular little arsenic-eaters'. Under such a doctor's care, the young patients fared well unless their parents took them to another practitioner. Then the juvenile Styrians, deprived of their life-sustaining drug, at once began to fall off and had to be taken back to the first doctor.[14]

British physicians as a whole dismissed tales of arsenic-eating as myths: 'what a mess of absurdity is here!' Christison scoffed. Had anyone actually seen an arsenic-eater in the act of swallowing the poison? Had anyone determined that what was swallowed was truly arsenic? Von Tschudi apparently had done neither. But through the 1850s and 1860s, others did. It would be demonstrated beyond question that the arsenic-eaters did indeed swallow sizeable amounts of a substance that was in fact arsenic, and that when they did so judiciously they suffered no injury. Eventually, it would be decided that the reason they escaped harm was that they ingested the poison in solid lumps instead of as a powder or in a liquid. The lumps did not dissolve to any significant extent, but rather passed through the digestive tract largely intact. Nevertheless, enough arsenic was absorbed to produce the beneficial effects on skin and weight commonly seen as the initial reaction to small doses. (In the 1850s, French missionaries in China reported that arsenic-*smoking* was common in the north of that country, the smokers enjoying exceptional health: 'their lungs acted like smith's bellows', it was said, and as to complexion, they were 'as red as cherubs. The southern Chinese alone have the yellow colour which is ascribed to the whole race.')[15]

Error is often more influential than fact, and the notion that arsenic-eating is Mother Nature's great beauty secret established itself firmly in popular imagination through the rest of the century. A best-selling popular-science text did much to sell the idea, painting the Styrian peasant girl as a winsome creature of 'blushing cheeks and tempting lips', with a 'winning lustre to her sparkling eye....She triumphs over the affections of all, and compels the chosen one to her feet.' It was hard to imagine a more potent formula for romantic success. Arsenic was 'a love-awakener...the harbinger of happiness, the soother of ardent longings, the bestower of contentment and peace!' Coquetry had a new weapon and, a French author predicted, 'all the known cosmetic preparations will pale beside it'.[16]

Stories began to circulate that in Florence society ladies had been taking arsenical beauty treatments since the 1830s, that in Germany both actresses and prostitutes used arsenic to increase their attractiveness, and that at a girls' school in Switzerland arsenic was given to all pupils for the same reason. Madeleine Smith had learned of the cosmetic use of arsenic during her three-year stint at Mrs Gorton's Academy for Young Ladies near London (she splashed arsenic solution over her skin, she told police), and by 1860,

British women generally were incorporating the practice into their 'esoteric mysteries of the toilet'. By the end of the decade, America's ladies had joined in. Arsenic, a physician disclosed in 1869, accounted for 'nearly all the brilliant complexions seen among the females of New York'. Thanks in particular to the inspiration of a recently emerging 'blonde fashion' among young women, 'arsenic eating has become almost a mania', no longer confined to *demi-mondaines* but common through the whole of society. Such a mania for so infamous a poison naturally stretched Styrian legend still further. When a German experimenter came up with preliminary indications that animals given arsenic expelled the poison in their breath and thereby contaminated neighbouring animals, the door was opened for imagining that arsenic-eaters would slowly destroy family members: 'What a prospect is this for the man whose wife is thus absurdly immolating herself on the altar of vanity!' an American doctor sputtered; 'what danger it intimates for the infant whose nurse shares in this ambition to be beautified'.[17]

Arsenical vapours could also produce fattening effects, it was supposed. In 1899, crewmen aboard a ship carrying 300 casks of arsenic from Britain to Philadelphia noticed that 'they were filling out their clothes to a much greater extent than when they shipped. Many became abnormally stout,' the crew's total weight-gain adding up to nearly 400 pounds by the time they reached port. The explanation offered was that the heat of the sun on the casks in the forecastle generated arsenic vapour that was inhaled by the men; that explained why the captain, whose quarters were far aft, did not add any poundage.[18]

Initially, beautification was pursued through small doses of Fowler's solution, or with arsenical mineral water. But it did not take long for patent medicine manufacturers to perceive the gold that lay buried in arsenic, and to set forth an enticing array of pills and tablets. Dr Simms' Arsenic Complexion Wafers, guaranteed to endow a woman's skin with 'beautiful transparency', was one such preparation. Dr Campbell's Arsenic Complexion Wafers (Fig. 7), a product that promised skin of 'unrivalled purity of texture, free from any spot or blemish whatever', was another. Such claims flew in the face of reality, of course, as Ambrose Bierce observed in his *Devil's Dictionary*: 'Arsenic, n. A kind of cosmetic greatly affected by the ladies, whom it greatly affects in turn.' A lady could, in fact, be affected to the point of death. In 1880, a woman died after taking arsenic to remove 'the spots in her face'.[19]

Arsenic-containing soaps were sold as well. Campbell offered a Medicated Arsenic Soap to supplement his wafers, though one could opt for Dr Mackenzie's or Jameson's soaps instead. None of the products contained much arsenic. The four-tablet daily dose of Campbell's Wafers contained only 0.0008 grain of the poison, and the soaps typically held only a hundredth of a grain

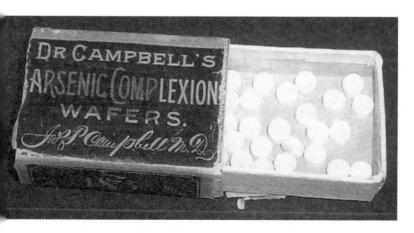

7. Campbell's Arsenic Wafers

per pound. The producer of one such soap admitted that he knew such a small amount had no effect, but included it to satisfy consumer demand. Some manufacturers marketed arsenical soaps that contained absolutely no arsenic at all. These last, interestingly, were the only ones to run afoul of the Sale of Food and Drugs Act, more than one being fined for mislabelling infractions. Finally, arsenic-containing preparations for removing unwanted facial hair were distributed widely.[20]

The ladies were not alone in risking health for vanity. A gentleman who had not seen a certain friend for some months, chanced to meet him on the street and was surprised by his 'blooming complexion, fullness of face, and bright sparkling eye', qualities the man had not previously possessed. His secret, the friend confessed, was arsenic pills. Men were likewise prone to experimenting with arsenical hair-washes advertised as baldness cures. But arsenic's chief appeal for the masculine was the promise of increased energy, endurance, and virility. Testimony at the Smith trial revealed that Émile had been an arsenic-eater, as did the man's appearance when exhumed five days after death for further chemical tests: 'the body was remarkably well-preserved', his physician recorded. This dual exploitation of arsenic-eating by men and women was a windfall for lawyers in cases of alleged spouse-murder, giving rise to what has been called 'the Styrian Defence'. As was done in the Smith case, attorneys could now argue that the deceased had arsenic in his (occasionally her) body because he had been an arsenicophagist, not because he had been murdered. Likewise, the accused had arsenic in her (occasionally his) possession because she was trying to make herself more alluring, not because she had poisoned her husband (husbands had to agree with Bierce: 'Eat arsenic? Yes, all you get, | Consenting, he did speak up; | 'Tis better you should eat it, pet, | Than put it in my teacup').[21]

The Styrian Defence seems to have first been used in Austria, when in 1851 a woman was acquitted of murder through the argument that the victim had been an arsenic-eater (it was this trial that drew von Tschudi into his investigation of the practice). In Britain, a twist on the defence was at least contemplated before Madeleine Smith was brought to trial. Throughout May and June of 1855, Mrs Wooler, a 38-year-old resident of County Durham, slowly declined with symptoms of vomiting, diarrhoea, tingling of extremities, and other signs of slow arsenic poisoning. Arsenic was found in her urine by Christison, and, after her death on 27 June, detected throughout her viscera by Alfred Taylor. Taylor also uncovered traces of arsenic in an enema syringe that had been used by Mr Wooler to administer supposedly nutritive 'injections' to his spouse. As this was, in Christison's phrasing, 'a species of service...very unusual for a non-professional husband to render to his wife', suspicion fell on Mr Wooler, and he was arrested and brought to trial. There it came out that in conversations with his wife's doctors the prisoner had displayed an unusual knowledge of poisons, that he had in his possession a bottle of Fowler's solution, and that the only time in her last weeks Mrs Wooler had been able to hold down her food was the one day her husband had been away. As Wooler's attorneys contemplated arguments they might make for his innocence, some consideration was given to maintaining that the wife had earlier become an arsenic-eater so as to be more attractive to her husband (who, it would seem, was not sufficiently beguiled), that when she realized she had become habituated to the poison she determined to leave it off, and then, in accord with Styrian pharmacology, had died when she stopped taking her arsenic. That line of argument was never advanced in court, nor was the wild hypothesis needed.

Testimony established that the Woolers had been an affection-
ate couple through all their eighteen years of marriage, and that
the husband had shown great tenderness toward his wife in her
final days, looking after her every day except the one on which
she didn't vomit. Swayed by those signs of devotion, the jury
voted for acquittal. Who did put the arsenic into Mrs Wooler's
body remains a mystery.[22]

*

Even if the Styrians were not dragged into the Wooler trial, the
fact that the strategy was considered indicates how quickly lawyers
latched onto the reports coming from Austria as a means of getting
clients off the hook. The defence would become a not infrequent
tactic in trials through the rest of the century (and be employed
even as late as 1937 in another case in Austria). One trial in particular, however, stood out from the rest with respect to notoriety, and
will serve as the best example of how arsenic-eating played into
judicial deliberations.[23]

Florence Chandler was an Alabama girl who in the spring of
1881 met James Maybrick, a Liverpool cotton merchant, on board
the boat taking them to England. She was 18, he was 42, but attraction was immediate, and by the end of July they had wed and settled in Liverpool. The union seems to have been happy enough at
first, but towards the end of the 1880s tensions began to surface.
Florence was a lavish spender and also given to placing bets on
slow horses. James, meanwhile, was not nearly so well off as he
had made himself out to be, partly because he spent somewhat
lavishly himself, bestowing £100 a year on a mistress who bore
him three children before his marriage and two more after. Eventually, Florence learned of her spouse's ongoing infidelity and
determined on a bit of extramarital activity herself. Early in 1889,

she became friendly with Alfred Brierley, a cotton merchant like her husband but of significantly lesser age. In March of that year, she spent a clandestine weekend with Brierley at a London hotel. Later that month, she wandered off with him briefly at the Grand National Steeplechase, a public act of indiscretion that enraged Mr Maybrick. On getting home that evening, the couple quarrelled violently, Mrs Maybrick getting the worse of it—a black eye and body bruises to match. Soon after this blow-up, her husband suffered an attack of vomiting. His physician diagnosed dyspepsia, a minor indisposition, and Maybrick recovered as expected. Soon, however, there were renewed attacks, accompanied with diarrhoea, running through April into May. Despite the most attentive nursing from his wife, James Maybrick died on 11 May.[24]

Three days before Maybrick's passing, a nursemaid in the house found a packet of white powder labelled arsenic. Later that same day, Florence wrote a letter to Brierley in which she made reference to their affair, and gave it to the maid to post. The maid, put on alert by the arsenic, opened and read the letter, then passed it on to Maybrick's brother. He was taken aback not just by the admission of adultery, but also by Florence's statement in the letter that her husband was 'sick unto death', when in fact the doctors were still predicting recovery. Did Florence know something the physicians didn't? A professional nurse was called in at once and Florence denied access to James. When he died, she was arrested. She had apparent motive—hatred of her husband, desire to be with her lover—and she had means. A thorough search of the house turned up not only the package of arsenic uncovered by the maid, but also varying amounts of the poison in her husband's medicine bottles and other containers, in a jar of 'meat-juice' (a type of bouillon tonic commonly administered to invalids), and in one of Florence's apron pockets. In all, 100 grains of arsenic were found. It also quickly came to light that Florence had made two sizeable purchases of arsenical fly-paper in recent weeks, and had been observed soaking the papers in water. The inquest jury wasted no time committing her to trial for murder.

Mrs Maybrick was represented by the ablest counsel of the day, Sir Charles Russell, who constructed a masterful case in her defence during the eight-day trial (in 1873, Russell had been the prosecutor when Mary Ann Cotton was found guilty). The fly-papers, he argued, had been obtained for an entirely innocent purpose. Florence had for years maintained her complexion by use of an arsenical preparation prescribed by an American physician. In April, she discovered she had misplaced it, and eager to remove a skin eruption on her face before attending a ball, she fell back on a practice she had seen used by young women in Germany. There, ladies soaked fly-papers in elderflower water and applied the water to their faces with handkerchiefs. The practice of beautifying with fly-poison was not uncommon, one of the chemists she had patronized testifying that he could verify 'that ladies came to buy fly-papers when no flies were about'. Florence had purchased the papers, moreover, from chemists to whom she was well known, and had made no effort to hide from the house staff her procedure of dissolving the arsenic from the papers. Those were hardly the behaviours one would expect from a woman plotting to kill her husband. The water prepared from the papers she put into bottles to prevent evaporation, and these weak solutions were among the samples of arsenic found in the house; the presence of arsenic in her apron could likewise be accounted for in this way.[25]

Further, how could one explain the facts that there was considerably more arsenic in the home than could have been removed from the fly-papers, yet there existed no other record of a sale of arsenic to Florence? To be sure, she might have obtained the additional arsenic illegally, but then there would have been no need to buy the fly-papers. What had happened instead, Russell submitted, was that the husband had obtained it for himself. For four years before meeting Florence, James had lived in the American city of Norfolk, Virginia, where he maintained a business office. After coming down with a fever in Norfolk's steamy climate, he was treated with Fowler's solution, and by that route acquired a habit of taking arsenic for health. A servant from the Norfolk days was brought in to testify that he had been sent to buy arsenic for his master a number of times, and had seen him take the substance in beef tea. Another Norfolk acquaintance revealed that Maybrick had told him he ate arsenic 'enough to kill you', taking it 'because I find it strengthens me'. The defence even introduced into evidence a box of arsenic pills found in Maybrick's possession bearing the name of a Norfolk chemist (in an affidavit filed after the trial, another man who had known Maybrick in Virginia described seeing him take a white powder; when asked what it was, Maybrick replied 'longevity and a fair complexion, my boy'). Closer to home, a Liverpool chemist related that Maybrick had been coming to his shop for years, on occasion several times a day, for an arsenical tonic he took for strength and virility. As with the ladies' dependence on fly-papers, he added, the practice was anything but rare: upwards of a dozen men daily came to him for arsenical boosters. Even Maybrick's own physician characterized him as 'hypochondriacal...distinctly so,' and stated the man was given to taking presumed aphrodisiacs. There was ample reason to conclude that the packet of arsenic powder, the largest sample of the poison by far, belonged to Mr and not Mrs Maybrick. He too might have come by it without making a registered purchase (four years after the trial, a chemist admitted that he had supplied arsenic to Maybrick surreptitiously). Finally, not to be disregarded was the comment Florence had made immediately on being told she was suspected of poisoning her husband: 'Why, if he is poisoned he poisoned himself—he made a perfect apothecary's shop of himself.' James Maybrick was, it seemed certain, an arsenic-eater.[26]

To observers of the trial, there was no question but that Mrs Maybrick would be acquitted. A group of women in attendance actually petitioned the court clerk for permission to present the prisoner with a congratulatory bouquet once the verdict was announced. But supporters had not given sufficient weight to a critical factor: the jury was, by the law of the day, composed entirely of men, and Florence Maybrick was by her own admission guilty of the greatest affront, short of murder, a wife could commit against a husband. Her adultery, even though of the two-night-stand variety, and even though engaged in as retaliation for years of adulterous behaviour by her husband, could be neither ignored nor pardoned. It provided a plausible motive, and implied a debauched character, as renowned Justice James Fitzjames Stephen observed in his charge to the jury: it was 'a horrible . . . thought that a woman should be plotting the death of her husband in order that she might be left at liberty to follow her own degrading vices'. Further intensifying jurors' suspicions was the memory of another highly publicized Liverpool trial just five years before, in which two sisters were convicted of killing one of their husbands with arsenic obtained from fly-papers. After a span of only thirty-eight minutes, the jury returned a guilty verdict and the sentence of death was pronounced.[27]

The verdict took nearly everyone by surprise, and stirred angry protests that Mrs Maybrick was being executed for adultery, not for the crime for which she had been tried. Petitions for clemency poured into the Home Office, some 5,000 in all, signed by nearly half a million people, including groups of physicians and nearly 100 MPs (there was no court of appeals at the time, but the case proved a powerful impetus in bringing about the establishment of the Court of Criminal Appeal in 1907). So great was the clamour, the Home Secretary acted with dispatch to commute the death sentence. He did not, however, exempt Maybrick from all punishment. Declaring that while there was 'reasonable doubt' her husband had died from arsenic poisoning (two medical witnesses at the trial had testified his death more likely to have come from gastroenteritis), there was still strong reason to believe that she had administered arsenic to him with intent to kill. She therefore deserved the sentence of penal servitude for life.[28]

Not surprisingly, efforts to secure her release continued, and for many years; so many years that the Maybrick case became known as 'the English Dreyfus Affair'. One Home Secretary after another reviewed the record and denied her pardon. Resistance to granting a full reprieve seems to have been fortified to considerable degree by royal opinion, Victoria making no secret of her belief that the adulterous tramp was guilty. The Queen expressed herself 'most upset' at the commutation of the hanging sentence, finding it most offensive that 'so wicked a woman should escape by a mere legal quibble'. Her Majesty was a formidable presence, and Home Secretaries were just as quick to 'yield in Queen Victoria's name' as the Pirates of Penzance. Not until 1904, three years after Victoria's death, was Florence Maybrick released from prison—on the intervention of Edward VII. Even then, her freedom was granted not by a pardon, but on grounds of good behaviour. She returned to the United States, where she lived until 1941, dying in penury, an aged woman with a houseful of cats.[29]

Belief in the benefits of arsenic-eating, incidentally, declined sharply by the end of the nineteenth century, but it did not disappear altogether for a while. A book published in 1937 praised the maidens of Styria for being 'more beautiful than others anywhere in Europe', and even added a new component to the story, claiming that Styrian babies were born with an inherited tolerance for arsenic because their ancestors had been eating the poison for generations. During that same decade there were reports of arsenic-eating among the inhabitants of the Forest of Dean in England. The practice seems to have died out soon after, or at least I have found no further references to it.[30]

*

The Styrian defence exemplifies a broader challenge faced by prosecutors in arsenic poisoning trials. The defence rested on the possibility that arsenic found in a person's evacuations or organs was of non-criminal origin. But arsenic-eating was hardly the only way in which the poison could innocently enter someone's body. 'How to convict of arsenical poisoning,' a physician asked in 1860, 'when ladies use arsenical cosmetics; when confectioners sell arsenical sweetmeats; when paperhangers clothe our walls with arsenical hangings, and impregnate all the air with fine arsenical dust?' How, indeed, to prove that arsenic detected in vomit or stomach came from the hand of an assassin, given that the poison was to be met with around virtually every corner? Remember that counsel for Mary Ann Cotton tried to convince jurors that one of her victims had actually died from exposure to arsenical soap applied to his bed to kill bugs. He also threw out the idea that poisoning might have occurred from the green wallpaper in the bedroom (the prosecutor punctured that trial balloon by pointing out the paper's pigment was a copper-containing arsenical, but there was no significant amount of copper present in the child's body). In different situations, crafty lawyers could build a defence around the fact that the supposed victim took Fowler's solution, or wore green muslin, or was exposed to arsenic in some other way than through intentional poisoning. In an 1860 case, a woman charged with murdering her husband got off even though it was proved that she had contemplated poisoning him. Her attorney was able to show that the husband regularly rubbed arsenic into his gums to relieve toothache, and succeeded in persuading the jury that that was the source of the poison found in his stomach—even though the arsenic in that organ totaled 150 grains. The ubiquity of arsenic in domestic products, one physician complained, 'complicates a hundredfold the already bewildering difficulties of toxicology in its juridical relations'. Sorting through and weighing all the possibilities was a tricky business—defence lawyers, prosecutors, judges, and jurymen were all put to the test to determine where the arsenic found in a dead man's body was most likely to have come from.[31]

The complications extended, moreover, to arsenic found in a dead man's grave. As has been seen, poisoning was often not suspected until after burial, and the presence of arsenic not demonstrated until after exhumation. But bodies often lay in the ground for months, even years, before being exhumed, long enough for coffins to deteriorate and for groundwater to infiltrate. Since arsenic was often a constituent of soil, one had to wonder if the poison found in an exhumed cadaver had been present before death or had gained entry after.

The question of 'cadaveric imbibition' of arsenic from cemetery soil first came up for serious discussion during the Lafarge trial, when the suggestion was made that the source of the poison finally detected in the exhumed Monsieur Lafarge was the burial ground's dirt. Consequently, the soil around his coffin was tested for the poison, but none was found. That determination said nothing, of course, about the possibility that arsenic might be absorbed from soil in which the poison *was* present. The chief medical authority involved with the trial, Orfila, soon undertook an experimental determination of the matter, presenting his results in 1842. Arsenic compounds found in soil, he concluded, are insoluble and therefore cannot penetrate into the interior of the body. In obliging confirmation of that conclusion, two years later a woman was exhumed from a different French cemetery on the suspicion she had been poisoned by either her husband or another woman who wished to have her husband. When the grave was opened, it was found that her body had been dislodged from the coffin, and that she was covered in soil, soil impregnated with arsenic. Yet no arsenic could be found in her body.[32]

The evidence of chemistry, however, could strike a jury as counterintuitive. In 1847, Elizabeth Johnson was tried for murder in Liverpool when her husband was exhumed three months after his sudden death and arsenic found in his viscera. There was no shortage of evidence to support the charge. The Johnsons were known to quarrel frequently, Elizabeth had been seen in bed with a lodger in their house, and had told a neighbour she did not care for her husband, saying she 'wished he was stiff'. Less than a week before her husband's death, moreover, she had made a purchase of arsenic. But during the course of the trial, it came out that the husband's coffin had been found to have a large crack through which groundwater had entered. This revelation prompted the judge to ask a medical witness if arsenic could have entered the body from the soil. The witness granted it was possible, although no one had examined the soil to determine if it did, in fact, contain the poison. The seed of reasonable doubt had nonetheless been planted in jurors' minds, and they quickly arrived at a not guilty verdict. Afterwards, dirt was taken from the cemetery and analysed—and found to be completely free of arsenic.[33]

Subsequent researches determined that arsenic compounds in soil were not completely insoluble, and that under the right conditions some quantity of the poison could enter human remains. Absorption depended on a number of variables: the nature and concentration of the arsenical material in the soil, the length of time since burial, the condition of the casket, the amount of rainfall, and the position of the grave with respect to drainage. Even under the most favourable conditions, however, only traces of the poison would be taken in. If any weighable amount of arsenic was found in the body, it meant some source other than the soil was responsible.[34]

One such source, it was recognized, might be the introduction of arsenic into the body after death as a means of raising a false accusation against an innocent person, a deed that one medical man disgustedly described as 'the acme of human depravity'. The possibility of such depravity opened another avenue to defence lawyers, of course. An attorney in an 1849 Irish case, for example, proposed that the presence of physical signs suggestive of a stomach pump having been introduced into the dead man's body indicated that the victim had died of natural causes and arsenic had been injected afterwards by someone other than the two accused men. The jury was not persuaded. But toxicologists appreciated that chemical analysis was a more reliable tool than visual inspection, and that it was therefore necessary to establish if post-mortem introduction resulted in the same distribution of the poison through the body as introduction during life. Orfila, who poisoned any number of live animals to study the effects of arsenic, tested the possibility on dead animals in 1840, hanging a dog till it expired, then injecting arsenic into the stomach. Leaving the animal suspended for eight days, he then dissected it and analysed its organs for arsenic. Viscera near the stomach were found to contain the poison.[35]

Nevertheless, prevailing toxicological opinion for several decades was that the presence of arsenic in internal organs was proof it had been administered before death. Then, in 1883, a Michigan man fell under suspicion of murdering his wife with arsenic. She had been buried more than three months when questions were raised, and when her body was exhumed arsenic was found in the stomach and liver. The husband's story was that he had introduced an arsenical solution into her mouth and rectum in an effort to preserve her remains until a special casket he had ordered arrived from Detroit; not surprisingly, he was arrested and charged. During the trial, the matter of whether arsenic put into the body after death could diffuse from the stomach to the liver was debated. To resolve the question, Victor Vaughan, one of the most respected professors of medicine in America, carried out a pair of experiments. A muskrat captured by one of his students was killed and arsenic squirted from a bulb syringe into its mouth and rectum. The animal was placed in a pine box and buried for twenty-five days, then dug up and analysed: arsenic was found not only in its stomach, but in the liver, kidneys, lungs, and heart as well. The test was repeated with a human cadaver, which was put away in a cellar for twenty-five days, then analysed. Arsenic was found in all the same organs as with the muskrat, as well as in the brain. At the same time, a colleague did the experiment with a cat he shot, with the same results. The presence of arsenic in parts of the body beyond stomach and intestines was therefore not proof that the poison had been administered during life and had caused death. The husband was convicted of murder, by the way, but acquitted on appeal—in part because medical witnesses had failed to demonstrate clearly the arsenic could not have been put into the body after death.[36]

If Mr Millard truly did inject his wife with arsenic, he was simply expanding on a procedure that had become commonplace by his day. Arsenic was employed to preserve stuffed animals as early as the eighteenth century, and by the beginning of the nineteenth, experience with exhumed poisoning victims was indicating it was effective at protecting humans from decay as well. Sooner or later, arsenic was certain to be applied intentionally to the preservation of human remains. In 1834, a Palermo physician published an account of his success at injecting cadavers intended for anatomical study with a solution of the poison. Soon British medical scientists were experimenting with arsenic as an embalming agent, one obtaining a patent for his method as soon as 1836. To professors and students of anatomy, long bedevilled by the need to move quickly, before bodies decomposed, arsenical preservation seemed something of a revolution. Typical was the excitement expressed by the faculty at a British medical school in Calcutta. In 1838, they reported on their experiments treating 'a favourable subject' with a water solution of white arsenic. The solution was injected under pressure into both carotid arteries, on one side upwards into the head, on the other downwards into the torso. More of the solution was introduced into the abdominal cavity, then the body was left undisturbed for ten days in hot weather. By the end of that period, the only noticeable external change was some shrivelling of fingers and toes; internally, all was 'as red and fresh as though the individual had died but an hour before'. Abdominal, thoracic, and cranial organs were all unchanged, the brain being 'so remarkably firm and fresh' that one of the experimenters took it with him to exhibit in his anatomy lecture that afternoon. Several more new corpses were then treated, 'and all have been preserved in a degree which has astonished those who have had an opportunity of observing them'.[37]

Yet as useful as arsenical cadavers were for anatomical studies, they also posed risks. The publication of the Calcutta experiments prompted London student John Snow to write to *The Lancet* with a warning that the cadavers were 'highly dangerous' (this was the John Snow who in 1854 would establish himself as the patron saint of epidemiologists through his statistical demonstrations of the water-borne nature of cholera). Over the past two years, he and fellow students had performed several dissections on bodies treated with arsenic, and on each occasion had been stricken with vomiting. On Snow's urging, the use of arsenic-injected corpses was discontinued at the school, though it would be maintained for some time at other institutions. In France, the use of arsenic in cadavers was outlawed in 1846, in part because of poisoning of dissectors. But while arsenic-preserved bodies were often observed to be covered with dead flies, I have found no reports of human fatalities from that source.[38]

In America, by contrast, arsenical injection of the dead was just about to take off, not as a facilitator of anatomical study but as a service provided by funeral directors. There was already a long history of attempts to postpone the decay of corpses to give family time to travel to view the remains before burial or to allow bodies to be transported home from a distance (or even to preserve them as mementos; in France in the early 1800s, a woman had her 10-year-old child embalmed so she might 'continually enjoy the sight of her'). Packing bodies in ice was the most common practice for postponing putrefaction; in America, there were even patents issued for 'corpse coolers'. Encasing in salt was another option, as was soaking in alcohol. When a young American woman died at sea in the 1850s, her father had her placed in a barrel of spirits and shipped home to be buried still in the cask. The most ingenious procedure, made possible after the process of canning meats and vegetables was introduced in the early 1800s, was to place corpses in airtight burial containers. Too often, however, the seal was imperfect and the 'meat' inside spoiled, generating gases that eventually exerted enough pressure to cause the container to burst.[39]

Preserving remains intact acquired new urgency with the onset of the Civil War, as suddenly many more bodies had to be transported home for burial. Given the inadequacies of earlier methods, along with the success of arsenic in preparing anatomical subjects, it was an obvious decision to adopt the poison for embalming dead soldiers. Concurrently, the traditional humble trade of undertaking was undergoing a transformation into the modern profession of funeral directing, with its encouragement of heightened ceremony and conspicuous display in sending loved ones into the hereafter. Plain pine boxes would no longer do. One had to exit the world in style, and to satisfy that manufactured need, coffin designers ran wild with creations offering every luxury for the sojourn in the afterlife. There were metal coffins, terracotta ones, even glass receptacles. A bronze case came in either an 'Ornamental' or a 'Cloth Covered' version, the latter being swathed with 'fine French cloth, trimmed with silk fringe'. And that was only the outside. Inside, one might rest, as did the editor of the *New York Herald* after his death in 1872, on a cushion 'upholstered with white satin, silk and Venetian lace, heavy silken tassels dropping from each corner'.[40]

Part of the new pageantry of burial, of course, was exhibiting the pampered corpse at its farewell service. As viewing of the deceased before interment acquired ritual status, effective preservation became essential—not just for deceased soldiers being shipped cross-country, but equally for civilians transported no further than from home to nearby funeral home. The preservative of choice was arsenic. By the end of the Civil War, three distinct patents had been issued for arsenical embalming mixtures, and for several decades, a toxicologist complained at the start of the twentieth century, 'a non-arsenified cadaver twenty-four hours after death was only met with when some accident or superior power had stayed the hand of the "funeral director" '. Embalming with arsenic was not nearly as common a practice in Britain as in America, but it was done, and was reason for concern. Embalming-fluid arsenic could not be distinguished from arsenic administered in tea or porridge during life, and so stymied the toxicologist and legal authorities from demonstrating the commission of the crime: as one physician saw it, embalming outdid even cremation as a way for a poisoner to cover his tracks (this was the second reason why France banned the practice). Where arsenical embalming was the rule, 'special instructions to the undertaker from the poisoner are not necessary'.[41]

But not only might poisoners get away with murder, some worried, embalming fluid might leak through the coffin into the soil and eventually be absorbed by a body that had not been embalmed. Then if that body were to be exhumed for some reason and arsenic detected in it, an innocent person might be convicted of poisoning. The odds against such a chain of events were considerable, but the mere possibility of contamination by 'artificial cemetery arsenic' was not lost on defence lawyers, who could now protest that arsenic found in their client's victim had in fact been supplied by another corpse. In America, three states (New York, New Jersey, and Michigan) prohibited the use of arsenic for embalming around the turn of the twentieth century, though by then formaldehyde was beginning to replace arsenical formulations. But until that time, physicians who suspected that a death might be due to arsenic had to insist that the body not be embalmed, and even appeal to the coroner to forbid any treatment of the body until a post-mortem could be performed. (It perhaps does not need saying that arsenical embalming fluid was also yet another source of accidental poisoning, though it was mostly the children of undertakers who were at risk.)[42]

There was another possible complication to be considered. What if a woman were buried in her favourite green dress, her head adorned with her treasured artificial flowers? In the presence of liquids from putrefaction, arsenical pigments could dissolve and enter the body. If she were exhumed on suspicion she had been poisoned, how could one be sure the arsenic found in her remains came from a killer and not her clothing? Sometimes the determination was easy. In a case in which arsenic was detected in a 6-year-old exhumed eight years after burial, the argument was made that the poison had come from four religious pictures containing green pigment that had been placed in his coffin. The amount of arsenic found in the remains, however, totalled four grains, too much to have come from the pictures.[43]

In other instances, the matter was far less clear-cut. Just as with women who used arsenic as a cosmetic, and men who took it for virility, and the many who took it as medication or otherwise imbibed it, wittingly or not, it was necessary to consider all the possible sources of contamination with the poison before passing judgment on an accused poisoner. It was impossible completely to insulate the category of arsenic administered with murderous intent from those of arsenic taken with beneficent intent or innocently absorbed from the domestic environment. When arsenic was involved, a juror's lot, no less than a policeman's, was not a happy one.

11

Poison in the Factory and on the Farm

In the fall of 1889, a Norwich woman was brought to hospital on a stretcher, 'totally unable to walk or even stand'. For several weeks she had been steadily deteriorating, going from a severe headache, to 'green vomiting...followed by copious watery diarrhoea', to premature labour (she was seven months pregnant) and delivery of a child that died three hours later. All this occurred during the first week. By the middle of the second week, her hands were numb and tingling, and soon her feet and lower legs were similarly affected. A burning sensation in the extremities followed ('intense pain' was caused by the slightest pressure applied to her limbs) and by the end of the third week she needed support to stand and could no longer hold anything in her hands. The only way she could account for her condition was that shortly before the headache began she was frightened by a thunderstorm.[1]

In hospital, the woman slowly improved, but even after three months she could stand for just a few minutes, and then only by supporting herself with the back of a chair. By now, her husband had joined her at the clinic, coming in with the same symptoms. They appeared to be classic examples of the nerve injury that afflicts alcoholics—except that neither was a serious drinker. In giving his history to the attending physician, however, the husband explained that he was a taxidermist and spent much time rubbing a mix of arsenic and plaster of Paris into birds. When his urine was analysed, arsenic was found in quantity. The wife, who cleaned the husband's workroom twice a week, had arsenical urine as well. Away from the preserved birds, both gradually recovered, but it was still several months before they were at last able to walk unassisted the mile between hospital and home.

From the late eighteenth century on, taxidermists protected specimens from decay and attack by moths and other insects either by kneading arsenical powder or paste into fur or feathers, or by dipping the animals into an aqueous solution of the poison. As a result, the artisans commonly suffered skin and eye irritation, and in some instances the neuritis symptoms of the couple described above. Earlier in the 1880s, for example, a New York woman was made 'a physical wreck' by her job assembling headdresses from preserved pheasant heads imported from England. There was risk as well for people who purchased the preserved animals, especially if they kept them in their bedrooms, where most time was spent. But the serious threat was to those who worked with arsenic in their daily employment. Taxidermists, like the artificial flower-makers of Chapter 7, were representative of a wide-reaching public health problem: people poisoned by arsenic to which they were exposed in their occupation.[2]

That health could be damaged by occupation had long been recognized. Soldiers and gladiators had always known it, and as the business of extracting ores from the earth developed in the ancient world, it was quickly learned by those forced to work the mines (almost all miners in antiquity were slaves). Long hours of strenuous labour in cramped quarters brought physical exhaustion and premature ageing; cave-ins crushed and maimed; dust damaged lungs; inadequate ventilation resulted in suffocation. Mining declined sharply with the collapse of Rome, but was revived from the 1100s onwards (in central Europe primarily) as the growth of industry and commerce generated new demands for metals for manufacture and coinage. Miners were now employed rather than enslaved, and they worked fewer hours, yet the old physical hazards continued. When Italian physician Bernardino Ramazzini published, in 1700, the first comprehensive treatise on occupational health (*De Morbis Artificum*, or *On the Diseases of Workers*), he devoted the opening chapter to the injuries and ailments suffered by miners, whom he considered the most unfortunate of labourers. Emerging from their pit each day 'looking as ghastly as the retinue of the god of the underworld', they were fated for early death: 'women who marry men of this sort', he remarked dryly, 'marry again and again'.[3]

But miners' travails did not end with dark and dust and close air, Ramazzini discovered; they were also beset by 'noxious pests that lie hidden in the veins of ore'. Mercury was one such pest; arsenic was another, hiding particularly in veins of iron, cobalt, copper, and tin. Commonly in the form of arsenopyrite ($FeAsS$) interlaced with the other metallic ores, arsenic was often released by the practice of 'fire-setting', the use of fire to break apart hard rock-faces. As the individual ores reacted to heat by expanding at different rates, rock fractured into chunks that could be easily collected. In the process, however, arsenic was vaporized and could be inhaled, sometimes with deadly effect. As early as the 1450s, a German text on mining described how poison generated by the fire overwhelmed workers. So toxic were the fumes, men who tried to escape 'fall back into the shafts [from the ladders] when the poison overtakes them'. Lower levels of exposure caused chronic injury to lungs, eyes, and skin; miners attempted to protect themselves by setting most fires on Friday, so the vapours would dissipate over the weekend.[4]

In Britain, the mining of metals was concentrated in south-west England, in the counties of Devon and Cornwall, and especially in the valley of the Tamar, the river that divides the counties. Tin had been mined there since antiquity, but the golden age for the industry dawned with the nineteenth century and lasted into the 1860s, with copper as the chief metal produced—at mid-century, the richest copper mine in Europe was the Devon Great Consols works in the Tamar Valley (officially, it was the Devonshire Great Consolidated Copper Mining Company). By the time copper deposits began to run thin after mid-century, there was such high demand for arsenic for its multitude of uses, and such large supplies of arsenical ore deposited in waste heaps around the mines, that refining of the poison became a major enterprise. By 1870, as much as half the arsenic utilized throughout the *world* was being provided by Devon Great Consols alone, a fact most agreeable to one of the firm's chief shareholders, William Morris, wallpaper designer/manufacturer. But as the end of the century neared, sources of the mineral dried up and arsenic production in Britain faded away in the early 1900s; Devon Great Consols shut down operations in 1903. (A brief revival of arsenic production occurred during the First World War, when the mineral came into demand, thankfully briefly, for the production of poison gases for the military.)[5]

During the 1800s, the old practice of fire-setting came to be replaced by drilling and blasting procedures that threw up great clouds of arsenical dust that must also have compromised the health of miners. But with the mid-century transition to extraction of arsenic from ores already removed from the earth, the dangers of poisoning shifted from mines to smelters. The extraction process involved crushing the ore, then roasting it to release fumes of white arsenic that condensed on the walls of furnace flues. From crushing to roasting to scraping the poison from chimney walls and grinding it into powder, workers repeatedly exposed themselves to arsenic—and suffered the consequences. Although smelter employees stuffed cotton into their noses and covered their mouths with handkerchiefs, they still inhaled enough 'smeech', as they called arsenical dust and gases, frequently to experience perforation of the nasal septum (holes as large as an inch in diameter being produced) and to develop the bronchitis and hoarseness of voice caused by arsenic's thickening of the vocal cords. Worse were the cuta-

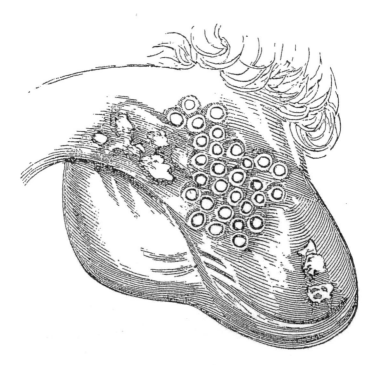

8. Scrotal skin eruptions caused by arsenic

neous effects produced. 'Arsenic pock' was the name workers gave to the eruptions resulting from the poison sticking to
sweat-moistened skin, pus-filled eruptions that could break out
anywhere on the body but were particularly common on the
scrotum (Fig. 8), the depression between the lower lip and chin,
along the border where the hat pressed upon the forehead, or,
simply, 'every crevice or fold where the arsenic can accumulate,
unless frequently and carefully washed out'.[6]

Physical debilitation had economic consequences. As late
as 1899, *The Lancet* called attention to 'the pauperism prevailing
among families of men formerly employed in arsenic works', poverty that could be attributed to early disability inflicted on them by
their jobs. Lung disease was the most frequent cause of disable-
ment; an 1899 survey determined that of the 100 deaths over the
past three years in the Cornwall mining town of Calstock, more
than 80 per cent were due to respiratory complaints. Epidemio-
logical studies conducted in the twentieth century would establish
that arsenic smelter workers were particularly prone to developing cancer of the lungs. Nevertheless, the breadth of individual
susceptibility to arsenic being as great as it is, there were men who
collected the poison from the chimneys for decades, 'literally wal-
low in it', a Cornish physician stated, without becoming visibly any
the worse for health.[7]

Smelter employment involved another potential hazard. The
large accumulations of arsenic on site presented a mighty temptation to anyone with a grudge against a fellow worker. In the
worst incident of its kind, in 1874, an unidentified malefactor
at the West of England Arsenic Works (an ancestor of the dis-
gruntled postal worker who periodically terrorizes American
post offices) added a large quantity of the poison to a storage
tank from which water was drawn for making tea for the morn-

ing shift. Within the half hour, all the tea drinkers were 'rolling about the ground writhing and crying out'. Two hundred were sickened, and more than a third of them 'narrowly escaped death'.[8]

One did not have to be a smelter employee, however, to be poisoned by the smelter's product. It was enough simply to live too close to a smelter. As far back as 1820, an arsenic plant near London was closed by court order because the smoke it released was judged 'pernicious to the inhabitants of the neighbourhood, producing very unpleasant sensations'. Thirty years later, it was determined that a young girl in Plymouth had died from inhalation of the fumes emitted by the arsenic works adjacent to the hospital where she was a patient. Animals in smelter neighbourhoods fared no better. There were numerous protests lodged by farmers that their horses and cattle were sickened, sometimes killed, by arsenic deposited on grazing land. Livestock were subject to losing their hooves, a Cornish doctor recorded in the 1820s, and cattle 'are often to be seen in the...pastures crawling on their knees' (it must be said that there are no corroborating witnesses for this repugnant scene). Donkeys, another Cornish practitioner reported, were particularly vulnerable to smelter emissions due to their fondness for thistles and similar plants with irregular surfaces that trapped arsenic dust and kept it from being washed away by rain. Apiculturalists lost bees to smelter fumes, and farm crops, fruit trees, and other vegetation were damaged. A Devonshire poet could lament by 1828, that

> Where the blossoming orchards bless'd the view
> Tremendous arsenic its fatal fumes
> Has breath'd and vegetative life has ceas'd
> And desolation reigns.[9]

Most of the output of arsenic smelters was passed on to workshops that converted the white arsenic into the various green pigments of commerce, chemicals that when poured into barrels for transport billowed into the air as a fine dust that was unavoidably inhaled by workers. Employees of pigment factories thus suffered the same as smelter workers, with nausea, headaches, inflammation of eyes and nose, skin rashes including pimples and boils, and scrotal eruptions that provoked near-constant scratching. Alfred Taylor reported the deaths of an entire family caused by the father's manufacture of arsenical greens adjacent to their living quarters.[10]

Once produced and packed, Scheele's green, Schweinfurt green, and the other arsenical pigments were shipped to any number of manufacturers for application to papers and fabrics; consequently, paper-stainers, paint-producers, those who printed wrappers, labels, shelf-liners and the like, seamstresses, and, of course, artificial flower-makers experienced all the signs of arsenic intoxication already outlined. There was seemingly no end of occupational opportunities for arsenic intoxication. During the period when composite candles were in vogue at least one worker died from mixing the poison with stearine. Those who wove green yarn were poisoned by their habit of biting through the ends of cotton strands before tying them off. An artisan who developed an improved method for enamelling watch dials that involved fusing arsenic with certain lead and tin compounds was sickened by fumes released in the process. Magenta dust used in coloured lithographic printing was sometimes contaminated with arsenic and poisoned printers. Men employed in tanneries could be injured by the orpiment applied to cattle hides to remove the hair. Even the hatters made mad by the mercury utilized in the felt hat trade could also be affected by the small amounts of white arsenic used in their manufacture. And in the United States, bank clerks sometimes fell prey to money coloured green with arsenic compounds.[11]

Not least among the victims of occupational arsenicism were those involved in the production of wallpaper, people who worked under much the same conditions as flower-makers. Injury extended even to those who merely hung the paper after it had been manufactured: 'a pale-faced, blear-eyed man' is how a physician described the typical wallpaper hanger, a man who 'suffered severely' every day the job involved green paper. His suffering was redoubled, furthermore, if a family decided that their paper was poisoning them and had to be taken down. When a vicar in the city of York had men strip his walls of paper he believed had sickened his children, the workers were within hours so ill that 'the reverend gentleman had to administer sundry doses of brandy and water to keep them at their work'. Among the many others similarly affected was the mother of the four Limehouse children, who was poisoned while removing paper after their deaths. The shop attendants who merely sold wallpaper, no less, could be injured, as happened to the man who developed diarrhoea and inflamed eyes during months in which he showed customers more than the usual number of samples of arsenical paper.[12]

Occupational damage was not limited to the ravages of white arsenic or green pigments. There was a still deadlier threat, arsine (AsH_3), the gas released in the Marsh test that sometimes killed analytical chemists. Taken in through the lungs, the colourless gas caused the same abdominal pain, vomiting, and diarrhoea as white arsenic. In addition, though, arsine attacked the liver, causing swelling and tenderness of the organ and in the process producing jaundice, the yellow colouration of the skin due to bile pigments absorbed into the blood. A 'deep copper bronze hue' of the entire body was a sign of arsine poisoning, as was darkening of the urine 'to all degrees up to a full port wine colour'. The latter was the effect of contamination of urine by haemoglobin released with the destruction of red blood cells (which, in turn, resulted in anaemia). Large quantities of haemoglobin interfered with kidney function, and could ultimately shut down urine secretion altogether and bring on death by uraemia (contamination of the blood with urinary waste products). Death might also come from acute liver damage. Either way, arsine inhalation was not a way anyone would choose to die. A worker employed in the manufacture of bleaching powder was poisoned by accidentally produced arsine: for the six days he lived after inhalation, he suffered from 'constant vomiting, coppery jaundice, lividity of the body, the mucous membranes of the lips almost black, suppression of urine—what little was drawn off consisting almost of blood'.[13]

Arsine had no industrial applications or economic importance. It nevertheless could be unintentionally generated whenever hydrogen came into contact with arsenic or arsenical ores. It was produced most commonly in commercial processes associated with the preparation of compounds of lead, copper, zinc, and bismuth, and posed a considerable risk to workers in chemical factories. Deaths from this source were first reported on the Continent in the 1870s; by 1900, several industrial arsine fatalities had been recorded in Britain. The poison could also be present in hydrogen manufactured with sulphuric acid contaminated with arsenic. A number of deaths occurred among soldiers filling military balloons, and at least three people who inflated balloons for sale to children were killed by arsine in their hydrogen. The most unusual instance of arsine poisoning occurred among steerage passengers on a boat from Antwerp to New York in 1905. Fifty were taken ill, and eleven died from arsine liberated by the action of water on an iron-arsenic ore stored in the hold below their quarters.[14]

*

Yet for most of the century, nearly all of it, workers had only scant protection from being poisoned by arsine, white arsenic, or green pigments. Some adopted makeshift precautions, such as the smelter employees who plugged their nostrils with cotton. Employers sometimes instituted preventive measures too, providing for arsenical powders to be packed into barrels in the open air, for example, or offering gauze masks to flower-makers. From the government, however, no help was forthcoming until the 1890s, despite repeated calls from medical practitioners for legislative enactments to protect workers in the arsenic industries.[15]

Neglect was due partly to the fact that the employees of chemical industries were next to invisible: constituting only a small percentage of the population, poor and uneducated, they were politically powerless. Physicians who tried to direct attention to the workers' plight similarly comprised only a minor segment of their profession, for occupational medicine was only just emerging as an established discipline. Parliamentary inaction was to an even greater degree an expression of laissez-faire abhorrence of checking the invisible hand believed beneficently to regulate the marketplace. The doctors who were attuned to occupational health hazards saw this as the great obstacle to establishing protections. In 1831, at a time when governments on the Continent were beginning to address questions of factory health and safety, *The Lancet* protested that 'in England alone is it that the principles of popular liberty are so sagely maintained that the people are allowed...to be suffocated in the asphyxiating vapours of manufactories, without the slightest concern being manifested by the rulers of the land'.[16]

The principle of non-interference with the liberty of manufacture cannot, however, account entirely for government's inattention to the dangers of arsenical employments, for there were, in fact, some occupational hazards regulated by law for most of the century. Statutes enacted in the 1840s, in particular, imposed significant requirements first upon textile factory owners, then colliery operators, to adopt measures to protect against accidents. But mechanical injury was quite a different thing from chemical poisoning. The injury was a distinct event with immediate effects and an obvious cause. Occupational poisoning, for the most part, was chronic, a drawn-out process whose cause was not so certain as that of a broken arm or fractured skull. A physician at a London hospital observed in the 1860s that men engaged in the manufacture of green wallpapers 'very frequently' came to his infirmary thinking they were suffering with a cold or similar ailment: 'few are anxious to believe that the work by which they live is killing them'. And even if a worker did realize the source of his illness, how eager would he be to complain, knowing that the work by which he lived might promptly be taken away from him by an offended boss? Like labourers throughout the chemical production business, arsenic workers were vulnerable to job blackmail; poisoning may not have been pleasant, but it beat starvation.[17]

For employers, there was no profit in calling attention to the dangers of their factories and workshops. Manufacturers nevertheless did feel compelled to respond to medical and lay critics, firing back not simply with denials that their workers were poisoned, but even with assurances that they positively benefited from their jobs. Not only were the workers 'who have been in our employment for thirty to forty years ... well and hearty', a wallpaper producer boasted, but they were 'longer lived than in most other trades'. Such statements only intensified medical scorn, of course. 'He might go a step further,' a doctor replied to another wallpaper manufacturer, and, 'as in the alleged arsenic-eaters of Styria ... be able to inform us that his men are in blooming health, remarkable for their florid complexions, strength of wind, and good appetites!'[18]

Chemical health hazards in the workplace were left completely unregulated until 1883, when Parliament passed a Factory and Workshop Act aimed at protecting workers engaged in the manufacture of lead carbonate, or white lead. Produced in enormous quantity for use in paints, as well as for glazing ceramic ware, white lead was responsible for an untold amount of occupational poisoning in the nineteenth century. It is difficult to determine if it caused more injury to workers than arsenic, but easy to understand why the substance was the first toxic industrial compound to be tackled by legislation in Britain. Lead carbonate had been manufactured since antiquity, and its poisonous effects recognized for nearly as long. Additionally, its dangers had long been dramatized in upper social strata by the reckless application of it as a cosmetic. Stylish ladies of ancient Rome had given their faces a pale finish with a dusting of white lead, and still in the Victorian era there were numerous lead-based complexion enhancers available from patent medicine houses. The Act strove to suppress white lead intoxication by requiring manufacturers to establish hygienic measures such as ventilation, protective clothing, washing facilities, and eating areas separated from the factory floor. Sadly, the law was honoured as much in the breach as the observance, and not until more stringent measures came into force at the end of the century did occupational lead poisoning begin to subside.[19]

Meanwhile, the situation of workers in arsenic industries, while not being completely overlooked, was not taken all that seriously either. As was discussed in Chapter 7, the London practitioner William Guy investigated the working conditions of artificial florists in the early 1860s and found poisoning to be common among them but not so grave as to require legislative intervention. In that same study, he had looked into the health of employees exposed to arsenic in the trades of paper-staining, wallpaper manufacture, and colour printing, and determined that while some suffered significant illness, their health overall was less compromised than that of the flower-makers. He did, it was noted, suggest that no one under the age of 18 be hired to make flowers, a proposal that many agreed with in principle, recognizing that minors were not competent to make informed decisions about the dangers of their work environment and so could not be supposed to be free agents like adults. Children, it turned out, would be the focus of the only governmental interest in arsenic workers for some time.[20]

In 1862, the government established a Royal Commission on Employment of Children (Royal Commissions, working through Parliament, were a centuries-old mechanism for investigating social problems and recommending remedial measures). Limited restrictions on the employment of children had already been imposed in some industries, most notably textile manufacture and mining. The 1862 Commission was charged with studying the conditions of labour of juveniles in industries not yet regulated by law. Among the first trades to be considered was paper-staining, the application of pigments and patterns to wallpapers. A review of the Commission's findings and conclusions for that occupation will further demonstrate just how vulnerable arsenic workers of all ages were to injury by their employment, and serve also as a reminder of how shamefully children were exploited for labour by Victorian industry—the Commission report reads like a chapter lifted from Dickens.[21]

The great majority of paper-staining operations were located either in London or in Lancashire. London manufacturers, it was hinted, were somewhat more high-minded than their northern brethren, for they hired only boys, and none under the age of 10 (girls were turned away in the capital's plants so 'their morals can't be corrupted'). Lancashire owners voiced no qualms about female workers, and were willing to take on boys as young as 8 (that is not to say they lacked scruples altogether: 'last year a boy only 6 years came to work here, but I sent him back'). The boys that were kept, and the girls too, typically worked fourteen-hour days, from six or seven in the morning to eight or nine at night, five days a week, half days on Saturdays (in slack periods, the day might end as early as six, but at peak times could stretch to eleven). Sundays the plants were closed. In London, the hours were marginally shorter, as employees were given an hour for a midday meal and half an hour for tea at five, a luxury denied Lancashire workers, who snatched what food they could while at their stations. The younger children, of course, had difficulty not falling asleep at their tasks, so inconveniencing foremen no end: 'I have to bawl at them to keep them awake', one complained, though another assured, unconvincingly, that 'there is no ill usage of the boys; just a lick of the head now and then, perhaps'.[22]

Many of the boys were probably already used to a lick of the head now and then, as they came from severely straitened economic circumstances, most of them trapped in poverty's brutal cycle. 'It is the young marriages that bring the children here so young,' it was explained to the Commission's investigators; 'the parents marry when they are children themselves', quickly produce a new brood, 'and send their children to work as soon as ever they can' so as to bring more income into the desperate household. Paper-staining, furthermore, was dirty work, the owner of a Leeds workshop pointed out, 'so that respectable people don't send their children'. His juvenile employees were drawn mostly 'from the lowest Irish on the other side of the town'; boys at other plants were similarly 'a very ignorant lot and very rough'.[23]

That ignorance was what most disturbed the Royal Commissioners, their report, published in 1863, being dominated by regrets that so few paper-stainers, the adult ones included, could read at even a rudimentary level. Without literacy, they could never hope to escape their degraded place in life. But while there was actually free education available to poor children, the 'ragged schools' set up by philanthropists to serve the disadvantaged, fourteen-hour days left little time or energy for the pursuit of learning. A 14-year-old at one wallpaper factory said he went to a ragged school 'sometimes from 8 to 9 ½ of a night [but] by the time we get home and have supper we are generally more ready for bed than school'. Even on Sunday, one plant manager reported, 'we can't get them to go to school... for they lie abed all day to rest'. Many owners professed to be ready to shorten children's hours to allow for education—on the provision that all companies be required to do so—but doubted parents would go along with such a scheme. 'The lot of parents don't care a screw about education, they are all for the money'; from parents' perspective, it made no sense to cram learning into their child's head if it meant the whole family 'would go short in their bellies'.[24]

Worse things could happen to their bellies, at least when colouring paper with arsenical pigments. The Commission heard numerous stories of the consequences of working with arsenic: ' I have a terrible pain in my belly; working amongst that green always makes me ill'; emerald green 'irritates in the nostrils and lips, and in the privates'; emerald green 'is bad, and no mistake'. Only one fatality among the child workers was uncovered, however, and the many cases of sickness were countered by the many who worked among the greens without incident. 'A boy here and there goes queer with the paint,' a worker acknowledged, 'but for one that does, there are 10 that don't.' Many of the stainers interviewed dismissed any threat from emerald and the other greens. A twenty-year veteran of the trade had 'never been sick a day', and while one man related how 'the irritation with some constitutions is so great that the whole skin peels off', he at once added that he had never known of 'any permanent injury from working the emerald green'. Ultimately, the Royal Commission's report downplayed the dangers of paper-staining and no action regulating arsenic ensued.[25]

From the 1860s onward, of course, consumer apprehension about arsenical products led to decreasing use of the poison in items such as wallpapers, flowers, and dresses. The threat to workers thus seemed to be receding, so even less in need of Parliamentary attention. Yet the employment of arsenical pigments in domestic items did not disappear altogether during the nineteenth century, and the degree of its decline varied considerably from one industry to another. The production of the pigments themselves still posed significant risks down to the closing years of the century: in 1888, a government visitor to a Schweinfurt green factory in Kent found 'the air was filled with it. I could hardly breathe and for some hours after my visit suffered from soreness in the throat.'[26] His, moreover, had been a brief encounter with the poison, far less exposure than that endured by employees day after day.

By the 1890s, the discipline of occupational health was reaching maturity in Britain, generating greatly heightened awareness of the 'dangerous trades' in which the nation's labourers were engaged. At the same time, traditional resistance to government interference with manufacture was relaxing somewhat, allowing a flurry of legislation imposing tighter regulation of industrial practice. The same provisions for ventilation, sanitation, and protective clothing previously applied to white lead production were now (1892) extended to arsenic employments. In 1895, another Factory and Workshop Act mandated regular inspection of industries involving three dangerous chemicals—arsenic, lead, and phosphorous—and required that cases of poisoning of workers be reported to the government. Over the first two decades of the law's administration, an average of only six cases of occupational arsenic poisoning per year were recorded; only nine fatalities occurred during that period (the introduction of automated procedures in handling arsenical dusts aided in the decline). There undoubtedly were cases of poisoning that escaped inspectors' attention, but even so, a problem that had once constituted a 'Dance of Death' inflicting 'suffering in the most terrible manner' (1860s descriptions of artificial flower production) had been reduced to an occasional misfortune. By the early 1900s, less than 1 per cent of all industrial poisoning cases could be attributed to arsenic.[27]

*

Among the workers covered by the 1895 Act were those engaged in the manufacture of arsenical sheep dip. Not included, however, were the men who applied the dips down on the farm. Their numbers were considerable, for the production of wool was one of Britain's chief industries. To ensure the health of their sheep, and thus the quantity and quality of their wool, sheep farmers periodically treated the animals with preparations meant to destroy lice, ticks, and other parasites that caused skin irritation. Not all sheep dips contained arsenic: carbolic acid, mercury salts, tobacco, and lime-and-sulphur were all utilized to some degree in arsenic's stead. But the great majority of shepherds and 'flockmasters' felt arsenic did the job best: 'so important is [arsenic] considered by most farmers, that they would listen to no arguments tending to divert them'; sheep owners 'have a rooted prejudice against the use of any other ingredient'. They therefore usually opted for Cooper's formulation, or Bigg's or Froom's compositions, or another of the many brand-name arsenical sheep washes, or simply stirred up their own mixtures of white arsenic, water, and soap (the 1851 Sale of Arsenic Act placed no restrictions on the purchase of the poison for agricultural or industrial purposes, and farmers bought it by the hundredweight).[28]

Sheep 'dressing', as it was also called, involved immersing each sheep in a vat of dipping mixture for a minute or so. The procedure was not one with which the animals were inclined to cooperate, of course, so the dipper was forced to wrap his arms around the sheep and hold it close against his body while working the liquid into the wool with his hands. His clothing was soon saturated with the mixture, its penetration to the skin guaranteed by 'the friction which must be caused by a living sheep half drowned in poison, trying to struggle out for its life'. An efficient dipper would dress more than a hundred sheep a day, thousands over the course of the year (as many as 40,000 for the busiest workers, it was estimated). That was a lot of contact with an irritant poison, and it showed in the appearance of skin eruptions ranging from pimple-like rashes to pus-filled blisters, and even large boils. Sheep workers, a physician commented, 'all have a salutary dread of the arsenical dipping liquor'.[29]

All parts of the body could be affected by the liquor, but injury was notably more common on the most exposed areas, the hands and forearms and, as in other arsenical trades, the scrotum. Conscientious dippers wore leather aprons to keep the poisonous solution away from their genitals, and washed the parts thoroughly at the end of the day. Those who neglected to wear a water-resistant apron or did not bother to wash learned a terribly painful lesson. A man who spent nine hours dressing sheep on a Friday was completely incapacitated by Tuesday, his testicles blistered and covered with pus-oozing eruptions. The skin of the scrotum had largely sloughed off, and though he was 'a man of great spirit and endurance', his suffering 'seemed to be exquisite...motion of the pelvis

or thighs was almost intolerable'. At least one dipper, reasoning
that what worked for the sheep should work for the person, foolishly tried to exterminate his own body lice by applying dip to his
pubic region and armpits; his skin peeled away too, leaving the
testicles raw and bleeding and the hair in both areas feeling as if it
were 'being pulled up by the roots'. These were far from isolated
cases. Serious skin irritation was the norm with shepherds, enough
of a likelihood that some (to their employers' displeasure) tried to
get away with applying the dip from kettles or teapots rather than
risk contact with the skin. Rural physicians likewise took skin damage to be a given element of the job. Madeleine Smith's claim that
she used an arsenic solution to *improve* her skin set off a barrage of
letters to medical journals from country doctors all too familiar
with the effects of sheep dip.[30]

The man who attacked his lice with sheep dip also complained
'that he felt as if his bowels were on fire', a sure indication that
arsenic had been absorbed into his system. Constitutional poisoning was in fact a frequent result of working with sheep dip, and
was occasionally severe enough to kill. But it was the sheep who
were more likely to die in the process, whether due to overzealous
application of the dip by operators, or to their leaving the animals
immersed in the wash too long, not rinsing them with water after
removal from the vat, and/or not wiping them dry with a sponge
before returning them to pasture. Doing the job properly was
time-consuming, shortcuts were taken, and sheep were poisoned
in consequence. Yet the fault for sheep deaths was not always with
farmworkers, for sometimes dip manufacturers carelessly put too
much arsenic into their product. In 1851, an outbreak of sheep
poisoning occurred on Devon farms that had all used a particular brand of sheep wash. Within three days of being dipped, the
sheep 'could scarcely walk—they seemed to be paralysed'; their

skin was found to be blistered, 'as if they had been scalded. After a week they would fall down, and were unable to rise again—the blisters became worse, and broke, abscesses were formed into the bone...' Many animals died ('they turned black, the dogs and the flies would not touch them'), while virtually all the remaining ones 'were injured more or less...the ewes lost their teats' and few were left fit for breeding. One of the farmers sued the manufacturer for selling a too-potent formulation, and the jury found in his favour, awarding damages of £1 per lamb and £1.10s. per ewe for the animals he had lost. Towards the end of the same decade, a farmer in the North of England purchased a 'Celebrated Sheepwash' he had seen advertised and treated all his 869 sheep with it. A week later, only nineteen were left alive. He was granted damages amounting to £1,400.[31]

The use of sheep dip also exposed other livestock to danger. In the 1840s, for example, a farmer had all eight of his horses fall ill. A veterinary surgeon was called, and while he was examining the animals, his own horse was fed by the farmer. Soon it too was showing signs of sickness. Like the first eight horses, it had been given linseed that had been boiled in a pot that, it was eventually realized, had been used several months before for mixing sheep dip. All the horses died.[32]

Poisoning of sheep with arsenic dip was of more than economic importance, for poisoned animals were sometimes slaughtered for sale as food to people. Was the meat from such animals dangerous for human consumption? The question was raised as early as the 1840s, and quickly answered: it depends. The lead in investigating the matter was taken by a French physician aptly named Danger (Ferdinand), who conducted a series of experiments in 1842. In summary, the trials determined that dogs fed the flesh of sheep freshly killed with arsenic suffered poisonous effects. Dogs fed meat from sheep that had been given a non-lethal dose of arsenic, then butchered several weeks later exhibited no signs of poisoning, nor were six human volunteers who subsisted on the meat for nearly two weeks harmed by it. So, it depended on allowing enough time between dipping and slaughter for sheep to eliminate the arsenic from their bodies. Could farmers be trusted to adhere to that rule? It would be naive to suppose arsenical mutton never made it to market, but I have been unable to find any instance of human poisoning being connected with that source. There was also potentially a problem with chickens, for during the second half of the century poultry growers began to add arsenic to their animals' feed in order to fatten them for market (following the example of the Styrian peasant girls who plumped themselves up for their lovers). Analyses found only insignificant quantities of arsenic in the birds' flesh, though, the poison being quickly excreted in their feathers. Consequently, arsenical compounds would be used well into the twentieth century to promote rapid growth in pigs as well as poultry.[33]

Although non-arsenical sheep dips were available, the preference for arsenic continued to the end of the century, eventually occasioning a good deal of debate about the potential danger to health of arsenic in clothing, carpets, and other domestic items produced from the wool of treated sheep. Might a man be killed by his cardigan? It was soon determined, fortunately, that the arsenic applied to the animals was bonded so tightly to the wool that even the washing, carding, combing, spinning, and dyeing of the fibre before it was woven failed to remove the poison. If it was not dislodged by all that, it seemed very unlikely that in the end it could suddenly lose its grip and drift out into the air and poison anyone.

A survey of the subject published by *The Lancet* in 1899 concluded no cases of poisoning from contact with items made from the wool of dipped sheep had been recorded.[34]

Sheep and chickens were not the only farm animals presumed to benefit from the application of arsenic. The discoverer of the arsenic-eaters, von Tschudi, announced that Styrians commonly mixed the poison into their horses' oats in order to improve the animals' endurance for pulling heavy loads up hillsides. As with people, the horse's 'complexion' improved as well, its coat soon acquiring a 'sleek, round, glossy appearance'. The practice spread from the villages to Vienna, where grooms began treating their masters' horses by placing a pea-sized ball of arsenic in a linen bag and tying it to the animal's bit. Gradually dissolved by saliva, the arsenic entered the horse's system and gave it an energy and beauty that were the envy of grooms not in on the secret. The frothing at the mouth that it also produced was soon established as a trademark of Viennese horses, a characteristic 'so much admired'.[35]

The 1850s publicity barrage that informed the British of the arsenic-eating habit and encouraged some of them actually to adopt it likewise ensured that British horses would be offered the benefits of the poison. As early as 1855, there were reports of arsenic being given to horses in England, accompanied by complaints that carelessness and ignorance of proper dosage had destroyed many of the animals. The following year, the first of numerous prosecutions for killing horses with arsenic was held in Norfolk, though the two young men responsible were acquitted on the grounds that the overdosing was an innocent mistake. Such mistakes would continue, so entrenched was the notion of arsenic as an equine tonic, and farmers in some districts eventually united to form associations 'for preventing the administration of arsenic…to horses'. Indeed, Styrian pharmacology was repeatedly called on to account for the experiences of yet other species, being put forth as the obvious explanation, for example, of the transformation of a cat who lapped up milk containing sheep dip, lost all its hair, but survived and soon grew a new coat of 'beautiful silky fur'. One reason for shepherds' preference for arsenical dip was that they supposed enough of the substance would be absorbed through the sheep's skin as to exert a cosmetic effect on its fleece and fetch a higher price for the wool.[36]

Arsenic was also used in great quantities on farms intentionally to poison animals that might be destructive to crops (everything from slugs to birds), the poison being spread about at the ratio of 1 lb to the acre. Inevitably, other creatures were killed: accounts of cats, dogs, and horses poisoned in this way appeared in newspapers and medical journals with regularity. Included among the unintentional victims, of course, were the workers who dusted the arsenic over the fields; although their exposure was not sufficiently intense to kill them, they suffered the usual cutaneous effects.[37]

There were also incidents, even into the early years of the twentieth century, in which partridges were killed by the arsenical dust spread on farms. But, as was explained in the Preface, partridges—and pheasants—were more likely to be poisoned by eating wheat seed that had been steeped in a solution of white arsenic to protect against wireworm destruction of the seed and smut attacks (a fungal infestation) on the plant. The wheat was sown either by being broadcast about the land or by using drills, implements that dropped seeds into furrows that were then covered. If employed carelessly, though, a drill could leave seed on the open ground. A rural doctor related often seeing accumulations of seeds on footpaths between fields, 'the poisoned wheat lying in such a quantity that a child might have picked up a pint in a very few minutes'. But birds were more likely to eat the seeds, and poisonings of wildfowl were common enough that some predicted they would 'at no distant day, become extinct in this country'. There were also frequent warnings of the effects of eating such birds. It was to be hoped that most people were smart enough not to consume a bird found dead on the ground. But what if they shot and ate the bird before it had succumbed to the arsenical seed it had ingested? A Worcestershire physician told of dining on a pigeon pie made with birds shot by a friend during the planting season; he and the four acquaintances who shared the delicacy all experienced poisoning from the pigeons' flesh. Then there was the additional threat of birds taken by poachers, a major source of wildfowl for many poulterers selling meat to the public. As they skulked about the woods in pursuit of live birds, poachers were sure sooner or later to come upon partridges, pheasants, or pigeons killed by wheat seed. Given their interest in harvesting as many birds as possible, they would probably not hesitate to sell them along with their untainted prey. It was advisable, one doctor suggested, that in all cases of digestive upset occurring during the sowing season physicians should ask the patients if they had partaken of game birds lately. Police and jurors should be equally alert, lest someone be convicted of murder for a death that was actually poisoning by partridge.[38]

*

Poisoning could also come from a pear tree. Towards the end of the century, arsenic compounds began to be applied in quantity to fruits and vegetables for the purpose of destroying insects such as the apple codling moth and the Colorado potato beetle. The new insecticides were used much more extensively in America than in Britain, for agriculture was a much larger enterprise in the United States and had already turned towards monoculture, cultivation of one crop on a massive scale. Extensive, unbroken fields canopied by the foliage of a single plant, be it wheat, cotton, or potatoes, afforded ideal feeding conditions for the insect pests of the plant and generated a huge demand for insecticides. The Devon Great Consols Mining Company managed to stay in business into the early twentieth century thanks in considerable part to the demand for arsenicals to fight the boll weevil outbreak in the cotton fields of America's South in the late 1800s.[39]

The difference in scale between the two nations' consumption of arsenical pesticides was dramatized in 1891 when an English agricultural magazine protested that apples imported from America often arrived with a visible coating of arsenic left from excessive spraying. The *British Medical Journal* then weighed in against 'the use of poisons for the treatment of food' in terms that implied the threat came only from America, eliciting suspicions from American pomologists that the British were impugning the quality of their apples purely to boost the sale of homegrown and Commonwealth-produced fruit.[40]

That tempest soon blew over, but it was in fact the case that American produce was often shipped bearing residues of arsenical spray, and agricultural trade relations between the two countries remained uneasy. The tension would be heightened from around 1900 on, as a new compound, lead arsenate, emerged as the insecticide of choice, meaning lead residues were now added to those of arsenic. All came to a head in the last weeks of 1925, when a family of four in the London borough of Hampstead was sickened by lead arsenate-coated apples from America. Newspapers played up the incident with scare headlines ('Arsenic Apples') and satiric commentary (one editor, referring to a recently launched 'Eat More Fruit' campaign, enjoined readers to 'EAT MORE FRUIT: YOU will be DEAD CERTAIN if YOU DO.'). Over the next few weeks, nearly a thousand articles, editorials, and cartoons warning against the dangers of American produce would appear in British papers. The authorities, in the meantime, threatened to impose a boycott on American fruit unless arsenic residues were reduced to clearly harmless levels, and although the threat was never carried out, the public cut back sharply on their purchases of produce imported from the United States. In the end, American consumers benefited from the contretemps as well, for the threat of loss of the British market was the catalyst that at last brought together American farmers and federal pure food enforcers, in the 1930s, to work out measures to minimize arsenic and lead residues on produce. Lead arsenate would nevertheless continue as the chief insecticide in the United States until the end of the Second World War, when DDT, discovered in 1939, was released to the civilian market as 'the atomic bomb of the insect world'. Prior to that time, the lead compound was so widely employed that an agricultural writer suggested revising the 'A is for Apple' opening of a child's reader to 'A is for Arsenate | *Lead* if you please | Protector of apples | From archenemies.'[41]

Insecticides did, in truth, constitute one arsenic problem that was much worse in America than in Britain, where the compounds were applied in smaller quantities and less frequently, and in less adhesive formulations. Further, the British climate surely removed spray from produce more thoroughly than did America's. In any event, a government investigation of sources of arsenic poisoning in Britain concluded in 1901 that no cases due to arsenic residue had been reported in the country (in France, where arsenicals were applied to wine grapes, people were sometimes poisoned by wine, and may have been affected as well by eating the escargots that fed on the vines, vineyard snails being found to contain arsenic in 'considerable quantities').[42]

Where agriculture was concerned, British scientists worried much more—for a while, at least—about the possible contamination of produce by arsenic introduced into the soil from treated wheat seed and from fertilizer. By the middle of the nineteenth century, farmers were being won over to the use of a new 'artificial manure', superphosphate, a preparation made by treating mineral phosphate salts with sulphuric acid. The most economical process for producing sulphuric acid utilized iron pyrites as the starting material, and since pyrites generally contained quantities of arsenic as an impurity, sulphuric acid was frequently contaminated with arsenic, which was carried through to the superphosphate fertilizer. Scientists had to wonder if plants treated with superphosphate might be made unwholesome as foodstuffs by absorbing arsenic from the soil. A Dublin professor of agricultural chemistry was sure it must happen, reporting in 1859 that he had detected the poison in turnips grown with superphosphate, and—what seems to have been the clincher for him—that sheep offered superphosphate turnips shunned them in favour of turnips produced with ordinary manure.[43]

The professor's alarm was soon quieted by other chemists who determined that normally only minute amounts of arsenic were absorbed from the soil by plants, and that if larger quantities were taken up they quickly killed the plant, effectively preventing it from being eaten. If superphosphate-soaked soil actually did present a 'lurking danger...what a dreadful state the cattle of the country must be in', being daily fed pounds and pounds of roots grown in arsenic. Yet British cows were to all appearances healthy and flourishing (except for those pastured in the vicinity of arsenic smelters). Similarly, it was demonstrated that the arsenic in treated wheat seeds did not make it into the mature grain in detectable amounts. There was no need for 'apprehension of death in the pot', one analyst reassured; the superphosphate 'scare' was 'without foundation'.[44]

So soil was safe, to people if not always to plants. But could the same be said of water? Much injury occurs today from arsenic occurring naturally in water supplies in various places around the world.

These sources were contaminated in the nineteenth century as well, though they were mostly overlooked. In Britain, attention went instead to the waters from certain European spas that, as was noted in Chapter 9, held relatively low levels of arsenic and thus were sometimes recommended as alternatives to Fowler's solution. England had its own arsenical spa of a sort, the Cumbrian hamlet of Whitbeck, which in the 1860s rose to brief fame as the 'village of arsenic-eaters'. The stream that passed through the town originated near a mine with veins of arsenical cobalt ore and carried low levels of arsenic. Its water was used for all common purposes by the villagers, yet far from causing harm was 'productive of the most sanitary effects!' As in Styria, 'the rosy looks of the Whitbeck children, and the old age which a large proportion of the inhabitants of the village attain' were to be attributed to the beck's arsenic, as was the 'sleekness of coat' of Whitbeck horses. Cattle prospered on the water too, indeed all animals apparently except ducks (which, a physician explained tautologically, must have 'less eliminating power than others') and fish ('no fins are ever found in the arsenicate stream').[45]

The salubrity of Whitbeck water was explainable in part by its rapid flow through the hilly region: it did not stand still and permit a build-up of arsenic to dangerous concentrations. Quite the opposite situation applied to well water, as was tragically demonstrated in the 1840s by boys at a military academy near Vienna. The students suddenly began to decline in vigour, some actually dying before the cause of distress was discovered. The well that supplied the academy's water was found to contain the remains of numerous rats that had been exterminated with arsenic some months before when they had overrun the school's food storehouse. When the students were provided rat-free water, they recovered.[46]

Warnings were issued to the British public that the same fate could befall them if arsenic was used to kill rats on premises in which drinking and cooking water was taken from wells. Arsenic's dehydrating effects cause rats to be 'tormented with thirst, and [to] burrow under ground to seek for water', ending up in wells. Despite such warnings, there are innumerable references to reliance on arsenic to control rat populations on farms, and doubtless well water must have at least occasionally been contaminated by poisoned rats. Nevertheless, there do not appear to be any authenticated cases of poisoning that way. Well water in the vicinity of arsenic industries is another matter. In the most disturbing instance, a manufacturer of coloured paper poisoned neighbours over a span of thirty years with arsenical refuse that made its way into the groundwater. Only after three decades was the cause of all the sickness and death discovered.[47]

If a single paper-maker could spread such injury, it would seem that arsenic smelters must have done severe damage. One undoubtedly did. In 1898, it was finally determined that the mysterious 'Reichenstein disease' that had plagued generations of residents of Reichenstein, Silesia stemmed from arsenic, discharged over centuries by the town's smelter, contaminating the spring that supplied the town's drinking water; when a new source of water was made available in 1928, the Reichenstein disease disappeared. The potential for a similar affliction certainly existed in Britain (Devon Great Consols disease?), but none was ever established. Potentially, poisoning could come from river water also, for English smelters discharged considerable quantities of arsenical waste into rivers, the Tamar especially. The refuse was flushed away, however, with large volumes of the water used to power equipment, and then it was diluted much further in the river. There was no lack of fretting over the possibility of smelters poisoning waterways, but dangerous levels of pollution could not be demonstrated.[48] And when all was said and done, for a true Englishman there was a much more worrisome question than what might happen if he swallowed a little arsenical water now and then. That was: what if arsenic gets into beer?

12

'Dangers that Lie Wait
in the Pint-Pot'

The 2-year-old child seen by John Brown, Medical Officer of
Health for the Lancashire town of Bacup, on 27 November 1900,
was 'a bonny-looking little girl'—except for a bright red rash on
her hands and lower legs, and dark brown splotches on the skin
of her thighs. In addition, she was experiencing burning pain in
her legs and feet (the latter were so tender that she refused to wear
shoes), and her patellar reflex, or knee-jerk reaction, had been lost.
For Brown, the diagnosis was obvious: the bonny little girl had
been drinking too much beer.[1]

Bacup lies about twenty miles north of the great industrial centre of Manchester, regarded at the time as the hardest-drinking
town in the realm. Alcohol, the adage ran, was 'the shortest route
out of Manchester', the labourer's quickest escape from the dreary
grind of daily existence. The route was heavily trafficked. Among
physicians, Manchester was notorious for having far the highest level of alcoholic neuritis in the nation, more than twice the
incidence of the ailment among Londoners, and up to ten times
the rate for other British cities (identified as alcoholic neuropathy
today, the condition is caused by chronic excessive consumption of
alcohol, and its multiple symptoms include burning sensations in

the legs and feet). So common was alcoholic neuritis in Manchester, the city's physicians had acquired the reputation of being national specialists in the disorder. But during the summer of 1900, there occurred a sharp rise in the incidence of alcoholic neuritis that took it to a level extraordinary even for that booze-sodden precinct; by November, cases actually 'flooded the out-patient departments of the hospitals,' at one institution comprising nearly half of all patients.[2]

At first, the spike in the illness seemed easy enough to explain. British forces were enjoying early successes in the Boer War while at home a national election had recently been held; both events were excuses for revelry, and instances of alcohol-fuelled public merriment had noticeably increased. There were, however, two difficulties with the explanation of a politically inspired upsurge of binge drinking. First, all the affected patients drank primarily beer rather than strong spirits, and many insisted they consumed only moderate quantities, too little to produce such serious effects. It was axiomatic, of course, that devoted drinkers would lie to doctors when asked how much they imbibed: a nurse who took care of many alcoholic neuritis patients said that whenever she enquired if they drank excessively they denied it, though, she added, 'they were naturally not believed'. For a while, it was possible simply not to believe Manchester patients' protestations of moderation. But as their numbers grew and they remained adamant that they were not sots, some physicians began to wonder if something other than alcohol was at work.[3]

Second, the typical case involved pathological signs not usually seen in alcoholic neuritis. In particular, victims exhibited rashes and pigmented patches of skin such as those observed on Dr Brown's young patient, complaints that, when accompanied by neuritis, had long been associated with chronic arsenic intoxication. Putting symptoms together with drinking habits, Ernest Reynolds, assistant physician to both the Manchester Royal Infirmary and the Manchester Workhouse Infirmary, analysed samples of beer from the city's breweries and determined that many, particularly the least expensive varieties, the 'fourpenny' ales favoured by working-class drinkers, held notable quantities of arsenic. He announced his discovery at the 21 November meeting of the Manchester Medical Society, and three days later in the *British Medical Journal*. In the meantime, the public press had picked up the story.[4]

It was less than a week after Reynolds's announcement that Dr Brown saw the young girl in Bacup, but already so much publicity had been given to arsenical beer poisoning in Manchester, he immediately suspected that, despite his patient's tender age, beer must be at fault. Brown questioned the child's father (who likewise was suffering with neuritis) and learned that he operated a public house in the town, at which he was accustomed to let his toddler roam free in the evenings among the clientele. These 'kindly disposed customers at the bar', as the doctor generously described them, did their best to amuse the girl by offering her 'sups', their term for small portions of beer. Taken individually, the sups amounted to little. But when given to her by nearly everyone in the pub, as they were, sups quickly added up to an injurious amount. Examination of the beer served at the father's establishment, as well as other products of the town's eleven breweries, determined that arsenic was present in nearly every one, thus explaining all the other cases of neuritis that had suddenly cropped up in Bacup the last few weeks. The publican's daughter therefore was far from alone in her misery; she was simply the most unusual victim in yet another instance of wholesale poisoning of the public by arsenic (she was not, however, the youngest victim, as several infants were poisoned by their beer-drinking mothers' milk).[5]

The 'Manchester beer epidemic,' as it was soon being called, provides a fitting capstone to our survey of arsenic among the Victorians. Occurring in the final year of the nineteenth century (and only weeks before the death of Victoria in the first month of the twentieth), it would exert significant influence on the way arsenic would be dealt with in the future. Nor is 'epidemic' too strong a word to apply to the incident. Several thousand cases of neuritis would be reported during its course, and some victims would meet with a much worse fate, for the concentration of arsenic in some batches of beer was potentially lethal. Reynolds found that in most samples he tested, arsenious acid was present in the range of one-tenth to one-seventh of a grain per gallon, though as much as a quarter grain per gallon was detected in one batch. Subsequent analyses of other brews would discover that contamination levels of three-quarters of a grain were not rare, that some samples contained as much as two grains per gallon, and that one extraordinary batch held three grains per gallon. Three grains could be deadly, and, as one worried physician pointed out, 'a gallon per day was not an uncommon amount to be drunk'. On average, the neuritis patients had been drinking a mere four to five pints daily, but more than a few admitted to ten to fifteen pints a day. One man claimed a thirty-pint per diem habit; yet even he was outdone by the stalwart who bragged of downing forty a day when 'on the spree'. Had the last gentleman taken a liking to the most heavily contaminated beer, he would have swallowed up to fifteen grains of arsenic in twenty-four hours, more than enough to put paid to his sprees for good.[6]

But a toper didn't need the thirst of Gargantua in order to be harmed by the poison. Symptoms appeared in people taking as little as one or two pints daily, and even among these models of restraint the damage was dreadful—and distinctive. Once a physician had treated a few cases, he would find 'there is no difficulty whatever in diagnosis. There is no other disease which will produce the same grouping of symptoms.' That grouping, moreover, was amazingly broad in its content, comprising a virtual textbook of the toxic versatility of arsenic. With the possible exception of an outbreak in Paris in the 1820s (to be discussed below), this was the largest mass poisoning with arsenic on record, so afforded opportunity for every manifestation of its action to be expressed and observed.[7]

Symptoms typically began with the trademark nausea and vomiting, regurgitation occurring in some victims after every meal, and in a few after every pint (these were in a way the fortunate ones, as they were eliminating most of the arsenic as quickly as they were taking it in). Indeed, many patients were no longer drinking any beer at all by the time they sought medical help, having given up the drink 'because it was not "agreeing" with them'. Diarrhoea, sometimes tinged with blood, was another early sign of arsenical beer consumption.[8]

Next came the standard running of the eyes and nose ('often with tears visibly overflowing', in some instances 'so marked that the sufferers are constantly mopping the running eyes'), along with bronchitis and hoarseness. Multiple skin problems appeared about this time as well, and in one form or another affected nearly all cases. In many victims, the skin developed a reddish hue ('as if stained with red ink'), which steadily darkened to copper, then to bronze, and in exceptional cases nearly to black, 'so that many of the patients resemble mulattoes'. 'Vagabond pigmentation' was another description of the darker colouring (there actually was a formal diagnostic category of 'vagabond's disease', *Morbus reorum*, applied to the dark, rough skin often found affecting homeless people infested with vermin). Among Salford drinkers affected by darkening of the skin, the condition came to be called 'khaki disease'. By whatever name, the discoloration tended to be more pronounced about the neck, in the armpits, on the nipples, around the abdomen, and on the genitals and buttocks, while the face was often only slightly affected (Fig. 9 shows an extreme example of this contrast). Poisoned drinkers were often believed at first examination to have Addison's disease, while at other times they were simply presumed to be uncommonly dirty: after all, 'the majority of these cases...belonged to the lower classes, in whom personal cleanliness is usually non-existent'. Some doctors found it impossible to distinguish between arsenical pigmentation and dirty skin 'without...a vigorous application of soap and water' (one of

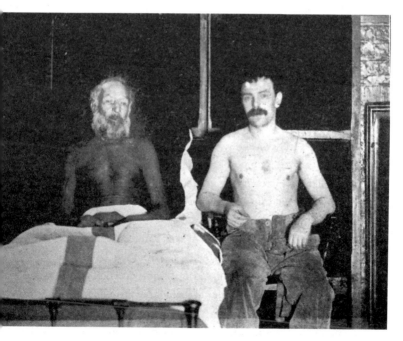

9. Man with contrasting skin colouration caused by arsenical beer

the nurses at the Salford Infirmary complained that one patient 'was washed three times without visible improvement'). Within those dirty areas, however, patches of normal skin could remain, resulting in a spotted appearance (Fig. 10). Most wondrous of all to behold was that not only did the skin colour resemble that of mulattoes, 'but the texture of the skin takes on the same beautifully soft velvety feel to the touch, quite different from that of normal English skin'.[9]

Eventually, however, the pigmented skin became scaly and often so loose that it could be removed easily by rubbing—or left to shed of its own accord. 'I have seen it so plentiful', one doctor reported, 'as to give rise to a conspicuous deposit on the bed-sheet.' Keratoses, often referred to as 'arsenical warts', often appeared on the skin, particularly on the hands and feet. 'Whoever has seen a well-marked arsenical palm', a Liverpool practitioner stated, 'is not likely to forget it.' The palm appeared 'simian rather than human', was 'clammy with excessive perspiration', deeply lined and red in colour, 'tough and resistant' in texture, and 'studded with little nodules'. An arsenical sole was even more unattractive, its nodules looking like 'pegs of horn driven through the thickened sole', pegs that 'at length break away and leave deep pits behind' (Fig. 11). Blister-like eruptions ranging in size from a pinhead to circles of several inches in diameter broke out on many, eventually rupturing and spilling their contents, and leaving scar-like marks behind. Finally, the once soft and velvety skin grew thicker, making it difficult to close the hands.[10]

Unfortunate as were the various skin conditions, the bulk of patients' suffering came from neurological damages, to both the sensory and the motor nerves. The onset of this stage was signalled by tingling in the fingers and toes (one patient reported that his hands felt as though 'he were about to take hold of a battery';

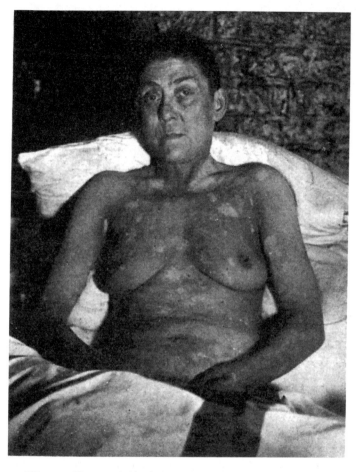

10. Woman with spotted skin due to arsenical beer

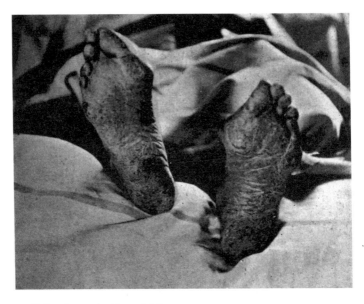

11. Soles of arsenical beer drinker

another joked he had foot and mouth disease, because his feet began
to tingle after beer passed through his mouth). Tingling soon grew
to pricking pains and burning sensations, bringing about severe
discomfort in the feet particularly (in one town near Manchester,
the local beer had come to be called 'tender-foot ale'). Some likened the sensation to a feeling that 'dogs were gnawing... the soles
of their feet', for others it seemed they were 'walking on hot bricks'.
In a few patients the pain was so severe as to require morphine.
Later, numbness would develop in the hands and feet, so that sufferers could be recognized by their habit of rubbing their fingers
together to restore feeling.[11]

But if fingers were numb, arms and legs became extremely
sensitive to pressure as nerves grew inflamed. Even 'light pressure

produced most exquisite pain and caused the patients to scream out';
many complained they could not stand the weight of their bedclothes
upon them. Reynolds maintained he could do an instant diagnosis
of arsenical neuritis simply by squeezing a patient's leg and observing the 'sudden expression of pain' on his or her face. This hyperaes-
thesia of the limbs proved the most enduring symptom, commonly
lasting three months or more after the end of exposure to arsenic; in
some cases the sensitivity continued for nearly a year.[12]

These sensory ailments were paralleled by motor disturbances
in an estimated 70 per cent of cases. The muscles of the limbs atro-
phied, making walking so 'painful and difficult [that] the patients
progress slowly in a gingerly and halting manner'; even when simply standing, 'the patient shuffles from one foot to another, and
seeks support by leaning against anything convenient'. Other muscles were similarly enfeebled, those of the trunk becoming so weak
patients could not lift themselves up in bed. Paralysis of certain
muscles supervened, most commonly those of the ankle, producing
a gait that in itself was diagnostic of arsenic poisoning: one had
merely to listen for 'the "double-rap" step...the heel coming
down first, quickly followed by a sudden (not gradual, as in health)
descent of the anterior part of the foot and so making the second
rap'. Some lost the ability to walk altogether and became confined
to bed, but even the upright victims were easy to spot 'from their
tearful expression as they...shuffle about the house and loiter at
street-corners'. The combination of muscular degeneration and
chronic pain surely accounts for the marked decline in the birth
rate observed in Manchester and other northern communities nine
months after the peak of the epidemic.[13]

Physical deterioration was likely to be accompanied by mental
decay. Patients commonly exhibited a 'peculiar waking dream-like
state', along with memory loss, first of time, then of place, leading

to what some physicians called 'confusional insanity'. In advanced cases, it was reported that 'any suggestion, however absurd, is at once accepted' by the patient: thus a paralysed man restricted to bed for weeks 'when asked if he has not been for a walk this morning will say that he has and will tell you with much circumstance where he has been'.[14]

Such sad cases of poisoning were not, moreover, confined to Manchester and Salford. They existed in Bacup, and by the end of the year reports of beer poisoning were flowing in from many other sites, from Liverpool, Lancaster, Leicester, Lichfield, Preston, and Chester, as well as from numerous smaller towns and villages spread through most of the counties of the Midlands and North. The outbreak remained known as the 'Manchester epidemic', though, not just because the first cases had been recognized in that city, but also because there had been more cases (upwards of 2,000) occurring there than anywhere else. By the time the epidemic had run its course, an investigative body determined, the cases totalled at least 6,000, 'and probably the number was in fact very considerably greater'. At least seventy ended in death, with 'an altogether disproportionate number' of fatalities occurring among women. This gender imbalance was accounted for by the fact that men took their beer in public houses and tended to frequent several different ones, some of which sold beers not contaminated with arsenic; thus their total intake of the poison was diluted. But women, bowing to the convention that ladies did not linger in the rowdy, masculine domain of the pub, drank their beer at home, and commonly obtained it from a single nearby tavern. Those who picked the wrong tavern took in arsenic with every glass. Often, moreover, they took many glasses. In Liverpool, at least, 'it was the custom for these women to congregate in each other's houses and send for cheap beer during the whole of the day'. By doing their drinking off premises, women received what publicans called 'the long pull', that is, 'a good deal more beer than they asked for'. In the end, this was not the bargain it appeared.[15]

*

The bad news was broken to the public on 23 November, through a *Manchester Guardian* headline announcing the appearance of 'A Peculiar Epidemic'. Lengthy stories followed daily in the press, unsettling the public with announcements of 'excitement and alarm' and of 'the dangers that lie wait for them in the pint-pot'. On 26 November, the first two deaths from arsenical beer were reported, and soon after it was observed that 'the consumption of fourpenny ale was not a fraction so great as it had been a fortnight previously'. Arsenic had become a godsend for anti-alcohol organizations, an opportunity to demonize drink in even darker hues. Thus when Sir Wilfred Lawson delivered his presidential address to the annual meeting of the United Kingdom Alliance, Britain's largest temperance society, serendipitously scheduled for Manchester only a fortnight after the discovery of contaminated beer, he opened with the reminder 'that sensible people abstained from alcohol and arsenic (laughter)', as if the two were sure to be found together. *Punch* expanded on his theme with a cartoon showing Sir Wilfred, 'A Gentleman of All Temperance', lifting a glass of the only proper beverage, water, while laying a Shakespearean curse on a stupefied drinker slouched by the tavern door: 'I would have him poisoned with a pot of ale,' he recites from *Henry the Fourth, Part 1* (Fig. 12). The loss of taste for beer, however, served not to stimulate a craving for water, but a thirst for whisky instead. A *Guardian* correspondent wrote from Edinburgh that the sudden surge in demand for spirits, coming as it did on top of the usual busy Christmas season, was 'taxing the energies of the whisky merchants to the utmost'. So often is one man's poison another's profit.[16]

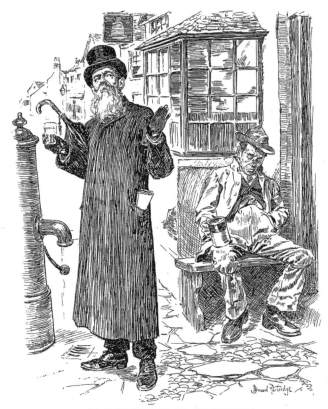

"A GENTLEMAN OF ALL TEMPERANCE."
Measure for Measure, Act III., Sc. 2.

Sir W-lfr-d L-ws-n (with his favourite, and, under certain conditions, harmless beverage, alluding to the beer-drinker). "'I WOULD HAVE HIM POISONED WITH A POT OF ALE!'—AHEM!—SHAKESPEARE!"   *(Vide Henry the Fourth*, Part 1, Act 1, Sc. 3.)

12. 'A Gentleman of All Temperance', Punch cartoon, 1901

The heightened demand for whisky would not last, for Manchester and area physicians had acted quickly to find the source of arsenic in regional beers and remove it. Within two days of Reynolds's announcement of the epidemic, Charles Tattersall, the Medical Officer of Health for Salford, succeeded in tracing the arsenic to the glucose sugar that producers of inexpensive brews substituted for malted barley, the proper source of carbohydrates for fermentation into beer. All the arsenical beers, furthermore, were found to be made with glucose from a single supplier, the Liverpool-area firm of Bostock and Co., sugar purveyor to approximately 200 breweries in the North and Midlands.[17]

Bostock manufactured its glucose by boiling starch in sulphuric acid, a material that, it will be recalled from the preceding chapter's discussion of superphosphate fertilizers, was most economically made using arsenic-containing iron pyrites. That was one of the methods of sulphuric acid manufacture employed by Nicholson's of Leeds, the company on which Bostock depended for its acid (the wide variation in concentration of arsenic in affected beers was due to different brewers replacing different percentages of malt with glucose, and to the mixing of other sugars with Bostock's product in varying proportions). The poisoning outbreak's concentration among the working class was now explained: cheap beer was being made with arsenical sugar in place of good barley malt. Twenty years earlier, interestingly, a notice in *The Times* had informed readers that American brewers often used sugar made with arsenical sulphuric acid, but then hastily assured that since British beer makers employed only natural cane sugar, 'British beer drinkers need not be alarmed.' Times had changed, so much so that consumers of other beverages also had reason for alarm. Just weeks before the first beer poisonings came to light in Manchester, London was set on edge by a brief episode of arsenic poisoning from soda fountain phosphates, an effervescent drink whose preparation involved sulphuric acid.[18]

While it is difficult to feel kindly towards any brewer who would use glucose in place of barley, respect does have to be granted to Manchester beer producers for their readiness to confront the problem they had created. 'Although they could not believe that beer by any possibility could be the cause,' Tattersall related, 'they threw open their breweries to me without the slightest reserve, and were most anxious that the whole matter should be cleared up ... as quickly as possible.' Indeed, by the end of the very day of Reynolds's announcement that arsenic had been found in beer, the Manchester Brewers' Central Association had appointed a committee, with representation from the medical profession as well as the brewing industry, to address the situation.[19]

The committee soon recommended two steps. First, all beers that had been made with Bostock sugar had to be recalled and destroyed if found to contain arsenic. Thousands of barrels of beer were soon being emptied into the sewers of Manchester (in the process introducing a new method of distributing arsenic as rat poison), as well as those of Salford, Liverpool, and other cities that quickly followed the lead. In the end, hundreds of thousands of gallons of beer were destroyed in this way, 267,000 in Liverpool alone. The largest brewer in Manchester, Groves and Whitnall, claimed that the value of the thousands of barrels the firm voluntarily poured out was no less than £15,000. Second, brewers were enjoined to stop using Bostock sugar and not to sell any new batches of beer until a professional analyst had certified them to be free of arsenic.[20]

Following the committee's recommendations was, of course, a matter of self-interest for brewers, and for publicans too: any retailer knowingly selling an injurious food product was liable to punishment under the 1875 Sale of Food and Drugs Act. Arsenical beer was still being discovered on occasion into the early months of the next year (and tavern owners involved prosecuted and fined), but by the end of January it was generally agreed that poisonous brew was no longer a serious worry. Anxiety was revived in mid-February, when twenty-two young men at a racing stable came down with arsenic poisoning after an evening of swilling ale. It was soon determined, however, that the fault was theirs, not the brewer's; somehow they had managed to contaminate their beer with arsenic stored in the stable for killing rats.[21]

In matters of negligence, however, the standard had already been set by Messrs. Bostock and Nicholson. At an inquest held in Liverpool in early 1901, to determine if either firm was criminally culpable of manslaughter, it was explained that Nicholson produced two grades of sulphuric acid, an arsenic-containing product and a 'dearsenicated' one: this latter, the company boasted, was 'the purest acid on the face of the earth'. It was also the acid they had supplied to Bostock for years, until March 1900, that is. At that juncture, Nicholson's found itself pressed to meet growing demands for dearsenicated acid. Hoping to free up increased amounts of the pure acid, the two brothers who ran the company reviewed all their contracts to see if anyone was receiving the pure product who had not specifically requested it, with the intent of replacing such orders with pyrite acid. Bostock, it was discovered, had never ordered arsenic-free acid, nor had the company stated what the acid was to be used for. Nicholson's would never 'have dreamt of sending them the unpurified acid' if they had known it was to be utilized in food products: 'It would have been murder to have sent it.' So it turned out to be.[22]

Nicholson's, of course, were not about to accept guilt, even though chemists determined their acid was contaminated with arsenic 'to an exceptional and enormous degree'. The Bostock people, they argued, should have told them they were using the acid to manufacture a foodstuff. They also should have noticed that the pyrite acid had a brownish tinge, quite different from the clear acid they had received previously, and that the glucose produced from it was similarly discoloured. Surely any responsible food manufacturer would follow a policy of analysing his products for contaminants, especially if their colour had changed. Yet Bostock had not only sold toxic sugar to brewers, the firm also used it to manufacture its own line of fruit-flavoured 'Table Syrups'. In 1900, the company sent trial samples of two-pound tins of the treacle-like concoction to retailers, unaware that each tin contained two grains of arsenic. In this instance, however, the public were spared, for Bostock had been careless in another manufacturing step, and the syrups had crystallized by the time grocers opened them; the samples were returned before falling into the hands of consumers. When the company came to be incriminated in the beer epidemic, its stock of 14 tons of poisonous syrups was uncovered—and burned.[23]

With respect to brewing glucose, the inquest jury agreed that Bostock 'were to blame for not notifying that the acid was required for food purposes'. That did not amount to a criminal degree of negligence, though, nor did Nicholson's behaviour: while the acid manufacturers had shown 'extreme indifference', it had not been 'reckless' indifference. Both companies received a scolding, but no punishment was levied, at least not by the court. The marketplace was less forgiving. There was a precipitous drop in Bostock's stock as sales evaporated. At the same time, the business was successfully sued by more than one brewer for recovery of the cost of beer poured down the drain (as well as for fees paid to chemical analysts and the expenses of circulars sent to pubs warning of arsenic in their beers). In a typical case, in Manchester in February 1901, Bostock was fined nearly £1,400. In the meantime, the glucose-maker's own legal action against Nicholson's failed. The company was insolvent by spring.[24]

The Manchester epidemic was not the first instance of mass poisoning by an arsenicated beverage. In 1828, the mysterious *épidémie de Paris* killed, according to one surely inflated estimate, 40,000 residents along the banks of the Seine over a period of several months; only years later was it decided the *épidémie* had been caused by arsenic-contaminated wine. More recently, in 1888, a wine merchant in Hyères, in the south of France, had mistaken arsenic for the plaster of Paris commonly used to clarify wine. As had happened when the same mistake was made with lozenges in Bradford, hundreds of people sickened, and three died.[25]

But those had been one-off contaminations confined to single locations. In Manchester and other stricken areas, poisoning had gone on for several months before it was recognized that arsenic, not alcohol, was responsible, and it now seemed likely to some physicians that the poison had been attacking beer drinkers for years. As early as 1879, Alexander Blyth, the nation's foremost food chemist, had warned that the growing use of glucose in place of malt could introduce arsenic into beer, but no heed had been taken. By the end of 1900, though, it was retrospectively evident that some of those many cases of *alcoholic* neuritis diagnosed over the years must actually have been attacks of *arsenical* neuritis. A few doctors were so taken by this possibility as to argue that perhaps all the cases had been misdiagnosed, that 'alcoholic neuritis' had never actually existed but had all along been low-level arsenic poisoning; only with the introduction of greater amounts of arsenic into beer in 1900, with many more people affected and the severity and scope of symptoms increased, did the arsenic disease become apparent. This was, however, a minority opinion, and a short-lived one too, for while diagnoses of alcoholic neuritis did drop significantly in frequency after arsenic was removed from beer, they did not disappear altogether: the disease was, in fact, real. Equally short-lived was the proposal of several Chester physicians that the 1900 epidemic was actually an outbreak of beriberi, soon after to be demonstrated to be a deficiency of the vitamin thiamine.[26]

*

However much it distressed the medical community, arsenical beer was music to the ear for another group. For twenty years before the Manchester outbreak, a national Pure Beer Movement had been pressing for legislation to prohibit the sale of beer that contained any ingredients other than the four fundamentals: barley malt, yeast, hops, and water. That recipe had been the standard in olden days, but in 1847 Parliament granted brewers permission to substitute sugar for malt, enabling them to produce beer at lower cost and thus increase their sales to the working classes. In 1880, the door was opened still wider, Parliament enacting the so-called 'free mash-tun' system, which allowed brewers to add to the mash—the mixture of fermentable starches to be transformed into beer—any materials desired providing they were not injurious. Rice and maize now came into common use, though in much smaller amounts than sugar. Even so, the free mash-tun crossed a line in the minds of ale traditionalists. It seemed to presage a complete abandonment of standards, a spiralling degeneration of quality. By 1900, grumbling over the degraded state of British ale was everywhere to be heard. 'Public taste has been educated to accept beers which would have been rejected by our forefathers,' one critic sniffed, while another opined that 'no persons now living have ever tasted' properly made ale, 'or would greatly relish [it] if it were unexpectedly placed before them'. The latter was something of an overstatement, as roughly half the nation's several thousand breweries still professed to turn out a substitute-free product. Nevertheless, that percentage was decreasing, and it was not unreasonable for those who did relish the genuine article to fear that in time it might be swept away entirely by the flood of cheap and inferior brew.[27]

This was a threat with profound cultural implications, for good beer was synonymous with Great Britain, the symbolic lifeblood of the greatest empire on earth, 'the very ark', as an MP proclaimed in 1896, 'of the British Constitution'. Ale was the historic sustenance of British yeomanry, a fact set forth most vividly in 1751 by Hogarth in 'Gin Lane' and 'Beer Street', engravings that contrasted the physical decay and moral dissipation of spirit drinkers with the robust health and bounding prosperity of those pledged to malt and hops. The latter picture was inscribed with a moral:

> Beer, happy Produce of our Isle
> Can sinewy Strength impart,
> And wearied with Fatigue and Toil
> Can chear each manly Heart....
> Genius of Health, thy grateful Taste
> Rivals the Cup of Jove,
> And warms each English generous Breast
> With Liberty and Love.

This Genius of Health, further, nourished the spirit as fully as the body. 'Inspired by thee,' mused John Gay,

> ...the warrior fights,
> The lover woos, the poet writes
> And pens the pleasing tale;
> And still in Britain's isle confest
> Nought animates the patriot's breast
> Like generous, nappy ale.

Ale was an inalienable part of the national patrimony. Only in Britain did crowds welcome in the New Year with hymns to beer, singing 'Up with the sale of it, Down with a pail of it, Glorious, glorious beer.' But beer could not be made glorious with glucose.[28]

Such was the fervent belief of gustatory and cultural purists, though they were, sadly, as much a minority then as today. The reality, as another MP pronounced in 1896, was that 'the average consumer is quite indifferent as to whether his beer comes from barley or from sugar. All that he wants is "good strong stuff" to make him drunk.' Spokesmen for the Pure Beer Movement appreciated that fact. They recognized the political value of rhetorical homage to tradition ('Englishmen are a beer-drinking race, and pure beer is a thing they always wish for'), but their tributes to ale as the quintessentially British beverage were at bottom only so much lip-service. Their hearts were elsewhere. The Movement should therefore not be mistaken for an early version of the Campaign for Real Ale that has so dramatically improved quality and choice in beers since the 1970s. Those who marched under the banner of Pure Beer were concerned much less about the flavour of ale and the satisfaction of discriminating drinkers than they were with the economic well-being of barley growers.[29]

By the last third of the nineteenth century, English agriculture was in a bad way, the importation of cheap grain from North America and Argentina having sharply depressed the demand for home-grown cereal crops; the price of barley actually dropped by a third during this period. The Pure Beer agitation, launched by Parliamentary representatives from agricultural constituencies in reaction to the free mash-tun law of 1880, aimed to force all brewers to employ barley malt exclusively for the purpose of increasing the demand for that grain, thereby raising its price, and consequently rescuing farmers from being driven off the land. Without a law banning the substitution of sugar, rice, and other materials for malt, British barley growers would, it was predicted, 'become as extinct as the dodo or the wooly-haired mammoth'.[30]

Yet while Pure Beer proponents brought bills before Parliament throughout the 1880s and early 1890s, they were consistently turned back by the brewing industry's position that the movement was not at all about pure beer and consumer welfare, but simply about 'barley beer', meaning the interests of barley farmers. Not until 1896 did their dogged efforts start to show some hope of success, yet even then sponsors were persuaded it would be best to withdraw their latest bill in favour of the appointment of an expert committee to investigate the question and issue a report and recommendations. The expectation was that this body would provide independent support to the cause and improve its chances of victory. The hope proved illusory. The committee, whose deliberations were protracted by the collection of testimony from numerous individuals in the brewing industry as well as the Pure Beer Movement, at last submitted its 428-page report in 1899. Its conclusions were that maintaining a government watch over all the ingredients added to the mash-tun in all the nation's breweries would be prohibitively expensive, and that once fermentation had been completed and a beer released onto the market, it was next to impossible to determine chemically if its alcohol had come from barley or glucose. A Pure Beer law, in short, was unaffordable and unenforceable and, a majority argued, unnecessary as well, for in the end, the only sense of 'pure' that really mattered was that beer be free of any injurious ingredients. None of the materials currently being used in the manufacture of beer were harmful, the committee determined, and even if deleterious ingredients did occur, they 'are so infrequent and unimportant that legislation is not required to deal with them'. The very next year came the Manchester epidemic.[31]

'Providence has intervened,' a Pure Beer campaigner rejoiced shortly before Christmas 1900, through the Manchester epidemic, an event that exploded the Parliamentary committee's conclusion that the materials in glucose beers were 'unimportant'. It seemed to barley beer's champions that the 'lamentable visitation' of arsenic had demonstrated beyond doubt the necessity of making beer free of substitutes. Had northern brewers been making ale as tradition decreed, the tragic epidemic would never have occurred. Seizing fortune by the forelock, the Pure Beer Movement's commander, Sir Cuthbert Quilter, MP for Sudbury, in the barley-growing county of Suffolk, hammered this point home again and again in the aftermath of the Manchester outbreak. The victims of arsenical beer should not be allowed to die in vain, he demanded, and they would not, if the people would stand up and 'impress unmistakably upon the Government how vitally their interests are concerned with the purity of the national beverage'.[32]

A cartoon printed in a Manchester newspaper reinforced Quilter's message (Fig. 13). Under the heading of 'Pro Bono Publico', two potent emblems of national identity confront one another. John Bull, the representative of traditional British values, is shown upbraiding John Barleycorn, the symbol of malt and its derivatives beer and whisky. While Barleycorn props himself idly against a cask of 'Ye Goode Olde Ale', Bull, holding a press account of the beer epidemic, demands that he 'stir up and give us a good old fashioned brew'. Through an archway behind can be seen a 'Modern Chemist' working at his lab bench concocting the new-fashioned brew made from sulphuric acid, saccharine, and—yes —arsenic. 'You are leaving too much to the youngster yonder,' the one John reproves the other, hoping to rouse him to fight back against the degradation of the national drink.[33]

Barleycorn did not actually stir up and get to work, but barley growers certainly did. By early January, agents of the Pure Beer League, led by Quilter, were busy circulating petitions throughout

Pro Bono Publico.

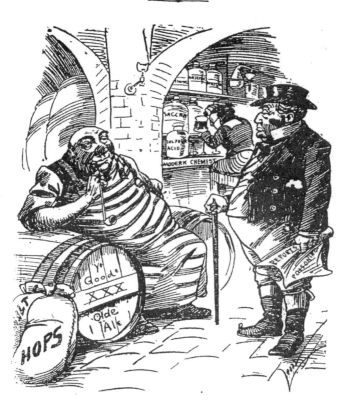

John Bull to John Barleycorn: "Come, John, stir up and give us a good old fashioned brew. You are leaving too much to the youngster yonder."

13. 'Pro Bono Publico', Manchester Evening Mail cartoon, 1900

the countryside, soliciting signatures calling on Parliament to enact a pure beer law. More than 200 of these documents were collected, and in some villages, it was reported, 'every elector has signed for pure beer'. Similar demands issued from Chambers of Agriculture in rural towns, and other organizations protective of farming interests. Yet if the battle was carried primarily by farmers, city labourers were hardly indifferent. They were upset by being the chief victims of toxic beer, of course, but were riled perhaps even more by the perception that neglect of pure beer legislation was yet one more instance of discrimination against the working classes. 'If the upper classes found their wines and beverages contained noxious things', it was put forth at a Shropshire rally, if 'they thought they were being poisoned, there would soon be a great uproar'. In February 1901, a new Pure Beer Bill was introduced for Parliamentary debate.[34]

The arsenic scare pumped new life into the Pure Beer Movement, but the rejuvenation was not to last. The Movement's vigour was undermined from the start by the fact that by 1900 many drinkers (some said most) had acquired a taste for the lighter beers made with glucose and other barley substitutes. They had been encouraged, further, by medical assurances that such beers were good for them, as they did not cause 'the heaviness, drowsiness, stupidity, and headache which so commonly follow the consumption of heavy ales'. There was scant political support to be gathered for denying drinkers what they wanted, and the framers of the newest Pure Beer Bill had little choice but to retreat to the principle that the consumer should at the minimum be informed of what ingredients had been used to make his beer. Hence it was now proposed only that brewers be required to label their product 'malt beer' (read 'Pure Beer') or, if malt substitutes were involved, 'part malt beer'. The concession was made grudgingly, Quilter sneering that a buyer of the latter could 'get a liquor made of anything, and will have to accept the risk'. Such a law also, of course, would do nothing to boost the demand for homegrown barley.[35]

Nor was the barley cause helped by the discovery made just a week before Christmas 1900. Less than a month after Bostock glucose had been identified as the source of arsenic in North-country beers, a Manchester chemist investigating the epidemic announced that he had also detected the poison in many samples of barley malt used by area brewers. He was at first uncertain of the origin of the arsenic in the malts, but soon determined it was introduced in the process of drying the grain. The time-honoured method of preparing malt was to dry it in an oast-house in which the material was spread across a floor of perforated tiles or netting above a room in which a coke or anthracite fire was maintained. The heat from the fire rose through the malt and out through a chimney in the cone-shaped roof. Coke was the preferred source of heat among northern brewers (it was cheaper in their region), but it contained large concentrations of pyrites (hence arsenic), and the poison was conveyed to the malt in the rising fumes. Arsenic 'in considerable quantities' was found in nearly half the fifty samples of malt tested, though nearly a third of the malts showed no trace of the poison.[36]

Similar findings were soon announced by other chemists, to the disgust of Pure Beer advocates, who smelled a rat. How fortunate it was, one commented in mock amazement, that those brewers who used sugar had made their discovery of arsenic in malt just 'in the nick of time' to save their debased product from being singled out as dangerous. Quilter saw arsenical malt as 'merely a red herring drawn across the path', for, he believed, concentrations of arsenic were so low that a person 'would have to drink a thousand bar-rels of beer' before he would have to worry about being poisoned.

To those capable of objectivity, however, it was evident that 'Pure Beer' would not necessarily be any more pure than glucose beer, and offering drinkers an all-malt beer would leave them 'just as far from getting rid of arsenic in beer as we are now'. Dramatic confirmation of that conclusion was provided in Yorkshire in January 1902, when—*pace* Quilter—several cases of poisoning, and two fatalities, were traced to arsenic in beer made entirely with malt—malt dried over coke.[37]

This turn of events prompted calls from some parties to develop other procedures for drying malt, though brewers by and large were convinced that the time-tested method was essential for flavour, so turned instead to the replacement of coke with low-arsenic anthracite, and to efforts to remove the arsenic from the dried barley. The poison was not absorbed into the grain, after all, but merely rested on the surface and ought to be easily brushed off. 'Scores of thousands of pounds', by one estimate, were soon invested in machinery to 'polish' malt free of arsenic before it went into the mash-tun, and with completely gratifying results—dried malt was soon free of arsenic. Brewers nevertheless worried that the poison might find its way into their tuns from other sources, and frantically instituted every measure they could think of to keep every trace of it away from their premises. Poor brewers, an industrial chemist sighed, 'at present arsenic was their *bête noir*'.[38]

The idea that beer made from barley and hops exclusively was the only pure beer nevertheless continued to unravel. Some worried that barley grown in soil that had been treated with superphosphate fertilizers might absorb at least traces of arsenic. Reports that hops, beer's other main ingredient, could be contaminated with arsenic, albeit in 'minute' amounts, began to appear (hops were treated with sulphur dioxide as a preservative, and the sulphur used to make the gas sometimes contained arsenic). From Bacup came another announcement from John Brown, that the rubber used for the tubes that conveyed beer from the barrel to the tap often contained arsenic, so that beer that stood overnight in the tubing could absorb appreciable quantities of the poison. It paid not to get to the pub too early in the day, before the previous night's leftovers had been dispensed to less-enlightened drinkers. There was, however, no time guaranteed safe from another form of contamination. 'The iniquitous and antiquated pump or pull system' used to serve beer was famously difficult to keep clean. 'Some beer pulls taken out the other day in the south-west of England', *The Times* announced, 'were actually found to be moving inside with bacteria, the smells being so bad when the pulls were dismantled that the men at work as well as the inmates of the publichouse concerned turned quite ill and had to go outside for a time.' Beer had nevertheless been served to patrons 'through these abominations up till the time they were dismantled'.[39]

The original goal of the Pure Beer movement—a traditional, all-barley brew—was now obscured by a swarm of new possibilities of injury: the meaning of pure beer had been reconfigured as beer free of arsenic or other contaminants from *any* source, not just glucose, and brewed from *any* non-toxic ingredients that produced an ale agreeable to consumers. But that was hardly the only reason for the failure of the Pure Beer Bill in the 1901 session of Parliament. Ultimately, what finished off the Pure Beer campaign was another by-product of the arsenic scare.

*

On 11 January 1901, the government announced the appointment of a Royal Commission 'to inquire into arsenical poisoning from the consumption of beer'. Chaired by the renowned physicist Lord Kelvin, the Commission interviewed four dozen physicians, chemists, and representatives of the brewing industry. Their collective testimony, presented in a 1903 report, came to more than 300 double-columned, small-print pages. Analysis of all that evidence led Commission members to the conclusion that injurious quantities of arsenic could readily be prevented in beer, and other foods, by conscientious manufacturers. Nevertheless, harmless trace amounts (such as sometimes found on hops) might occasionally be introduced despite producers' best efforts. Indeed, when small quantities of arsenic were present in the very air of cities, thanks to the burning of coal, how could any product be kept completely free of the poison? As was pointed out by a chemist, 'one could find arsenic in almost anything if one only took enough of it'. Thus if retailers were to be spared unjust prosecution under the Sale of Food and Drugs Act for selling beer (or any food) containing a deleterious ingredient, the government could not require 100 per cent purity. Rather, it was necessary to set an upper limit on the concentration of arsenic that would be recognized as safe for consumers and attainable by manufacturers. Any product found to hold a higher level could be acted against as deleterious.[40]

This idea of establishing a 'tolerance' for arsenic was not new with the Royal Commission. In the early 1880s, the Swedish government enacted a statute relating to fabrics that prohibited the sale of items containing more than 0.0009 per cent arsenic by weight, or roughly an ounce of arsenic per seventy pounds of material. In one instance, a carpet was condemned for having a thousandth of a grain of arsenic per sixteen square yards of fabric. Such stringency caused 'great trouble and annoyance', naturally, for British wool producers doing business with Sweden. Their attachment to arsenical sheep dips made it next to impossible to manufacture wool that could pass the Swedish requirement, and there was much muttering among sheep-men over the unreasonableness of Scandinavians. In 1900, the American state of Massachusetts adopted a broader law, one that restricted the concentration of arsenic in woven fabrics and wallpapers to a tenth of a grain per square yard, and in dress fabrics to a hundredth of a grain per yard.[41]

Yet while proposals for a comparable standard for wallpaper had been presented in Britain as early as 1883 (by the National Health Society committee discussed in Ch. 8), it was left to the Royal Commission twenty years later to lay down an arsenic tolerance that would be officially accepted. Determining precisely what the tolerance should be, however, was not the most straightforward procedure. The concentration of arsenic in beer and other foods that might be considered a safe level was affected, after all, by a number of variables. Age, sex, body size, and general state of health were all factors in influencing whether or not an individual would suffer injury. So was a person's drinking and eating proclivities: the ten-pint-a-day beer drinker was at notably more risk than the man who took only the occasional glass. Not least among the uncertainties was the nebulous entity of individual susceptibility. Some people were by nature much more disposed to damage from arsenic than others, and if all members of society were to be protected, a figure that was harmless to even the most vulnerable had to be adopted.

These considerations were much debated by physicians in the aftermath of the beer epidemic, and aired even more thoroughly in the hearings of the Royal Commission. In the end, it was decided by the Commission that 1/100 grain of arsenic per gallon or pound was adequate to protect consumers from poisoning. The Commission's recommendation was at once adopted in Britain for purposes of enforcement of the Sale of Food and Drugs Act, and was so quickly accepted by other European countries it was soon being recognized as the 'world tolerance'. In 1927, it would be made the American standard as well, and ultimately would be embraced by the World Health Organization. Further, the setting of tolerances for many other potentially harmful substances would become standard policy among food regulatory agencies in Western countries during the twentieth century. The arsenical beer epidemic was also the stimulus for the 1905 establishment within the British government of a 'Foods Section' charged with stricter monitoring of all aspects of food purity.[42]

In the meantime, the Pure Beer Movement had been derailed. The meetings of the Royal Commission, presided over by its prestigious scientific members, were widely publicized. Physicians were kept abreast of the deliberations by regular reports in *The Lancet*, while the public was informed of the goings-on at every session by articles in the popular press. The notice and respect accorded the Commission meant that once it framed the investigation to include all sources of arsenic in beer, not just glucose, public and Parliamentary attention would be diverted from Pure Beer's fixation on all-barley brews. The Commission's inquiry was the final stroke in redefining purity to mean absence of harmful amounts of arsenic rather than presence of malt and malt only. Pure Beer protagonists would struggle on for another quarter-century, but never again come close to victory.

*

In the aftermath of the Manchester beer epidemic, Britain's Society of Chemical Industry met for a lengthy discussion of the ongoing threat of arsenical sulphuric acid. The nation produced more than a million tons of the material every year, and since nearly all of it was derived from pyrites, some 1,800 tons of arsenic annually found its way into the marketplace. As one Society member cautioned, it was imperative to purify the acid in order to preclude any 'possibility of mischief in the future'.[43]

Sulphuric acid would in fact soon be cleaned up, but that hardly prevented all future mischief from arsenic. First, the poison continued in use for homicide and suicide, not nearly as extensively as in the previous century, to be sure, and only rarely after the 1920s. Nevertheless, there has been a conviction for arsenical murder in Britain as recently as 1992, when Zoora Shah was found guilty of killing her abusive husband in—where else?—Bradford. Still more recently, in 2007 a California woman was convicted of using arsenic to kill her husband for insurance benefits. The verdict was overturned the following year, however, when, in echo of the Smethurst trial, it was discovered that chemists had botched the analysis of the dead man's viscera and wrongly reported arsenic. The original conviction clearly was influenced as well by revelations of a degree of sexual promiscuity by the accused that scandalized even a twenty-first-century jury—much as Eliza Fenning and Florence Maybrick had been convicted partly as punishment for sexual impropriety.[44]

Arsenical homicide also continued as a plot device in literature, the most entertaining example being Dorothy Sayers's *Strong Poison* (1930). There the villain, Urquhart, is cast as an arsenic-eater in the Styrian mould, immune to ordinary lethal doses of the poison. Thus when he kills his victim with a toxic omelette, he appears above suspicion because he too has partaken of the dish and not been affected. But then detective Lord Peter Wimsey notices Urquhart's clear complexion and sleek hair, applies the Marsh test to some strands of that hair, and exposes the killer's clever scheme.[45]

Arsenic poisoning through accident also became much less common as crude white arsenic was replaced as a vermin-killer by commercial preparations in liquid form not mistakable for flour or sugar. Mishaps nevertheless do still occur from time to time, as in St Andrew's in 1943, when two people died and more than 150 were made ill by contaminated sausages. Soon after, in France in 1952, a replay of the violet powder poisonings of the 1870s took place when more than seventy infants were killed and nearly 300 injured when arsenic was confused with zinc oxide in the manufacture of talcum powder. Three years later in Japan, some 12,000 babies were poisoned and 130 killed by powdered milk. The manufacturer of the milk preparation used sodium phosphate as a stabilizer and, as had happened with Manchester glucose, some batches of phosphate had not been rid of arsenical impurity.[46]

Clothing is no longer made with arsenic-containing fabrics, but museum curators nevertheless have to wear protective gloves and masks when handling Victorian gowns, or wallpapers, taxidermy specimens, and other historical artefacts. Arsenical wallpaper production has likewise ceased, yet there remains an enormous amount of toxic paper, and paint, in houses dating to Victorian times. In 1931, two Gloucestershire children were killed by arsenical paper applied decades earlier, and in 1954, the American ambassador to Italy, Clare Booth Luce, was sickened by green paint that flaked off the ceiling of her residence in Rome (a villa once described all too accurately as one of 'Borgian splendour'). Within the past decade, a *Lancet* author has estimated that hundreds of thousands of pounds are still being spent annually for removal of arsenical papers and paints by people renovating nineteenth-century houses.[47]

In the meantime, a new residential application of arsenic developed, that of preserving wood intended for outdoor use with chromated copper arsenate, or CCA. Since the 1970s, most verandas (decks), playground equipment, and picnic furniture have been made from CCA-treated wood. Not until the end of the century, however, did it become evident that CCA-arsenic can be rubbed off in small amounts by contact and liberated in somewhat greater quantities by sanding, sawing, and the action of the elements. A number of non-fatal cases of poisoning similar to those suffered by Victorians in green gowns and green rooms have been recorded in recent years. Although manufacture of arsenicated wood was halted at the end of 2003, more than sixty million homes in America still have a deck or veranda built with the material, which, environmental scientists assure, 'will be a health hazard for generations to come'.[48]

A far more serious hazard is posed by water. Arsenic at harmful levels occurs naturally in water sources in various parts of the world, particularly in sections of Argentina, Chile, and Taiwan. The most heavily exposed population, however, is in Bangladesh and the Indian state of West Bengal, unfortunate victims of the best of intentions. The region has long experienced high childhood mortality from intestinal infections caused by polluted surface water. In 1972, the United Nations Children's Fund (UNICEF) launched a programme of well construction to provide access to non-infectious ground water. The method promoted was tube well drilling, which involves sinking roughly two-inch-diameter metal tubes into the ground to a depth of several hundred feet, and installing a hand pump in the top. UNICEF provided nearly a million tube wells in the early years, and private industry quickly followed, until there are now around ten million wells in Bangladesh alone. Child mortality has been halved.[49]

The unintended consequence is that germs have been replaced by poison, by arsenic taken into the water from deep-lying iron ore deposits. Present at levels as high as 2,000 parts per billion, 200 times the recognized safe concentration, arsenic is now causing an increase of skin and other cancers that an epidemiologist studying the problem has declared 'the largest mass poisoning of a population in history'. Given the average twenty-year interim between the initiation of consumption of arsenical water and the appearance of cancer, the epidemic will only get worse: it is estimated that a minimum of 350,000 arsenical cancer fatalities will occur in Bangladesh. Efforts are being made to develop new water supplies free of both micro-organisms and arsenic, but the endeavour is expensive; even if it does succeed eventually, there is already a guarantee of an 'environmental disaster...greater than any seen before'.[50]

From the non-CCA-treated veranda of my home in Washington State, I can look across Puget Sound to the former site of one of the largest arsenic smelters in the world. As arsenic production came to a close in Britain at the turn of the twentieth century, American mining companies took over much of the business. For the first half of the 1900s, arsenic manufacture was dominated by the Anaconda Copper Mining Company of Butte, Montana, whose toxic emissions despoiled the landscape and destroyed livestock every bit as thoroughly as the fumes from Devon Great Consols had done. All the while, the company denied causing any injury to health, and even took credit for the beauty of Butte's womenfolk: 'the ladies are very fond of this smoky city...because there is just enough arsenic there to give them a beautiful complexion'.[51]

Anaconda's arsenical ores ran low by mid-century, and the firm was supplanted by the American Smelting and Refining Company (ASARCO) in Ruston, Washington, whose world's-tallest smokestack belched forth hundreds of thousands of pounds of arsenic a year until finally closing (due to falling copper prices) in 1985. By then, ASARCO had spread arsenic over a 1,000-square-mile area, with the bulk of it deposited in the soil of nearby neighbourhoods and the waters of Commencement Bay, an arm of Puget Sound (the toxicity of sediment in this part of the Sound is the inspiration for a local joke about the 'Commencement Bay Salmon Derby': the winner is the person who lands the fish with the most heads).[52]

Since 1983, the area around the smelter has been designated a priority toxic waste clean-up site by America's Environmental

Protection Agency, with more than thirty million dollars being spent thus far on residential soil removal and dredging and capping of sediments in Puget Sound. To be fair, a good bit of the clean-up cost has been paid by the company, though federal regulators have had to hound the firm every step of the way and ASARCO continues to resort to one evasion after another to escape contributing to the considerable work left to be done. In the end, most of the expense of alleviating ASARCO's toxic legacy will fall to taxpayers. Meanwhile, as the ruins of the smelter have been cleared away, the land on which it rested, with stunning views of water and mountains, has become prime real estate. Luxury condominiums have been built, though on grounds that will remain without shade, as any trees would be killed when their roots reached the arsenical subsoil.[53]

*

This book concentrates on arsenic in the nineteenth century, but in doing so it provides a backdrop against which one can consider the myriad chemical threats facing the world today. Every year, new chemical products are welcomed into our domestic, working, and recreational environments, products whose possible toxic effects cannot be clearly foreseen (often they are substances that have never before existed). As with arsenical candles and papers and fabrics, these items will become established in commerce before their dangers are recognized, ensuring that any attempt to curtail their use will be resisted by manufacturers with vested interests in their continuation and fought or ignored by politicians ideologically opposed to government interference with business and/or beholden to powerful lobbying groups. It is a familiar story, one that has been repeated all too often over recent decades. Its first full telling, however, came much earlier, with arsenic's poisoning of Victorian Britain.

ABBREVIATIONS

The following abbreviations are employed for periodicals and newspapers cited in the notes:

AAP	*Allergy and Asthma Proceedings*
ADS	*Archiv für Dermatologie und Syphilis*
AIH	*AMA Archives of Industrial Health*
AJE	*American Journal of Epidemiology*
AJMS	*American Journal of Medical Sciences*
AM	*Archives of Medicine*
AMJ	*Association Medical Journal*
AYR	*All the Year Round*
BJD	*British Journal of Dermatology*
BJIM	*British Journal of Industrial Medicine*
BMJ	*British Medical Journal*
BMSJ	*Boston Medical and Surgical Journal*
BWHO	*Bulletin of the World Health Organization*
CB	*Chemistry in Britain*
CD	*Caduceus*
CEJ	*Chambers's Edinburgh Journal*
CH	*Chemical Heritage*
CJPLSA	*Chambers's Journal of Popular Literature, Science and the Arts*
CN	*The Chemical News*
CS	*Critical Survey*
CTJ	*Chemical Trade Journal and Oil, Paint and Colour Review*
EHP	*Environmental Health Perspectives*
EHR	*Economic History Review*
EMJ	*Edinburgh Medical Journal*
EMSJ	*Edinburgh Medical and Surgical Journal*

EN	*Endeavour*
ENHR	*English Historical Review*
EWJ	*The English Woman's Journal*
FP	*Federation Proceedings*
GH	*Good Housekeeping*
GHR	*Guy's Hospital Reports*
GM	*Gentlemen's Magazine*
HW	*Household Words*
JA	*Journal of Allergy*
JAAD	*Journal of the American Academy of Dermatology*
JAMA	*Journal of the American Medical Association*
JCD	*Journal of Chronic Diseases*
JCE	*Journal of Chemical Education*
JCM	*Journal de Chimie Médicale*
JFH	*Journal of Family History*
JHMAS	*Journal of the History of Medicine and Allied Sciences*
JPET	*Journal of Pharmacology and Experimental Therapeutics*
JRSM	*Journal of the Royal Society of Medicine*
JSCI	*Journal of the Society of Chemical Industry*
LD	*Literary Digest*
LL	*London Lancet*
LMJ	*London Medical Journal*
MG	*Manchester Guardian*
MH	*Medical History*
MLJ	*Medico-legal Journal*
MAPC	*Medical and Philosophical Commentaries*
MPC	*Medical Press and Circular*
MR	*Medical Record*
MSR	*Medical and Surgical Reporter*
MTG	*Medical Times and Gazette*
NEJM	*New England Journal of Medicine*
NG	*National Geographic*
NR	*The Northwest Reporter*
NYT	*New York Times*
PAAAS	*Proceedings of the American Academy of Arts and Sciences*

PH	*Public Health*
PHH	*Pharmaceutical Historian*
PIH	*Pharmacy in History*
PJ	*Pharmaceutical Journal*
PJT	*Pharmaceutical Journal and Transactions*
PMJL	*Provincial Medical Journal Leicester*
PP	*Parliamentary Papers*
PSLT	*Pathological Society of London: Transactions*
PU	*Punch*
RH	*Rural History*
RIM	*Rhode Island Medicine*
RR	*Residue Reviews*
RRPE	*Review of Radical Political Economics*
SC	*Science*
SLS	*Social and Legal Studies*
SPI	*Seattle Post-Intelligencer*
SR	*Sanitary Record*
SSH	*Social Science History*
SU	*Surgery*
TA	*The Analyst*
TE	*The Economist*
TL	*The Lancet*
TM	*Time Magazine*
TNT	*Tacoma News Tribune*
TP	*The Practitioner*
TPMSA	*Transactions of the Provincial Medical and Surgical Association*
TT	*The Times (of London)*
USNWR	*US News and World Report*
WKW	*Wiener Klinische Wochenschrift*
WMW	*Wiener Medizinischer Wochenschrift*

In the notes, the first time a source is referenced within a chapter, a complete citation will be given, e.g.: 7. John Marshall, *Remarks on Arsenic, Considered as a Poison and a Medicine* (London: Callow, 1817). If the reference occurs in a later note within that chapter, the citation will be simply to the author, with an indication of the note in which the full reference is given, e.g.: Marshall (n. 7).

The quotations preceding the Introduction are from Robert Christison, *A Treatise on Poisons* (Edinburgh: Black, 1829), 172; and Mathieu Orfila, *A General System of Toxicology: or, a Treatise on Poisons* (Philadelphia: Carey, 1817), 46.

NOTES

Preface

1. Leonard de Vries, '*Orrible Murder* (London: Book Club Associates, 1974), 27, 35, 73; Henry Fuller, *TT*, 13 December 1848: 8 (the article was originally published in *MTG* 19 (1848–9), 151); Michael Harris, in W. F. Bynum et al. (eds.), *Medical Journals and Medical Knowledge: Historical Essays* (London: Routledge, 1992), 108–25.

2. Fuller (n. 1), 8.

3. J. A. Paris and J. S. M. Fonblanque, *Medical Jurisprudence*, 3 vols. (London: Phillips, 1823), ii. 212; James Tunstall, *Observations Upon the Sale of Arsenic and the Prevention of Secret Poisoning* (London: Simpkin, Marshall, 1849), 4, 11–12; *TL*, 1889 (ii): 1357.

4. *TT*, 6 January 1875: 3; J. T. Arlidge, *The Hygiene, Diseases and Mortality of Occupations* (London: Percival, 1892), 430.

5. Henry Povall, *Arsenical Poisoning by Means of Wall Papers, Paints and Other Articles* (Mount Morris, NY: n.d., pamphlet held by Countway Medical Library, Boston), 1.

6. *BMJ*, 1862 (ii): 268; J. Alfred Wanklyn, *Arsenic*, 2nd edn. (London: Kegan Paul, Trench, Trübner, 1901), 15; *TL*, 1879 (ii): 96; Jabez Hogg, *SR* 10 (1879), 261.

7. Ralph Hennebach, *NYT*, 27 July 1983: A22.

8. Henry Carr, *Our Domestic Poisons*, 2nd edn. (London: Clowes, 1884), 14–15; Frank Draper, *CN* 26 (1872), 103.

9. Henry Carr, *Our Domestic Poisons* (London: Ridgway, 1879), 6.

10. Anthony Thomson, *TL*, 1836–7 (ii): 449.

11. John Gay, *MTG*, 1859 (i): 95.

12. *TL*, 1849 (ii): 305.

13. *BMJ*, 1871 (ii): 393.

Chapter 1

1. William Roughead (ed.), *Trial of Mary Blandy* (Edinburgh: Hodge, 1914), 75, 134; William Jackson, *The New and Complete Newgate Calendar; or, Villainy Displayed in all its Branches*, 6 vols. (London: Hogg, 1795), iv. 10.

2. Oliver Goldsmith, 'The Double Transformation', in *The Complete Works of Oliver Goldsmith* (London: Oxford University Press, 1906), 54; Roughead (n. 1), 34; Jackson (n. 1), 11; Axylus, *GM* 22 (1852), 117.

3. Roughead (n. 1), 66, 68.

4. Sylvanus Urban, *GM* 22 (1752), 112; S. T., *GM* 22 (1752), 152–5.

5. Roughead (n. 1), 71.

6. Ibid. 65, 72, 81–2.

7. Urban (n. 4), 110, 114–15.

8. Roughead (n. 1), 73–6, 109; Anon., *The Fair Parricide: A Tragedy in Three Acts Founded on a late Melancholy Event* (London: n.p., 1752), 19, 40. Also see Susan Heinzelman, in Heinzelman and Zipporah Wiseman (eds.), *Representing Women: Law, Literature, and Feminism* (Durham, NC: Duke University Press, 1994), 309–36.

9. Roughead (n. 1), 64, 134, 157, 206; Urban (n. 4), 9.

10. Jackson (n. 1), 23; *GM* 22 (1752), 188–9; 'Mary (Molly) Blandy before her execution', Wellcome Images, Wellcome Library, London.

11. Roughead (n. 1), 46, 48, 76, 187, 195; Axylus (n. 2), 116–17.

12. Henry Schroeder and Joseph Balassa, *JCD* 19 (1966), 85–106; W. D. Buchanan, *Toxicity of Arsenic Compounds* (Amsterdam: Elsevier, 1962), 1–2; *TNT*, 24 September 2007: A6.

13. John Stillman, *The Story of Alchemy and Early Chemistry* (New York: Dover, 1960), 19, 29, 46.

14. Philip Ball, *Bright Earth: Art and the Invention of Colour* (Chicago: University of Chicago Press, 2001), 80; Buchanan (n. 12), 2; Louis Lewin, *Die Gifte in der Weltgeschichte* (Berlin: Springer, 1920), 158; Paul Stecher (ed.), *The Merck Index of Chemicals and Drugs*, 7th edn. (Rahway, NJ: Merck, 1960), 103; D. M. Jolliffe, *JRSM* 86 (1993), 287.

15. Kenneth DuBois and E. M. K. Geiling, *Textbook of Toxicology* (New York: Oxford University Press, 1959), 133; Lewin (n. 14), 106–7, 320; Robert Christison, *A Treatise on Poisons*, 2nd edn. (Edinburgh: Black,

1832), 292; *MTG*, 1885 (ii): 60; *AJMS* 91 (1886), 689; *BMSJ* 119 (1888), 70; R. A. Witthaus, *Manual of Toxicology*, 2nd edn. (New York: Wood, 1911), 522.

16. Roughead (n. 1), 80; Witthaus (n. 15), 402; Buchanan (n. 12), 16.

17. Alfred Taylor, *GHR* 6 (1841), 21; Taylor, *On Poisons, in Relation to Medical Jurisprudence and Medicine* (Philadelphia: Lea & Blanchard, 1848), 256; Henry Baker, *Employment for the Microscope* (London: Dodsley, 1753), 133.

18. Nathaniel Potter, *An Essay on the Medicinal Properties and Deleterious Qualities of Arsenic* (Philadelphia: Woodward, 1796), 51; Mathieu Orfila, *A General System of Toxicology: or, a Treatise on Poisons* (Philadelphia: Carey, 1817), 11.

19. Witthaus (n. 15), 448, 484; Joseph Kesselring, *Arsenic and Old Lace* (New York: Dramatists Play Service, 1942); W. B. Ryan, *TL*, 1851 (i): 410–11; John Johnstone, *An Essay on Mineral Poisons* (Evesham: Agg, 1795), 22; Roughead (n. 1), 80; Philip Holland, *A Report of the Trial and Acquittal of Mary Hunter* (Manchester: Gillett, 1843), 12.

20. Johnstone (n. 19), 22; Roughead (n. 1), 82; *TT*, 19 March 1858: 12; John Marshall, *Remarks on Arsenic, considered as a Poison and a Medicine* (London: Callow, 1817), 13, 43; *TL* 3 (1824), 175; Taylor (n. 17), 259.

21. Witthaus (n. 15), 457–9; *TT*, 5 September 1846: 7; Henry Dermott, *TL*, 1851 (ii): 552; Marshall (n. 20), 1, 13; *Trial of Miss Madeleine H. Smith Before the High Court of Justiciary, Edinburgh* (Edinburgh: Mathers, 1857), 72.

22. *Trial of Mary Elder, or Smith, Before the High Court of Justiciary* (Montrose: Smith, 1827), 9; Urban (n. 4), 112.

23. Roughead (n. 1), 81; Ryan (n. 19), 411; Orfila (n. 18), 53; John Prestwich, *Prestwich's Dissertation on Mineral, Animal, and Vegetable Poisons* (London: Newberry, 1775), 21; Baker (n. 17), 133.

24. Marshall (n. 20), 13; *TT*, 6 August 1889: 9; Roughead (n. 1), 83.

25. Marshall (n. 20), 17; Johnstone (n. 19), 22–3; *TL*, 1844 (i): 507.

26. William Guy and David Ferrier, *Principles of Forensic Medicine*, 4th edn. (London: Renshaw, 1875), 469, 471; National Research Council, *Arsenic in Drinking Water* (Washington, DC: National Academy Press, 1999), 229–50; *PJT* 3 [3rd series] (1872–3), 472.

27. Witthaus (n. 15), 452–3; S. W. Abbott, *BMSJ* 120 (1889), 480; John Morley, *BMJ*, 1873 (i): 88; Potter (n. 18), 53–4; *TL*, 1844 (i): 507; *MG*, 4 November 1858: 2.

28. Frederick Peterson and Walter Haines (eds.), *A Text-book of Legal Medicine and Toxicology* (Philadelphia: Saunders, 1904), 409; Witthaus (n. 15), 484.

29. *PJT* 3 [3rd series] (1872–3), 472; Potter (n. 18), 57–8; Mathieu Orfila, *Directions for the Treatment of Persons Who Have Taken Poison* (London: Longman, Hurst, Rees, Orme, & Browne, 1820), 17, 33–4; Hugh Ward, *EMSJ* 33 (1830), 61–6.

30. Andrew Meharg, *Venomous Earth: How Arsenic Caused the World's Worst Mass Poisoning* (New York: Macmillan, 2005), 38–41; Gaius Suetonius Tranquillus, *The Twelve Caesars*, trans. Robert Graves (Baltimore: Penguin, 1957), 226–7; Johan Beckmann, *A History of Inventions and Discoveries*, 3 vols. (London: Bell, 1797), i. 75.

31. C. J. S. Thompson, *Poisons and Poisoners* (New York: Macmillan, 1931), 91; Lewin (n. 14), 159; *BMJ*, 1929 (ii): 588.

32. Carlo Beuf, *Cesare Borgia: The Machiavellian Prince* (New York: Oxford University Press, 1942), 306–7; Sarah Bradford, *Lucrezia Borgia: Life, Death, and Love in Renaissance Italy* (New York: Viking, 2004), 193; Cathy Newman, *NG* 207 (May 2005), 20; Thompson (n. 31), 143–4, 160.

33. Beckmann (n. 29), i. 75, 84; Thompson (n. 31), 144–5; Anthony Thomson, *TL*, 1836–7 (ii): 451; Christison (n. 15), 35; William Shakespeare, *Twenty-three Plays and the Sonnets* (New York: Scribner, 1953), 1018.

34. Thompson (n. 31), 144–5.

35. Ibid. 145–7.

36. Albert Borowitz, *Innocence and Arsenic: Studies in Crime and Literature* (New York: Harper & Row, 1977), 65; Peter Shaffer, *Amadeus* (New York: French, 1981); *TT*, 14 August 1815: 3.

37. Frances Mossiker, *The Affair of the Poisons* (New York: Knopf, 1969), 142–8; The Earl of Birkenhead, *More Famous Trials* (New York: Doubleday, Doran, 1929), 265–80; Edward Bulwer Lytton, *Lucretia or the Children of Night* (Boston: Estes & Lauriat, 1892), 170, 375–8, 419.

38. Beckman (n. 30), 75; Newman (n. 32), 20; Thompson (n. 31), 116–17, 124, 148–59; William Johnson, *The Age of Arsenic* (London: Chapman & Hall, 1931), 55–7, 127; George Male, *Elements of Juridical or Forensic Medicine*, 2nd edn. (London: Cox, 1818), 21; Edward Cooke, *EMSJ* 3 (1807), 20; Henry Morley, *HW* 13 (1856), 220–4; Prestwich (n. 23), 23.

39. Baker (n. 17), 135; Torbern Bergman, *Physical and Chemical Essays*, 3 vols. (London: Murray, 1784), ii. 308.

Chapter 2

1. Henry Morley, *HW* 13 (1856), 221.

2. Michael Harris, in W. F. Bynum et al. (eds.), *Medical Journals and Medical Knowledge: Historical Essays* (London: Routledge, 1992), 120; I.R., *CEJ* 12 (1849), 209–11; *MTG* 23 (1851), 331.

3. Katherine Watson, in José Bertomeu-Sánchez and Agustí Nieto-Galan (eds.), *Chemistry, Medicine, and Crime: Mateu J. B. Orfila (1787–1853) and His Times* (Sagamore Beach, Mass.: Science History Publications, 2006), 187; *TT*, 22 August 1859: 6; Harris (n. 2), 120.

4. Katherine Watson, *Poisoned Lives: English Poisoners and Their Victims* (London: Hambledon & London, 2004), 33; Ian Burney, *Poison, Detection, and the Victorian Imagination* (Manchester: Manchester University Press, 2006), 21; *MTG*, 1858 (i): 429–31.

5. Richard Altick, *Victorian Studies in Scarlet* (New York: Norton, 1970), 55; David Mitch, *The Rise of Popular Literacy in Victorian England* (Philadelphia: University of Pennsylvania Press, 1992), pp. xvi, 48–9; Judith Knelman, *Twisting in the Wind: The Murderess and the English Press* (University of Toronto Press: Toronto, 1998), 35–43.

6. Ferdinand Danger and Charles Flandin, *De l'Arsenic* (Paris: Bachelier, 1841), p. ix; Kari Konkola, *JHMAS* 47 (1992), 186–209.

7. *TT*, 25 August 1849: 8; Anthony Thomson, *TL*, 1836–7 (ii): 449; Howard Taylor, *EHR* 51 (1998), 587; Lionel Rose, *The Massacre of the Innocents: Infanticide in Britain 1800–1939* (London: Routledge & Kegan Paul, 1986), 8.

8. Terence O'Donnell, *History of Life Insurance in its Formative Years* (Chicago: American Conversation Company, 1936), 247–302; Morley

(n. 1), 224; Edward Bulwer Lytton, *Lucretia or the Children of Night* (Boston: Estes & Lauriat, 1892), 309.

9. J. M. Baernreither, *English Associations of Working Men* (London: Swan Sonnenschein, 1889); P. H. J. H. Gosden, *The Friendly Societies in England 1815–1875* (Manchester: Manchester University Press, 1961).

10. Gosden (n. 9), 14–16; James Riley, *Sick, Not Dead: The Health of British Workingmen During the Mortality Decline* (Baltimore: The Johns Hopkins University Press, 1997), 40.

11. Baernreither (n. 9), 188–98; P. H. J. H. Gosden, *Self-Help: Voluntary Associations in the 19th Century* (London: Batsford, 1973), 130–1.

12. *TT*, 20 September 1848: 4; 12 May 1846: 7; John Clay, *TT*, 18 January 1849: 3; Paul Johnson, *Saving and Spending: The Working-Class Economy in Britain 1870–1939* (Oxford: Oxford University Press, 1985), 43–6.

13. Clay (n. 12); Josephine McDonagh, *Child Murder and British Culture 1720–1900* (Cambridge: Cambridge University Press, 2003), 112–13; *TT*, 12 December 1853: 6; J. D. Havard, *The Detection of Secret Homicide* (London: Macmillan, 1960), 51–5.

14. *TT*, 29 March 1819: 3; Watson (n. 4), 34, 89–111; Morley (n. 1), 224.

15. *MTG*, 1872 (ii): 435; *TT*, 7 October 1872: 10; 15 October 1872: 3; 16 October 1872: 8; 8 March 1873: 11; 20 March 1873: 7; George Poore, *A Treatise on Medical Jurisprudence* (New York: Longmans, Green, 1901), 170; John Glaister, *The Power of Poison* (New York: Morrow, 1954), 81. There is some disagreement over the total number of Cotton's victims, estimates ranging from twenty-two down to fourteen. A thorough recent account of Cotton's crimes is to be found in Watson (n. 4), 211–17: there she argues that some of the fifteen children died from natural causes.

16. *TT*, 7 October 1872: 10; 8 March 1873: 11; 20 March 1873: 7; Arthur Appleton, *Mary Ann Cotton: Her Story and Trial* (London: Michael Joseph, 1973), 121–2.

17. Geoffrey Abbott, *William Calcraft: Executioner Extra-ordinaire!* (Barming, UK:Dobby, 2004); William Calcraft, *The Groans of the Gallows* (London: Hancock, 1846).

18. Burney (n. 4), 21; *TT*, 6 October 1842: 6; 12 December 1853: 6; 26 April 1843: 7.

19. Burney (n. 4), 21; George Robb, *JFH* 22 (1997), 176–90; Watson (n. 4), 45, 58.

20. Robb (n. 19), 177.

21. *TT*, 4 October 1842: 6; Robb (n. 19), 186. Also see Margaret Hallissy, *Venomous Woman: Fear of the Female in Literature* (New York: Greenwood, 1987).

22. *TT*, 8 March 1851: 4; 23 September 1850: 2; 26 September 1846: 4; 22 September 1848: 4; 7 March 1851: 6.

23. *TT*, 20 August 1846: 5; 26 September 1846: 4; 8 March 1851: 4.

24. *TT*, 8 March 1851: 4; 5 September 1850: 5.

25. *TT*, 29 August 1848: 5; 7 March 1851: 6; 5 September 1848: 8; 31 August 1848: 7; 25 July 1848: 7; 1 September 1848: 4.

26. *TT*, 14 September 1848: 6; 31 August 1848: 7; 7 March 1851: 6; 10 March 1849: 6.

27. *TT*, 8 March 1851: 4; 12 December 1853: 6.

28. Robb (n. 19), 187; Watson (n. 4), 58; *TT*, 22 September 1848: 4.

29. *TT*, 5 September 1850: 5; 14 September 1848: 6; 8 March 1851: 4; 21 September 1848: 5; 22 September 1848: 4; 20 September 1848: 4; 5 September 1848: 8.

30. *TT*, 7 March 1851: 6; 26 March 1851: 6; 22 August 1859: 6.

31. *TT*, 22 September 1848: 4.

32. Taylor (n. 7).

33. *TT*, 22 September 1848: 4.

34. Ian Burney, *Bodies of Evidence: Medicine and the Politics of the English Inquest 1830–1926* (Baltimore: The Johns Hopkins University Press, 2000), 3; John Jervis, *A Practical Treatise on the Office and Duties of Coroners* (London: Sweet, Maxwell, Stevens, & Norton, 1854), pp. iii, 1; John Glaister, *A Text-book of Medical Jurisprudence and Toxicology* (Edinburgh: Livingstone, 1931), 14; R. Henslowe Wellington, *The King's Coroner* (London: Clowes, 1905), 1–34.

35. Burney (n. 34), 3–5; Glaister (n. 34), 14; Jervis (n. 34), 258.

36. Mary Beth Emmerichs, *SSH* 25 (2001), 93–100.

37. Charles Dickens, *Bleak House* (London: Oxford University Press, 1948), 146; Burney (n. 34), 80–3.

38. *TT*, 18 October 1847: 5; Olive Anderson, *Suicide in Victorian and Edwardian England* (Oxford: Clarendon, 1987), 33.

39. Watson (n. 4), 179–86; Jonathan Toogood, *TL*, 1845 (i): 509; *BMJ*, 1857: 304.

40. *TL*, 1841 (i): 411; Watson (n. 4), 157; *TL*, 1846 (i): 693; *BMJ*, 1857: 304; Havard (n. 13), 38–66.

41. *TL*, 1846 (i): 589–90.

42. *TT*, 8 March 1851: 4; 22 June 1846: 4; Watson (n. 4), 43.

43. *TT*, 22 June 1846: 4; *TL*, 1846 (i): 642, 693; *BMJ*, 1857: 304.

44. Toogood (n. 39).

45. Emmerichs (n. 36), 94; Watson (n. 4), 159; Thomas Forbes, *Surgeons at the Bailey: English Forensic Medicine to 1878* (New Haven: Yale University Press, 1985), 12–14.

46. Burney (n. 4), 15–17; *TT*, 23 August 1860: 8.

47. John Tuck, *PJT* 4 [series 2] (1862–3), 458; *TT*, 22 June 1846: 4; George Male, *Elements of Juridical or Forensic Medicine*, 2nd edn. (London: Cox, 1818), 19; Mathieu Orfila, *A General System of Toxicology: or, a Treatise on Poisons* (Philadelphia: Carey, 1817), p. vi.

48. *TT*, 25 August 1849: 8.

49. *TT*, 26 March 1851: 6.

50. *TT*, 7 March 1851: 6; 26 March 1851: 6.

51. *TT*, 30 December 1844: 7; 22 July 1847: 7; 7 August 1847: 5.

Chapter 3

1. *TT*, 8 March 1851: 4; 7 March 1851: 6.

2. George Male, *Elements of Juridical or Forensic Medicine*, 2nd edn. (London: Cox, 1818), 21, 23; 7 March 1851: 6; 22 August 1859: 6.

3. 22 August 1859: 6; Judith Knelman, *Twisting in the Wind: The Murderess and the English Press* (University of Toronto Press: Toronto, 1998), 75.

4. I.R., *CEJ* 12 (1849), 209.

5. *TT*, 8 March 1851: 4.

6. I.R. (n. 4), 209–10; *TT*, 17 December 1846: 7.

7. Newspaper article quoted by Ian Burney, *Poison, Detection, and the Victorian Imagination* (Manchester: Manchester University Press, 2006), 122; *TT*, 22 August 1859: 6.

8. John Paris and J. S. M. Fonblanque, *Medical Jurisprudence*, 3 vols. (London: Phillips, 1823), i. pp. iii–xxv; Thomas Forbes, *Surgeons at the Bailey: English Forensic Medicine to 1878* (New Haven: Yale University Press, 1985), 49–108.

9. Paris (n. 8), pp. xxiv–xxvi; Forbes (n. 8), 4–9; Burney (n. 7), 40–5.

10. *BMJ*, 1857: 587; Ian Burney, *Bodies of Evidence: Medicine and the Politics of the English Inquest 1830–1926* (Baltimore: The Johns Hopkins University Press, 2000), 108; *TT*, 5 September 1846: 7.

11. *BMJ*, 1857: 587.

12. *BMJ*, 1859 (i): 703.

13. John Smith, *An Analysis of Medical Evidence* (London: Underwood, 1825), 38; Michael Ryan, *A Manual of Medical Jurisprudence* (London: Renshaw & Rush, 1836), 460; *AMJ* 3 (1855), 1114–15.

14. José Bertomeu-Sánchez and Agustí Nieto-Galan, in Bertomeu-Sánchez and Nieto-Galan (eds.), *Chemistry, Medicine, and Crime: Mateu J. B. Orfila (1787–1853) and His Times* (Sagamore Beach, Mass.: Science History Publications, 2006), pp. ix–xx; Allen Debus (ed.), *World Who's Who in Science* (Chicago: Marquis, 1968), 1288; Mathieu Orfila, *A General System of Toxicology: or, a Treatise on Poisons* (Philadelphia: Carey, 1817), pp. xlvii–xlviii. Also see Marina Stajic, in Samuel Gerber and Richard Saferstein (eds.), *More Chemistry and Crime* (Washington, DC: American Chemical Society, 1997), 137–48.

15. Joseph Ince, *PJT 4* [series 2] (1862–3), 450–8.

16. Louis Casarett, in Casarett and John Doull (eds.), *Toxicology: The Basic Science of Poisons* (New York: Macmillan, 1975), 5; John Johnstone, *An Essay on Mineral Poisons* (Evesham: Agg, 1795), 25; Alfred Taylor, *On Poisons, in Relation to Medical Jurisprudence and Medicine* (Philadelphia: Lea & Blanchard, 1848), 99; W. D. Chowne, *TL*, 1839 (ii): 737–43; *TT*, 27 March 1848: 7; Robert Christison, *A Treatise on Poisons*, 2nd edn. (Edinburgh: Black, 1832), 311; Jürgen Thorwald, *The Century of the Detective*, trans. Richard and Clara Winston (New York: Harcourt, Brace & World, 1964), 273.

17. Robert Christison, *The Life of Sir Robert Christison*, 2 vols. (Edinburgh: Blackwood, 1885–6); Bertomeu-Sánchez (n. 14), 125–52; Robert Christison, *A Treatise on Poisons* (Edinburgh: Black, 1829), 175;

Christison, *A Treatise on Poisons*, 1st American edn. (Philadelphia: Barrington & Haswell, 1845), 200–1; Taylor (n. 16), 254.

18. Christison (n. 16), p. v.
19. *BMJ*, 1857: 586–7.
20. R. A. Witthaus, *Manual of Toxicology*, 2nd edn. (New York: Wood, 1911), 481; George Bottomley, *TL*, 1854 (i): 289–90.
21. William Whitford, *TL*, 1884 (i): 419–21; Witthaus (n. 20), 478.
22. Anthony Thomson, *TL*, 1838–9 (i): 180–1.
23. John Glaister, *A Text-book of Medical Jurisprudence and Toxicology* (Edinburgh: Livingstone, 1931), 713; Robert Harvey, *MTG*, 1876 (i): 581; Male (n. 2), 73. A colour illustration of the stomach of an arsenic victim is provided in Frederick Peterson and Walter Haines, *A Text-Book of Legal Medicine and Toxicology*, 2 vols. (Philadelphia: Saunders, 1904), volume 2, 412. Yellow deposits in the digestive tract were also often due to bile.
24. Glaister (n. 23), 713; Robert Christison, *EMJ* 3 (1857–8), 481; Witthaus (n. 20), 496; Christison (n. 16), 304.
25. William Roughead (ed.), *Trial of Mary Blandy* (Edinburgh: Hodge, 1914), 84; Taylor (n. 16), 267; Glaister (n. 23), 713; Harvey (n. 23), 581.
26. Christison (n. 16), 309; Anthony Thomson, *TL*, 1836–7 (ii): 449–57; Henry Baker, *Employment for the Microscope* (London: Dodsley, 1753), 137.
27. *TT*, 31 January 1848: 3; G. D. Hedley, *TL*, 1842–3 (ii): 801; William Whitford, *BMJ*, 1884 (i): 505; Alfred Taylor, *On Poisons, in Relation to Medical Jurisprudence and Medicine*, 2nd edn. (Philadelphia: Blanchard & Lea, 1859), 381.
28. Christison (n. 16), 312–15.
29. Hedley (n. 27), 801; Whitford (n. 27), 505.
30. *MTG*, 1885 (i): 838; Frederick Lowndes, *BMJ*, 1884 (i): 555–6; R. A. Witthaus and Tracy Becker, *Medical Jurisprudence, Forensic Medicine, and Toxicology*, 2nd edn. (New York: Wood, 1911), 504–5.
31. *TT*, 7 February 1857: 12; 15 May 1857: 10; 21 May 1857: 12; 27 July 1857: 10; 29 July 1857: 9.
32. *TT*, 14 September 1840: 6; W. A. Campbell, *CB* 1 (1965), 200.
33. Campbell (n. 32), 198–202.

34. Robert Christison, *EMSJ* 22 (1824), 61; Christison (n. 16), 250; George Fownes, *A Manual of Elementary Chemistry* (Philadelphia: Blanchard Lea, 1860), 311. For details on the development of chemical analysis, see Ferenc Szabadvary, *History of Analytical Chemistry* (Oxford: Pergamon, 1966).

35. Roughead (n. 25), 81–6.

36. Baker (n. 26), 133; George Sigmond, *TL*, 1837–8 (i): 400; Thomson (n. 26), 452; Glaister (n. 23), 22.

37. John Marshall, *Remarks on Arsenic, considered as a Poison and a Medicine* (London: Callow, 1817); John Watkins, *The Important Results of an Elaborate Investigation into the Mysterious Case of Elizabeth Fenning* (London: Hone, 1815), 1; Anonymous, *Circumstantial Evidence: The Extraordinary Case of Eliza Fenning* (London: Cowrie & Strange, 1829), 2–3; Knelman (n. 3), 182–8.

38. Marshall (n. 37), 11, 31–3; Watkins (n. 37), 59; Anonymous (n. 37), 6; *TT*, 13 August 1821: 3.

39. Katherine Watson, in Bertomeu-Sánchez (n. 14), 186; *TT*, 12 April 1815: 3. For commentary on the fairness of her trial, see Watkins (n. 37), Anonymous (n. 37), and V. A. C. Gatrell, *The Hanging Tree: Execution and the English People 1770–1868* (Oxford: Oxford University Press, 1994), 359–60.

40. Tim Marshall, *CS* 13 (2003), 98; John Marshall, *Five Cases of Recovery From the Effects of Arsenic* (London: Chapple, 1815), 35; *TT*, 27 July 1815: 3; 1 August 1815: 3.

41. Gatrell (n. 39), 353; Charles Dickens, *AYR* 18 (1867), 72; Anonymous (n. 37), 6; *TT*, 27 July 1815: 3; 1 August 1815: 3; Tim Marshall (n. 40), 109; Watkins (n. 37), 98.

42. Tim Marshall (n. 40); Dickens is quoted by Gatrell (n. 39), 368, who also outlines the decades-long debate over the Fenning case, 353–70; Anonymous (n. 37), 6; C. J. S. Thompson, *Poisons and Poisoners* (New York: Macmillan, 1931), 253; *TT*, 21 July 1857: 5.

43. Marshall (n. 37), 11–14, 36–7; John Marshall (n. 40), 24–8; Anonymous (n. 37), 3–4; *EMSJ* 13 (1817), 507–20.

44. Marshall (n. 37), 37; letter from T. W. Wansborough to Thomas Wakley, 31 August 1830, British Library; Male (n. 2), 85; Witthaus (n. 30), 503.

Chapter 4

1. *PJT, 1* (1841–2), 278.
2. Henry Morley, *HW* 13 (1856), 224; *PJT* 9 (1849–50), 162; *PJT* 1 (1841–2), 277.
3. Anonymous, *The Trial of Robert Sawle Donnall* (Falmouth: Lake, 1817).
4. *TT*, 9 April 1817: 3; 3 April 1817: 3; Anonymous (n. 3), 104; George Male, *Elements of Juridical or Forensic Medicine*, 2nd edn. (London: Cox, 1818), 79.
5. Anonymous (n. 3), 121.
6. *TT*, 4 August 1834: 6.
7. *TT*, 11 November 1833: 3; Katherine Watson, in José Bertomeu-Sánchez and Agustí Nieto-Galan (eds.), *Chemistry, Medicine, and Crime: Mateu J. B. Orfila (1787–1853) and His Times* (Sagamore Beach, Mass.: Science History Publications, 2006), 188–90; Watson, *MH* 50 (2006), 383; *TT*, 20 February 1844: 7; A. G. Madge, *PHH* 15/2 (1985), 12–14.
8. Watson, in Bertomeu-Sánchez (n. 7), 192–4.
9. J. Alfred Wanklyn, *Arsenic*, 2nd edn. (London: Kegan, Paul, Trench, Trübner, 1901) 40–2; *AMJ* 2 (1854), 1060; *MTG*, 1868 (i): 316.
10. W. A. Campbell, *CB* 1 (1965), 199.
11. Campbell (n. 10), 199–200; Henry Baker, *Employment for the Microscope* (London: Dodsley, 1753), 133; Alexander Blyth and Meredith Blyth. *Poisons: Their Effects and Detection* (London: Griffin, 1920), 557; John Glaister, *Poisoning by Arseniuretted Hydrogen or Hydrogen Arsenide* (Edinburgh: Livingstone, 1908), 13; Frederick Peterson and Walter Haines (eds.), *A Text-book of Legal Medicine and Toxicology* (Philadelphia: Saunders, 1904), 429.
12. Campbell (n. 10), 200.
13. José Bertomeu-Sánchez, in Bertomeu-Sánchez (n. 7), 218; Jürgen Thorwald, *The Century of the Detective* (New York: Harcourt, Brace & World, 1964), 278; *PJT* 1 (1841–2), 278.
14. Bertomeu-Sánchez (n. 13), 218; Thorwald (n. 13), 279.
15. *TT*, 8 September 1840: 6; 10 September 1840: 6; Mary Hartman, *Victorian Murderesses* (New York: Schocken, 1977), 10–50; Joseph Ince, *PJT* 4 [series 2] (1862–3), 454; *TL* 1840–1 (i): 479–82.

16. *TT*, 10 September 1840: 6; *TL*, 1840–1 (i): 481; Thorwald (n. 13), 284–6.

17. Bertomeu-Sánchez (n. 13), 214–15, 250; Alfred Taylor, *On Poisons, in Relation to Medical Jurisprudence and Medicine* (Philadelphia: Lea and Blanchard, 1848), 121.

18. Ince (n. 15), 456; *TT*, 14 September 1840: 6; 10 September 1840: 6; 15 September 1840: 6; Thorwald (n. 13), 286–8.

19. *TT*, 15 September 1840: 6; 16 September 1840: 3; Bertomeu-Sánchez (n. 13), 221; Thorwald (n. 13), 289–90; Campbell (n. 10), 200; *TL*, 1840–1 (i): 481; Hartman (n. 15), 46.

20. Taylor (n. 17), 292.

21. Campbell (n. 10), 201.

22. Robert Goldsmith, in Samuel Gerber and Richard Saferstein (eds.), *More Chemistry and Crime* (Washington, DC: American Chemical Society, 1997), 154–5; Alfred Taylor, *PJT* 2 [2nd series] (1860–1), 261–70; Wanklyn (n. 9), 59; Robert Christison, *TL*, 1842–3 (ii): 870–1.

23. Arthur Appleton, *Mary Ann Cotton: Her Story and Trial* (London: Michael Joseph, 1973), 100; *TT*, 1 September 1848: 4; Ian Burney, *Poison, Detection, and the Victorian Imagination* (Manchester: Manchester University Press, 2006), 154.

24. Noel Coley, *MH* 35 (1991), 420–1; Campbell (n. 10), 201–2; Humphry Sandwith, *Minsterborough: A Tale of English Life*, 3 vols. (London: Chatto & Windus, 1876), iii. 109; Wellcome Images, Wellcome Library, London.

25. Anonymous, *The Domestic Chemist* (London: Bumpus & Griffin, 1831), 16.

26. Katherine Watson, *MH* 50 (2006), 375–83; Coley (n. 24), 416; Coley, *EN* 22 (1898), 143–7.

27. Taylor (n. 17), 89.

28. Ibid. 268.

29. Ibid. 138; *MTG*, 1882 (i): 147.

30. Thorwald (n. 13), 287–8; *MTG*, 1878 (i): 653–4.

31. Taylor (n. 17), 92; Robert Christison, *EMSJ* 27 (1827), 454.

32. *TT*, 22 August 1859: 6; *PJT* 1 (1841–2), 278.

33. Coley (n. 24); Katherine Watson, *MH* 50 (2006), 383–7; *TT*, 7 March 1851: 6; Burney (n. 23), 158; *TT*, 23 August 1848: 7; 29 August 1848: 7.

34. *TT*, 8 July 1859: 12.

35. *TT*, 21 May 1859: 12; 22 August 1859: 6; Leonard Parry (ed.), *Trial of Dr. Smethurst* (Edinburgh: Hodge, 1931), 112, 159–62.

36. *TT*, 8 July 1859: 12; Parry (n. 35), 59.

37. Parry (n. 35), 12–13; W. Tyler Smith, *TT*, 26 August 1859: 9.

38. Parry (n. 35), 27, 84–9, 164; *TT*, 16 August 1859: 8; 14 November 1859: 8.

39. *MTG*, 1859 (ii): 217; *BMJ*, 1859 (i): 702–3; *TT*, 22 August 1859: 10.

40. *TT*, 29 August 1859: 9; Parry (n. 35), 19–21; *BMJ*, 1859 (ii): 726; Mary Smethurst, *TT*, 27 August 1859: 8.

41. *TT*, 5 September 1859: 9; *BMJ*, 1859 (ii): 742; *TT*, 10 September 1859: 5; 18 November 1859: 11; Parry (n. 34), 22.

42. *TT*, 1 December 1859: 9; 2 December 1859: 8; 6 December 1859: 5; Parry (n. 35), 29–31.

43. Parry (n. 35), 87–8, 162; William Herapath, *TT*, 26 August 1859: 9.

44. Parry (n. 35), 18–19; Taylor (n. 17), 119.

45. Taylor (n. 22), 312; William Herapath, *PJT* 2 [2nd series] (1860–1), 377–8; *BMJ*, 1859 (ii): 725.

46. R. Nagle, *MLJ* 38 (1970), 51–3; J. F. Fielding, *BMJ* 290 (1985), 47–8.

Chapter 5

1. W. H. Wills, *HW* 2 (1850), 155–7.

2. *PJT* 9 (1849–50), 206; Wills (n. 1), 156.

3. *TL*, 1839 (i): 597–9; *PJT* 13 [3rd series] (1882–3), 1005; *BMJ*, 1874 (i): 355–6; *PJT* 11 [3rd series] (1880–1), 830.

4. Robert Christison, *A Treatise on Poisons*, 2nd cdn. (Edinburgh: Black, 1832), 83.

5. *PJT* 17 (1857–8), 436; Robert Barnes, *TL*, 1847 (ii): 651–3; *PJT* 13 [3rd series] (1882–3), 98; *TT*, 20 September 1855: 6; 28 September 1855: 5; 2 March 1872: 5; Charles Markham, *TT*, 7 March 1872: 11.

6. *TL*, 1897 (i): 845; *PJT* 3 [2nd series] (1861–2), 342.

7. *BMJ*, 1857: 397; J. Ivor Murray, *EMSJ* 4 [NS], (1858–9), 13–16.

8. *PJT* 9 (1849–50), 283; *PJT* 1 [3rd series] (1870–1), 596–7.

9. *PJT* 1 [3rd series] (1870–1), 66; *PJT* 10 [3rd series] (1879–80), 656.

10. *MTG* 19 (1848–9), 205; *PJT* 18 (1858–9), 578–9; *PJT* 10 [3rd series] (1879–80), 32; *PJT* 17 (1857–8), 42–3.

11. Charles Tidy, *LL*, 1878: 505–7.

12. *BMJ*, 1878 (ii): 669; *SR* 8 (1878), 343, 390, 408; *PJT* 8 [3rd series] (1877–8), 996, 1009, 1015–16, 1057; Alexander Blyth, *A Manual of Practical Chemistry* (London: Griffin, 1879), 380; *TT*, 14 June 1878: 11; 8 August 1878: 10; *SR* 9 (1878), 121; *SR* 8 (1878), 312; *BMJ*, 1878 (i): 795–6; ibid. 833–4.

13. *TT*, 8 March 1873: 11.

14. Parl. Debs. (series 3), vol. 152, col. 209 (1859); R. A. Witthaus, *Manual of Toxicology*, 2nd edn. (New York: Wood, 1911), 430; S. W. Abbott, *BMSJ* 120 (1889), 480.

15. Flaubert quoted by Andrew Meharg, *Venomous Earth: How Arsenic Caused the World's Worst Mass Poisoning* (New York: Macmillan, 2005), 120; John Marshall, *Remarks on Arsenic, Considered as a Poison and a Medicine* (London: Callow, 1817), 162.

16. John Jervis, *A Practical Treatise on the Office and Duties of Coroners* (London: Sweet, Maxwell, Stevens, & Norton, 1854), 140, 357; Michael Macdonald and Terence Murphy, *Sleepless Souls: Suicide in Early Modern England* (Oxford: Oxford University Press, 1990), 15; Olive Anderson, *Suicide in Victorian and Edwardian England* (Oxford: Clarendon, 1987), 269–82.

17. Anderson (n. 16), 20; *TL*, 1839 (i): 597; 1842–3 (ii): 588; Robert Paterson, *EMJ* 3 (1857–8), 393; Thomas Bryant, *TL*, 1852 (ii): 299–300; *PJT* 16 [3rd series] (1885–6), 161–2; *TL*, 1862 (i): 325; Alfred Taylor, *On Poisons, in Relation to Medical Jurisprudence and Medicine* (Philadelphia: Lea & Blanchard, 1848), 151.

18. Mathieu Orfila, *A General System of Toxicology: or, a Treatise on Poisons* (Philadelphia: Carey, 1817), 49–51; Taylor (n. 17), 151–2; *PJT* 9 (1849–50), 354; W. T. Fewtrell, ibid. 358; *TT*, 3 March 1849: 7.

19. *TT*, 31 October 1811: 3.

20. John Glaister, *A Text-book of Medical Jurisprudence and Toxicology* (Edinburgh: Livingstone, 1931), 678; Taylor (n. 17), 73.

21. Taylor (n. 17), 73–4; W. Allison, *TL*, 1845 (i): 414.

22. *TL*, 1834–5 (i): 126–7; Henry Dermott, *TL*, 1851 (ii): 552–3; Albert Brundage, *A Manual of Toxicology*, 7th edn. (New York: Harrison, 1911), 98; Kenneth DuBois and E. M. K. Geiling, *Textbook of Toxicology* (New York: Oxford University Press, 1959), 135.

23. Louis Lewin, *Die Gifte in der Weltgeschichte* (Berlin: Springer, 1920), 164–6; John Glaister, *The Power of Poison* (New York: Morrow, 1954), 87; *TL*, 1848 (i): 193; George Lefevre, *TL*, 1844 (i): 442; *TT*, 3 April 1851: 6.

24. Lefevre (n. 23), 442.

25. *TT*, 6 August 1849: 7; 30 April 1849: 8; 2 May 1849: 8.

26. *TT*, 30 April 1849: 8; 6 August 1849: 7; 4 May 1849: 8.

27. Taylor (n. 17), 252; Liza Picard, *Victorian London: The Life of a City 1840–1870* (London: Weidenfeld & Nicolson, 2005), 310; *TT*, 23 September 1850: 2; 5 September 1846: 7.

28. James Tunstall, *Observations Upon the Sale of Arsenic and the Prevention of Secret Poisoning* (London: Simpkin, Marshall, 1849), 4, 5, 9, 11.

29. *PJT* 9 (1849–50), 353.

30. Peter Bartrip, *MH* 36 (1992), 59; *PJT* 9 (1849–50), 207.

31. *PJT* 9 (1849–50), 302–3.

32. *TL*, 1844 (ii): 63; Thomas Cattell, *TL*, 1851 (i): 89–90, 116–17; Cattell, *TL*, 1847 (ii): 385–6; Cattell, *TL*, 1850 (i): 15–16.

33. *TT*, 25 March 1851: 4; *PJT* 10 (1850–1), 578–9; Bartrip (n. 30).

34. *MTG* 23 (1851), 652; A Magistrate's Clerk, *The Arsenic Act, with Full Instructions to Sellers of Arsenic*, 3rd edn. (London: Longman, Brown, Green, & Longmans, 1851); *PJT* 16 [3rd series] (1885–6), 262.

35. *PJT* 10 (1850–1), 578–9; *PJT* 7 (1848), 561; *PJT* 9 (1849–50), 249–50; Hugh Linstead, *Poisons Law* (London: Pharmaceutical Press, 1936), 20–2; Bartrip (n. 30), 61–6.

36. Tunstall (n. 28), 4; Linstead (n. 35), 22–3.

37. *TT*, 15 January 1852: 3; *MTG* 24 (1851), 268; 258–9; *TT*, 21 August 1856: 10; 26 August 1856: 6; 22 August 1856: 8.

38. *TL*, 1856 (ii): 258; *PJT* 1 [2nd series] (1859–60), 618–20; *PJT* 4 [2nd series] (1862–3), 535; *PJT* 11 [3rd series] (1880–1), 465–6; *PJT* 16 [3rd series] (1885–6), 181–4; *PJT* 15 [3rd series] (1884–5), 300.

39. *PJT* 24 [3rd series] (1893–4), 701–2, 826–7.

40. G. Latham Browne and C. G. Stewart, *Reports of Trials for Murder by Poisoning* (London: Stevens & Sons, 1883), 294.

Chapter 6

1. Robert Elliot, *MG*, 6 November 1858: 6.
2. *MTG*, 1858 (ii): 657–9; *TT*, 6 November 1858: 8–9.
3. Frederick Filby, *A History of Food Adulteration and Analysis* (London: Allen & Unwin, 1934).
4. Friedrich Accum, *A Treatise on Adulterations of Foods and Culinary Poisons* (London: Longman, Hurst, Rees, Orme, & Brown, 1820), pp. vi, 131, 224, 244–5, 300, 313; Liza Picard, *Victorian London: The Life of a City 1840–1870* (London: Weidenfeld & Nicolson, 2005), 153; Charles Browne, *JCE* 2 (1925), 829–51, 1008–34, 1140–9.
5. Accum (n. 4), 30, 306, 315.
6. Ibid. 157, 159–60, 179–204.
7. Torald Sollman, *A Manual of Pharmacology*, 7th edn. (Philadelphia: Saunders, 1948), 204; Louis Goodman and Alfred Gilman, *The Pharmacological Basis of Therapeutics* (New York: Macmillan, 1941), 263; *Adulteration of Food, Drink, and Drugs: Being the Evidence Taken Before the Parliamentary Committee* (London: Bryce, 1855), 71, 182.
8. Accum (n. 4), 98–9.
9. Ibid. 95–111; One of the Old School, *Wine and Spirit Adulterators Unmasked*, 3rd edn. (London: Robins, 1829), 75; An Enemy of Fraud and Villainy, *Deadly Adulteration and Slow Poisoning* (London: Sherwood, Gilbert, & Piper, *c.*1830), 23.
10. Accum (n. 4), 111–14; Alfred Taylor, *GHR* 6 (1841), 36; Robert Christison, *EMSJ* 33 (1830), 67–76.
11. *TT*, 12 August 1815: 3.
12. *GM* 22 (1752), 112; *TT*, 12 August 1815: 3; J.C., *TT*, 14 August 1815: 3; An Enemy (n. 9), 13.
13. Accum (n. 4), 292–7.
14. Browne (n. 4), 1031.
15. One of the Old School (n. 9); Anonymous, *The Domestic Chemist* (London: Bumpus & Griffin, 1831); An Enemy (n. 9).
16. An Enemy (n. 9), 4–6; *MG*, 12 November 1858: 2.

17. *MG*, 12 November 1858: 3; Parl. Debs. (series 3), vol. 156, col. 2027 (1860); *MG*, 11 November 1858: 4; Thomas Fuller quoted by Emily Cockayne, *Hubbub: Filth, Noise and Stench in England 1600–1770* (New Haven: Yale University Press, 2007), 88.

18. W. B. O'Shaughnessy, *TL*, 1830–1 (ii): 193; Edwy Clayton, *Arthur Hill Hassall: Physician and Sanitary Reformer* (London: Baillière, Tindall & Cox, 1908), 11–14.

19. Arthur Hassall, *TL*, 1851 (i): 20–1; *TL*, 1881 (ii): 638–9.

20. Arthur Hassall, *TL*, 1854 (i): 316–19.

21. O'Shaughnessy (n. 18), 197.

22. *TL*, 1833 (ii): 280; Walter Fergus, *TL*, 1849 (i): 191; *AMJ* 1 (1853), 105; John Glaister, *The Power of Poison* (New York: Morrow, 1954), 148.

23. Arthur Hassall, *TL*, 1854 (i): 428–9, 581–5; Anonymous, *The Tricks of Trade in the Adulteration of Food and Physic* (London: Bogue, 1856), 45; *Adulteration* (n. 7), 245.

24. Alfred Taylor, *On Poisons in Relation to Medical Jurisprudence and Medicine*, 2nd edn. (Philadelphia: Blanchard & Lea, 1859), 386; *TT*, 20 July 1848: 7.

25. Arthur Hassall, *Adulterations Detected* (London: Longman, Brown, Green, Longmans, & Roberts, 1857), 35; *TL* 1851 (i): 472–3.

26. *PU* 20 (1851), 27, 65; *TL*, 1881 (ii): 638–9.

27. David Caruso, *TNT*, 24 February 2007: A4.

28. *TNT*, 2 July 2007: A4; Jennifer Steinhauer, *TNT*, 26 July 2008: A3.

29. *Adulteration* (n. 7), 26, 35, 245.

30. *PU* 29 (1855), 45–7.

31. Anonymous (n. 23), 40, 42–5; Charles Shrewsbury (ed.), *Meliora, or, Better Times to Come* (London: Parker, 1852), 81; *TT*, 20 July 1848: 7.

32. Parl. Debs. (series 3), vol. 154, cols. 848–9 (1859); ibid. col. 847; ibid. vol. 156, col. 2026 (1860).

33. Ibid. vol. 156, col. 2026 (1860); ibid. vol. 154, col. 848 (1859).

34. *BMJ*, 1858 (i): 952; *Adulteration* (n. 7), 112.

35. Accum (n. 4), 7, 10–11, 14; the details of the Bradford poisonings recounted in this and subsequent paragraphs were gleaned from a number of articles in *MG*: 2 November 1858: 3; 3 November 1858: 3; 4 November 1858: 2, 3; 5 November 1858: 3; 6 November 1858: 5; 7 November 1858: 3; 15 November 1858: 3.

36. *TT*, 6 November 1858: 8–9.

37. *PJT* 18 (1858–9), 342.
38. *PU* 35 (1858), 206, 211, 216, 231.
39. *TT*, 23 December 1858: 8.
40. *MG*, 4 November 1858: 4; *TL*, 1858 (ii): 536–8; Ingeborg Paulus, *The Search for Pure Food* (London: Robertson, 1974), 27–8.
41. James Harvey Young, *The Medical Messiahs* (Princeton: Princeton University Press, 1967), 34, 184–90.
42. *PJT* 4 [2nd series] (1862–3), 243–4; Charles Kingsley, *The Water-Babies* (New York: Dodd, Mead, 1916), 234; Arthur Hassall, *Food: Its Adulterations, and the Methods for Their Detection* (London: Longmans, Green, 1876), 252, 453, 636. For surveys of British adulteration legislation, see Michael French and Jim Phillips, *Cheated not Poisoned? Food Regulation in the United Kingdom, 1875–1938* (Manchester: Manchester University Press, 2000), Paulus (n. 40), and Alexander Blyth, *Foods: Their Composition and Analysis*, 4th edn. (London: Griffin, 1896), 26–8.
43. Parl. Debs. (series 3), vol. 150, col. 1508; ibid. vol. 152, col. 206; *MTG*, 1858 (ii): 476; *MG*, 5 November 1858: 4; *PJT* 5 [2nd series] (1863–4), 89–90; *BMJ* 1863 (i): 567.

Chapter 7

1. *TL*, 1837 (i): 556–7, 640; 1837–8 (i), 321–3.
2. *TT*, 30 June 1837: 6; *TL*, 1837 (i): 556–7; Robert Hunt, *TL*, 1837–8 (i): 324.
3. James Scott, *Report of the Committee Appointed by the Westminster Medical Society, to Investigate the Subject of Adulterating Candles With Arsenic* (London: Painter, 1838), 5–6, 57–61; *TL*, 1837–8 (i): 424–8.
4. *TL*, 1837–8 (i): 426–7; Scott (n. 3), 30–1.
5. Scott (n. 3), 7, 35.
6. Ibid. 3–4; Hunt (n. 2).
7. Scott (n. 3), 9–10; *TL*, 1837–8 (i): 426.
8. Scott (n. 3), 12–13.
9. Ibid. 15–25.
10. Ibid. 27.

11. Ibid. 26–7.

12. Ibid. 33–4; *TT*, 9 November 1837: 3.

13. *TL*, 1845 (i): 139–40; 1837–8 (i): 674; *TT*, 20 December 1837: 8; 2 December 1837: 8; *MTG* 33 (1856), 129.

14. *PJT* 1 [2nd series] (1859–60), 408; Stevenson Macadam, *PJT* 10 [3rd series] (1879–80), 612; Alfred Taylor, *On Poisons in Relation to Medical Jurisprudence and Medicine*, 2nd edn. (Philadelphia: Blanchard & Lea, 1859), 385; *PU* 20 (1851), 65.

15. Ian Bristow, *Interior House-Painting Colours and Technology 1615–1840* (New Haven: Yale University Press, 1996), 22–8; Philip Ball, *Bright Earth: Art and the Invention of Colour* (Chicago: University of Chicago Press, 2001), 154; M. P. Crosland, *Historical Studies in the Language of Chemistry* (London: Heinemann, 1962), 70; J. A. Stoeckhardt, *PJT* 6 (1846–7), 138–40; William Guy, *PP*, 1863: XXV. 129; A. Hill, *BMJ*, 1872 (ii): 219.

16. Taylor (n. 14), 387–8; Frederick Barrett, *PJT* 3 [3rd series] (1872–3), 641–2; William Swift, *BMSJ* 124 (1891), 185–6; Edward Wood, *Arsenic as a Domestic Poison* (Boston: Wright & Potter, 1885), 45–6; H. C. Bartlett, *SR* 10 (1879), 267–8; *TL*, 1879 (i): 571; Alfred Taylor, *MTG* 8 [NS] (1854), 326.

17. Henry Carr, *Our Domestic Poisons*, 2nd edn. (London: Clowes, 1884), 29; Wood (n. 16), 7–9, 42, 46; *PJT* 8 [3rd series] (1877–8), 57; *PJT* 3 [2nd series] (1861–2), 198; Joseph Farrar, *BMJ*, 1877 (i): 8; Guy (n. 15), 133–4; *MPC*, 1879 (i): 474; Edward Dwyer, *TL*, 1862 (i): 23; Jabez Hogg, *BMJ*, 1879 (ii): 746.

18. Frank Draper, *CN* 26 (1872), 41; Carr (n. 17), 29; Macadam (n. 14); R. Bateman, *TL*, 1857 (ii): 378; *BMJ*, 1877 (ii): 672; *LL*, 1873: 560.

19. Hogg (n. 17); *BMJ*, 1879 (ii): 630.

20. *BMJ*, 1879 (i): 118; *TT*, 13 August 1861: 7; Henry Carr, *Our Domestic Poisons* (London: Ridgway, 1879), 11; *BMJ*, 1875 (ii): 590; Alfred Taylor, *Medical Jurisprudence*, 5th edn. (London: Churchill, 1854), 62; R. Biggs, *TL*, 1860 (i): 8.

21. R. R. Cheyne, *BMJ*, 1874 (ii): 644; A.B., *TT*, 14 September 1863: 9; Macadam (n. 14), 611; G. Owen Rees, *TT*, 16 June 1877: 6; Draper (n. 18), 31; *BMJ*, 1862 (i): 177; Francis Image, *TP* 24 (1880), 110.

22. Macadam (n. 14), 611; *BMJ*, 1862 (i): 215; *TT*, 11 February 1862: 6.

23. Carr (n. 20), 33; *BMSJ* 124 (1891), 392–3; Jabez Hogg, *MPC*, 1879
    (ii): 61–2, 84–5; *TL*, 1901 (i): 1220–1; F. W. Tunnicliffe and Otto
    Rosenheim, *TL*, 1901 (i): 1199–200; *TT*, 7 January 1869: 9; *BMJ*,
    1878 (ii): 265; *SR* 10 (1879), 407; Wood (n. 16), 11–12; *BMJ*, 1879 (i):
    559.

24. W. Harding, *TL*, 1892 (i): 525; *TL*, 1888 (i): 177–8; Carr (n. 20), 36;
    Henry M'Clure, *TL*, 1889 (i): 1237–8; Hogg (n. 23), 84–5; *BMJ*, 1901
    (ii): 129; *TT*, 7 January 1869: 9.

25. *BMJ*, 1862 (i): 177; Draper (n. 18), 31; *TT*, 20 October 1862: 10;
    Frederick Barrett, *PJT* 3 [3rd series] (1872–3), 641–2.

26. Arthur Hassall, *TL*, 1860 (ii): 535; *Royal Commission on Employment of
    Children in Trades and Manufactures Not Regulated by Law. Fourth Report*
    (London: Her Majesty's Stationery Office, 1865), 109–10; Hogg
    (n. 23), 85; *PJT* 3 [2nd series] (1861–2), 391; *BMJ*, 1861 (ii): 598; *TL*,
    1861 (i): 530; Draper (n. 18); Guy (n. 15), 138, 152.

27. Hassall (n. 26); Guy (n. 15), 138, 146–8, 150.

28. *TL*, 1861 (i): 530; *BMJ*, 1861 (ii): 584.

29. R. A. Witthaus, *Manual of Toxicology*, 2nd edn. (New York: Wood,
    1911), 419, 580; Alfred Taylor, *PJT* 2 [2nd series] (1860–1), 317; *Final
    Report of the Royal Commission Appointed to Inquire into Arsenical Poisoning
    from the Consumption of Beer and Other Articles of Food and Drink* (London:
    His Majesty's Stationery Office, 1903), 34; *BMJ*, 1902 (ii): 891;
    Louis Siebold, *PJT* 20 [3rd series] (1889–90), 278; Robert Peck, in
    Sue Ann Prince (ed.), *Stuffing Birds, Pressing Plants, Shaping Knowledge:
    Natural History in North America, 1730–1860* (Philadelphia: American
    Philosophical Society, 2003), 11–25; Frederick Peterson and Walter
    Haines (eds.), *A Text-book of Legal Medicine and Toxicology* (Philadelphia:
    Saunders, 1904), 429; *TL*, 1848 (ii): 697.

30. Wood (n. 16), 15–16; Witthaus (n. 29), 422, 579; Taylor (n. 14), 390–1;
    PJT 8 [3rd series] (1877–8), 1039–40; Harry Draper, *PJT* 1 [2nd
    series] (1859–60), 262–3; R. A. Witthaus and Tracy Becker, *Medical
    Jurisprudence, Forensic Medicine and Toxicology*, 2nd edn. (New York:
    Wood, 1911), 384.

31. Carr (n. 20), 21; Francis Brown, *Arsenical Paper-hangings* (1876
    pamphlet, Countway Medical Library, Boston), 4; *MTG*, 1862
    (i): 139.

32. Draper (n. 18), 91; Walter Fergus, *TL*, 1862 (i): 598–9; J. J. Putnam, *BMSJ* 124 (1891), 291; Carr (n. 20), 16; Hogg (n. 23), 84; *TL*, 1896 (ii): 1778.

33. Charles Sanger, *PAAAS*, *29* (1893–4), 148–77; J. J. Putnam, *BMSJ* 124 (1891), 623.

34. Putnam (n. 33), 624; *BMJ*, 1871 (ii): 393.

35. John Gay, *MTG*, 1859 (i): 95; *SR* 8 (1878), 166; Carr (n. 20), 41; *SR* 5 (1876), 312.

36. William Hinds, *MTG*, 1857 (i): 522; Brown (n. 31), 4.

37. Arthur Hassall, *PJT* 1 [2nd series] (1859–60), 191; Carr (n. 17), 4.

38. *BMJ*, 1861 (ii): 584; *TL*, 1837–8 (i): 427; Carr (n. 17), 5; *TL*, 1862 (ii): 451; *TT*, 12 September 1884: 6.

39. *BMJ*, 1862 (i): 474.

40. Carr (n. 20), 2–4.

41. *MTG*, 1861 (ii): 560; Peter Bartrip, *The Home Office and the Dangerous Trades: Regulating Occupational Disease in Victorian and Edwardian Britain* (Amsterdam: Rodopi, 2002), 141–2; Guy (n. 15), 126.

42. Guy (n. 15), 144–56.

43. Ibid. 158–61; Georgina Cowper and Elizabeth Sutherland, *TT*, 1 February 1862: 12.

44. Guy (n. 15), 160.

45. *BMJ*, 1861 (ii): 584.

46. B. R. P., *EWJ* 3 (1859), 73–85; *EWJ* 3 (1859), 380–7; Cowper (n. 43); *EWJ* 7 (1861), 191–7.

47. Cowper (n. 43).

48. *TE*, 23 December 2006: 93–4; M. N., *EWJ* 7 (1861), 308–14.

49. M.N. (n. 48), 314; S.E.M., *EWJ* 7 (1861), 428; *TT*, 7 February 1862: 10; *BMJ*, 1863 (ii): 435.

50. *TL*, 1888 (i): 178; Sanger (n. 33), 166; J. K. Haywood, *Arsenic in Papers and Fabrics* (Washington: Government Printing Office, 1904), 16–20.

51. Henry Povall, *Arsenical Poisoning by Means of Wall Papers, Paints and Other Articles* (Mount Morris, NY: Countway Medical Library, Boston, n.d.), 3; Peterson and Haines (n. 29), 429; R. R. Cheyne, *BMJ*, 1874 (ii): 643–4; Wood (n. 16), 10–13; Carr (n. 20), 12; *BMJ*, 1875 (i): 817; *TT*, 12 September 1884: 6; *BMJ*, 1877 (ii): 507; Carr (n. 17), 42; *MTG*, 1870 (i): 617; Simon Garfield, *Mauve: How One Man Invented a Colour that Changed the World* (New York: Norton, 2000).

Chapter 8

1. *BMJ*, 1862 (i): 474–5; 1862 (i): 507; *TT*, 23 April 1862: 6; Thomas Orton, *TT*, 29 April 1862: 8; *TT*, 1 May 1862: 10.

2. *BMJ*, 1871 (ii): 101.

3. Stevenson Macadam, *PJT* 10 [3rd series] (1879–80), 611–12; Alfred Taylor, *On Poisons in Relation to Medical Jurisprudence and Medicine*, 2nd edn. (Philadelphia: Blanchard & Lea, 1859), 388.

4. Alan Sugden and John Edmondsen, *A History of English Wallpaper 1509–1914* (London: Batsford, 1926), 8–52; Charles Oman and Jean Hamilton, *Wallpapers: An International History and Illustrated Survey from the Victoria and Albert Museum* (New York: Abrams, 1982); Andrew Meharg, *Venomous Earth: How Arsenic Caused the World's Worst Mass Poisoning* (New York: Macmillan, 2005), 66–7; Peter Bartrip, *ENHR* 109 (1994), 897–8; Liza Picard, *Victorian London: The Life of a City 1840–1870* (London: Weidenfeld Nicolson, 2005), 136.

5. Meharg (n. 4), 67; Alfred Fletcher, *TT*, 9 January 1858: 11; Bartrip (n. 4), 896; Alfred Taylor, *PJT* 17 (1857–8), 555.

6. Charles Sanger, *PAAAS* 29 (1893–4), 113; William Hinds, *MTG*, 1857 (i): 177. There was a brief article in a medical journal as early as February 1849 that suggested that green wallpaper might poison, but it seems to have attracted no serious attention: *MTG* 19 (1848–9), 330.

7. William Hinds, *PJT* 18 (1858–9), 222–4; Hinds, *MTG*, 1857 (i): 520–2.

8. Hinds, *MTG*, 1857 (i): 521.

9. *PP*, 1857: XII. 676; Alexander Halley, *TT*, 11 January 1858: 10; 9 June 1859: 9.

10. Manufacturer quoted by Peter Bartrip, *The Home Office and the Dangerous Trades: Regulating Occupational Disease in Victorian and Edwardian Britain* (Amsterdam: Rodopi, 2002), 151; David Michaels, *Doubt is Their Product: How Industry's Assault on Science Threatens Your Health* (New York: Oxford University Press, 2008), p. x.

10. Arthur Hassall, *PJT* 1 [2nd series] (1859–60), 190–1.

11. Jabez Hogg, *SR* 10 (1879), 260; R. C. Kedzie, *Shadows From the Walls of Death* (Lansing, Mich.: George, 1874), 3; Alfred Taylor, *PJT* 18 (1858–9), 419; T. Lauder Brunton, *BMJ*, 1883 (i): 1218.

12. A. F. Abel, *PJT* 17 (1857–8), 556–7; William Hinds, *PJT* 18 (1858–9), 223. J. K. Haywood, *Arsenic in Papers and Fabrics* (Washington: Government Printing Office, 1904), 8–14 provides a detailed account of experiments testing for arsenic vapour in the air of papered rooms.

13. Henry Carr, *Our Domestic Poisons*, 2nd edn. (London: Clowes, 1884), 18.

14. Thomas Traill, *PJT* 11 (1851–2), 84; Joseph Stephens, *TL*, 1879 (i): 686.

15. Taylor (n. 12); J. B. Metcalfe, *TL*, 1860 (ii): 535–6; Henry Letheby, *TL*, 1860 (ii): 536.

16. Hogg (n. 12), 260; Taylor, (n. 3), 743; Frederic Miggy, *TL*, 1862 (ii): 22; George Morris, *TL*, 1862 (i): 499; Jabez Hogg, *BMJ*, 1879 (i): 891–2; Hogg, *MPC*, 1879 (ii): 61–2, 84–5.

17. Walter Fergus, *TL*, 1862 (i): 598–9; Alfred Taylor, *PJT* 17 (1857–8), 554; David Dalzell, *MTG*, 1871 (i): 674.

18. *CJPLSA* 18 (1862), 165–72.

19. Anonymous, *The Green of the Period; or, the Unsuspected Foe in the Englishman's Home* (London: Routledge, 1869); *BMJ*, 1871 (ii): 101–2.

20. Humphry Sandwith, *Minsterborough: A Tale of English Life*, 3 vols. (London: Chatto & Windus, 1876), iii. 103.

21. Ibid. iii. 167.

22. Ibid. i. 188; iii. 116, 137.

23. Ibid. iii. 161, 251–4.

24. *PJT* 4 [2nd series] (1862–3), 243–4; Horatio Donkin, *BMJ*, 1881 (i): 681; R. A. Witthaus, *Manual of Toxicology*, 2nd edn. (New York: Wood, 1911), 581; William Clarke, *BMJ*, 1873 (i): 701; Edward Wood, *Arsenic as a Domestic Poison* (Boston: Wright & Potter, 1885), 5; R. C. Kedzie, *Shadows From the Walls of Death* (Lansing, Mich.: George, 1874); Francis Brown, *Arsenical Paper-hangings* (1876 pamphlet, Countway Medical Library, Boston); Carr (n. 14), 6–7.

25. Jabez Hogg, *BMJ*, 1879 (i): 891–2.

26. Henry Carr, *Our Domestic Poisons* (London: Ridgway. 1879), 4, 42–50.

27. Hogg (n. 12), 262; H. C. Bartlett, *SR* 10 (1879), 267–8; *TL*, 1879
(i): 777; Malcolm Morris, *BMJ*, 1880 (i): 275; *TP* 24 (1880), 235–9;
T. Lauder Brunton, *BMJ*, 1883 (i): 1218; Bartrip (n. 4), 906–7; Edward
Willoughby, *Correspondence Respecting the Presence of Arsenic and Other
Poisonous Pigments in Wall-papers and Textile Fabrics* (London: Harrison,
1883); *PJT* 14 [3rd series] (1883–4), 647–8; Carr (n. 14), 5.

28. William Guy, *PP*, 1863: XXV. 156; Meharg (n. 4), 69, 80; *TL*, 1863 (i):
77.

29. Morris quoted by Meharg (n. 4), 82; Sugden (n. 4), 159; Fletcher
(n. 5); Charles Harrington, *BMSJ* 118 (1888), 215.

30. *PJT* 3 [3rd series] (1872–3), 473; H. C. Bartlett, *SR* 10 (1879), 267–8;
Bartrip (n. 10), 154; Carr (n. 14), 6; Meharg (n. 4), 80–1.

31. Carr (n. 14), 9; Witthaus (n. 25), 582; Harrington (n. 30), 216; *SR 9*
[NS] (1887–8), 383; *SR* 2 [NS] (1880–1), 31–2.

32. Harrington (n. 30), 215; *BMJ*, 1872 (ii): 49; Carr (n. 14), 9; Henry
M'Cormac, *TL*, 1862 (i): 691; Brown (n. 25), 4; W. Everett Smith,
BMSJ 117 (1887), 476–7.

33. *SR* 1 (1874), 51; John Glaister, *A Text-book of Medical Jurisprudence and
Toxicology* (Edinburgh: Livingstone, 1931), 708; J. T. Arlidge, *The
Hygiene, Diseases and Mortality of Occupations* (London: Percival, 1892),
434; *SC* 9 (1887), 219–20; *BMSJ* 124 (1891), 217–18.

34. George Hale, *SC* 19 (1892), 104–6; Sanger (n. 6); Meharg (n. 4), 71;
Donald Hunter, *The Diseases of Occupations* (Boston: Little, Brown,
1969), 349; John Emsley, *Elements of Murder* (Oxford: Oxford
University Press, 2005), 125; Charles Thom and Kenneth Raper,
SC 76 (1932), 548–50; A. F. Lerrigo, *TA* 57 (1932), 163–4; B. L. Valee
et al., *AIH* 21 (1960), 143; *BMJ*, 1871 (ii): 392–3; James Putnam, *BMSJ*
120 (1889), 253–6.

35. Bartrip (n. 4) gives a compelling analysis of the role played
by the press, consumer preference, and the operation of the
marketplace.

36. Ben Weider, *The Murder of Napoleon* (New York: Congdon & Lattes,
1982); Weider, *Assassination at St. Helena Revisited* (New York: Wiley,
1995); Emsley (n. 35), 126–32; Cathy Newman, *NG* 207 (May 2005),
10–11.

37. W. B. Kesteven, *AMJ*, 1856 (ii): 810; Meharg (n. 4), 117–20.

38. William Broad, *NYT*, 10 June 2008: F2.

Chapter 9

1. William Rothstein, *American Physicians in the Nineteenth Century: From Sects to Science* (Baltimore: The Johns Hopkins University Press, 1972), 49.

2. William Shakespeare, *Twenty-Three Plays and the Sonnets* (New York: Scribner, 1953), 181; Thomas Fowler, *Medical Reports of the Effects of Arsenic* (London: Johnson, 1786), 109.

3. John Haller, Jr., *PIH* 17 (1975), 87–8; Dioscorides, *The Greek Herbal of Dioscorides* (Oxford: Johnson, 1934), 642.

4. Joseph Clutton, *A True and Candid Relation of the Good and Bad Effects of Joshua Ward's Pill and Drop* (London: Clutton, 1736), pp. v–vi.

5. Fowler (n. 2), preface.

6. Ibid.

7. Ibid. 108.

8. Ibid. 42–5, 62–6, 78, 115.

9. Ibid. 2–3, 45, 128.

10. Robert Willan, *LMJ* 8 (1787), 191, 198; John Jenkinson, *EMSJ* 5 (1809), 309.

11. J. Turner, *TL*, 1861 (ii): 112; Haller (n. 3), 98.

12. William Murray, *TL*, 1893 (i): 407; Daniel Bampfylde, *TL*, 1854 (ii): 441; Adolphe Wahltuch, *BMJ*, 1877 (ii): 253; *BMJ*, 1862 (i): 76; *TL*, 1863 (i): 181; Sheldon Cohen, *AAP* 17 (1996), 164; Frederic Julius, *TL*, 1861 (ii): 138; Duncan McNab, *AMJ* 4 (1856), 730.

13. James Begbie, *EMSJ* 3 (1857–8), 972; George Gaskoin, *BMJ*, 1875 (i): 747; Murray (n. 12), 406.

14. Frank Foster (ed.), *Reference-book of Practical Therapeutics*, 2 vols. (New York: Appleton, 1897), i. 143; Kurt Wiener, *Systemic Associations and Treatment of Skin Diseases* (St Louis: Mosby, 1955), 429–30; D. M. Jolliffe, *JRSM* 86 (1993), 287–9; Thomas Hunt, *TL*, 1846 (i): 543; ibid. 78; 1878 (i): 866–7.

15. Fitz-James Molony, *BMJ*, 1887 (ii): 939; G. N. Hill, *EMSJ* 5 (1809), 19–27, 312–19; *TL*, 1897 (ii): 197–9; Samuel Watson, *AMJ* 4 (1856), 56; Foster (n. 14), i. 143, 146; *TL*, 1842–3 (ii): 579; Henry Hunt, *TL*,

1838 (ii): 93–4; J. H. Aveling, *BMJ*, 1871 (ii): 247; Owen Rees, *TL*, 1864 (ii): 436–7; *TL*, 1861 (i): 330; *MSR* 18 (1868), 261; *TP* 20 (1878), 213; 22 (1879), 43; Benjamin Travers, *AMJ* 1 (1853), 812–13; James Braid, *BMJ*, 1858 (i): 135; David Livingstone, *BMJ* 1858 (i): 360–1; *TL*, 1892 (ii): 1274.

16. Wiener (n. 14), 429–30; *TL*, 1829–30 (i): 744; F. T. Wintle, *TL*, 1846 (ii): 678–9; Andrew Meharg, *Venomous Earth: How Arsenic Caused the World's Worst Mass Poisoning* (New York: Macmillan, 2005), 98.

17. A. F. Haseldon, *PJT* 18 (1856–7), 541–3; Lloyd Bullock, *TL*, 1850 (ii): 674-5; T. P. Lowe, *TL*, 1887 (i): 100; *TL*, 1848 (i): 193; *AMJ* 2 (1854), 1059–60; *TL*, 1891 (ii): 33; W. J. Beatty, *BMJ*, 1883 (ii): 1015; Foster (n. 14), 146; Haller (n. 3), 88; Begbie (n. 13), 964.

18. William Clarke, *BMJ*, 1873 (i): 699; *TL* 1837–8 (i): 674.

19. Worthington Hooker, *Physician and Patient* (New York: Baker & Scribner, 1849), 37.

20. D. W. Cathell, *The Physician Himself*, 4th edn. (Baltimore: Cushings & Bailey, 1885), 123–4.

21. J. Wheatcroft, *AMJ* 4 (1856), 17; *TL*, 1889 (i): 441.

22. Oliver Wendell Holmes, *Medical Essays* (Boston: Houghton, Mifflin, 1899), 185; Hill (n. 15), 315; Thomas Hunt, *TPMSA* 16 (1849), 406.

23. Mathieu Orfila, *Directions for the Treatment of Persons Who Have Taken Poison* (London: Longman, Hurst, Rees, Orme & Brown, 1820), 33; Hooker (n. 19), 37; Holmes (n. 22), 183, 203.

24. Thomas Hunt, *TL*, 1847 (i): 91; Hunt (n. 22), 403, 409; Begbie (n. 13), 961–2.

25. Fowler (n. 2), 82–98.

26. William Murray, *TL*, 1893 (i): 406–7; Hunt (n. 24), 91.

27. Jonathan Hutchinson, *TP* 43 (1889), 458.

28. Thomas Hunt, *TL*, 1846 (i): 77; Jabez Hogg, *MPC*, 1879 (ii): 62; *MTG*, 1885 (ii): 60.

29. B. H. Nicholson, *TL*, 1893 (i): 297; Percy Barker, *BMJ*, 1900 (i): 961; *TL*, 1899 (ii): 353.

30. *TL*, 1898 (i): 208; *BMJ*, 1898 (i): 215.

31. John Astbury, *EMSJ* 15 (1819), 415; F. A. Macpherson, *BMJ*, 1883 (i): 546; Meharg (n.16), 98.

32. John Winslow, *Darwin's Victorian Malady: Evidence for its Medically Induced Origin* (Philadelphia: American Philosophical Society, 1971).

33. John Ayrton Paris, *Pharmacologia* (New York: Lockwood, 1822), 209; Jonathan Hutchinson, *BMJ*, 1887 (ii): 1280–1; Hutchinson, *PSLT* 39 (1888), 352–63; Stuart Arhelger and Arnold Kremen, *SU* 30 (1951), 977–86; Michael Bates et al., *AJE* 135 (1992), 462–76.

34. Thomas Benedek and Kenneth Kiple, in Kiple (ed.), *The Cambridge World History of Human Disease* (Cambridge: Cambridge University Press, 1993), 102–10.

35. Anthony Thomson, *TL*, 1838–9 (i): 178.

36. Richard Meade, *An Introduction to the History of Surgery* (Philadelphia: Saunders, 1968), 150–5; Owen Wangensteen and Sarah Wangensteen, *The Rise of Surgery* (Minneapolis: University of Minnesota Press, 1978), 23, 455; Fanny Burney, *The Journals and Letters of Fanny Burney (Madame d'Arblay)*, 12 vols. (Oxford: Clarendon, 1975), vi. 596–616.

37. *MAPC* 4 (1776), 54–61; Louis Goodman and Alfred Gilman. *The Pharmacological Basis of Therapeutics* (New York: Macmillan, 1941), 738; Foster (n. 14), i. 144; George Sigmond, *TL*, 1837–8 (i): 400–5.

38. R. A. Witthaus, *Manual of Toxicology*, 2nd edn. (New York: Wood, 1911), 484; Sigmond (n. 37), 404.

39. W. Marsden, *TL*, 1862 (i): 319; ibid. 220–1; Foster (n. 14), i. 144.

40. Nathaniel Potter, *An Essay on the Medicinal Properties and Deleterious Qualities of Arsenic* (Philadelphia: Woodward, 1796), 32; Sigmond (n. 37), 403.

41. Hill (n. 15), 313; William Guy and David Ferrier, *Principles of Forensic Medicine*, 4th edn. (London: Renshaw, 1875), 476; *LL*, 1867: 57; *BMJ*, 1866 (ii): 395; *TL*, 1890 (i): 1190.

42. Haller (n. 3), 88; Fowler (n. 2), preface; Donald Hood, *TL*, 1890 (i): 595–6; *BMJ*, 1864 (i): 276–7; *PJT* 5 [series 2] (1863–4), 520; ibid. 379; Daniel Dougal, *BMJ*, 1863 (ii): 357.

43. Alfred Taylor, *On Poisons in Relation to Medical Jurisprudence and Medicine*, 2nd edn. (Philadelphia: Blanchard & Lea, 1859), 383; Witthaus (n. 38), 414, 421, 427–31; William Guy, *PP*, 1863: XXV. 133; Thomas Brown, *AMJ* 1 (1853), 878; H. G. Trend, *BMJ*, 1858 (i): 725–6; *TL*, 1885 (ii): 127; Louis Siebold, *PJT* 20 [3rd series] (1889–90), 277–80; 24 [3rd series]

(1893–4), 588; J. B. Barnes, *PJT* 8 [3rd series] (1877–8), 327; *PJT* 8 [3rd series] (1877–8), 404–5.

44. J. D. White, *TL*, 1850 (ii): 514; F. A. Sass, *TL*, 1859 (i): 82–3.

45. W. E. Harding, *BMJ*, 1881 (ii): 1056; N. Stevenson, *BMJ*, 1880 (i): 362; *TL*, 1851 (i): 382; George Ward, *PJT* 10 [3rd series] (1879–80), 400; George Waite, *TL*, 1858 (ii): 462–3.

46. W. D. Buchanan, *Toxicity of Arsenic Compounds* (Amsterdam: Elsevier, 1962), 5; Wiener (n. 14), 430.

47. Sheldon Cohen, *AAP* 17 (1996), 164; John Harter and Mark Novitch, *JA* 40 (1967), 327–36; Harold Novey and Stuart Martel, *JA* 44 (1969), 315–19; Jolliffe (n. 14); Stanley Aronson, *RIM* 77 (1994), 234.

Chapter 10

1. John Morison, *A Complete Report of the Trial of Miss Madeleine Smith* (Edinburgh: Nimmo, 1857), p. v; G. Latham Browne and C. G. Stewart, *Reports of Trials for Murder by Poisoning* (London: Stevens & Sons, 1883), 294; Douglas MacGowan, *Murder in Victorian Scotland: The Trial of Madeleine Smith* (Westport, Conn.: Praeger, 1999), 128; Nigel Morland, *That Nice Miss Smith* (London: Muller, 1957).

2. Quotations from Madeleine Smith's letters are taken from MacGowan (n. 1), which reproduces all the letters she wrote to Émile. L'Angelier was an Anglicization of the family name l'Angelier.

3. *Trial of Miss Madeleine H. Smith Before the High Court of Justiciary, Edinburgh* (Edinburgh: Mathers, 1857), 3; MacGowan (n. 1), 97–145.

4. *TT*, 2 July 1857: 5; 9 July 1857: 7; *Trial* (n. 3), 22–3.

5. MacGowan (n. 1), p. i; Wilkie Collins, *The Law and the Lady* (New York: Harper, 1875).

6. Robert Christison, *EMJ* 3 (1857–8), 481–3.

7. *TT*, 11 December 1863: 10.

8. MacGowan (n. 1), 145, 149–55; *TT*, 10 July 1857: 12; Morison (n. 1), p. viii; Morland (n. 2), 184–5; Richard Altick, *Victorian Studies in Scarlet* (New York: Norton, 1970), 190.

9. MacGowan (n. 1), 91–2, 132.

10. J. J. von Tschudi, *WMW* 1 (1851), 453–5; Craig Maclagan, *EMJ* 10 (1864–5), 669–70; Charles Heisch, *PJT* 1 [series 2] (1859–60), 556–60.

11. von Tschudi (n. 10), 454; John Emsley, *Elements of Murder* (Oxford: Oxford University Press, 2005), 97.

12. von Tschudi (n. 10), 454; Craig Maclagan, *EMJ* 10 (1864–5), 201; *MTG*, 1876 (i): 121; D. M. Parker, *EMJ* 10 (1864–5), 123.

13. *PJT* 6 [3rd series] (1875–6), 326; Heisch (n. 10), 558–9; *MTG*, 1876 (i): 121; *TL*, 1860 (i): 580; *PJT* 2 [2nd series] (1860–1), 287.

14. von Tschudi (n. 10); *CEJ* 14 (1851), 391; T. Lauder Brunton, *Lectures on the Action of Medicines* (London: Macmillan, 1897), 620.

15. Robert Christison, *EMJ* 1 (1855–6), 709–10; Heisch (n. 10); *PJT* 2 [2nd series] (1860–1), 337–9; Maclagan (n. 12), 200–7; *MTG*, 1876 (i): 121; Erich Schwartze, *JPET* (1922), 181–203; Kenneth DuBois and E. M. K. Geiling, *Textbook of Toxicology* (New York: Oxford University Press, 1959), 134; *AMJ* 3 (1855), 429.

16. James Johnston, *The Chemistry of Common Life*, 2 vols., 8th edn. (New York: Appleton, 1856), ii. 171–2; A. Chevallier, *JCM* (1854), 439.

17. R. A. Witthaus, *Manual of Toxicology*, 2nd edn. (New York: Wood, 1911), 518; *Trial* (n. 3), 29, 45, 71; G. Cadogan-Masterman, *PMJL* 8 (1889), 534–5; *TL*, 1860 (ii): 592; *MSR* 20 (1869), 474; *MSR* 39 (1878), 193–4.

18. *MR* 5 (1899), 215.

19. Emsley (n. 11), 104; Dr Campbell's advertisement in author's collection; Ambrose Bierce, *The Devil's Dictionary* (Owings Mills, Md.: Stemmer House, 1978), 18; *PJT* 10 [3rd series] (1879–80), 477.

20. *TL*, 1897 (i): 52, 1356; 1896 (ii): 1700, 1774; *TT*, 6 August 1889: 9.

21. Charles Boner, *CJPLSA* 5 (1856), 91; Donald Hood, *TL*, 1890 (i): 595–6; *Trial* (n. 3), 18; Emsley (n. 11), 103; Bierce (n. 19), 18.

22. von Tschudi (n. 10); R. A. Witthaus and Tracy Becker, *Medical Jurisprudence, Forensic Medicine, and Toxicology*, 2nd edn. (New York: Wood, 1911), 514; Christison (n. 15); *TT*, 10 December 1855: 10; 12 December 1855: 8; Alfred Taylor, *On Poisons, in Relation to Medical Jurisprudence and Medicine*, 2nd edn. (Philadelphia: Blanchard & Lea, 1859), 96; M., *TT*, 27 December 1855: 4.

23. Emsley (n. 11), 103.

24. Details of the Maybrick case can be found in a number of sources: H. B. Irving (ed.), *Notable British Trials* (London: Hodge, 1912); Nigel

Morland, *This Friendless Lady* (London: Muller, 1957); Mary Hartman, *Victorian Murderesses* (New York: Schocken, 1977), 215–54; Richard Altick, *Victorian Studies in Scarlet* (New York: Norton, 1970), 252–8; The Earl of Birkenhead, *More Famous Trials* (New York: Doubleday, Doran, 1929), 119–30; and C. Ainsworth Mitchell, *Science and the Criminal* (Boston: Little, Brown, 1911), 206–13.

25. Altick (n. 24), 253.
26. Hartman (n. 24), 246–7; Morland (n. 24), 13, 70, 130–1.
27. Irving (n. 24), 343; William Whitford, *TL*, 1884 (i): 419–21; *TT*, 18 February 1884: 12; Morland (n. 24), 13. A recent argument for Mrs Maybrick's guilt has been made by Emsley (n. 11), 171–93.
28. *TT*, 8 August 1889: 7, 10; 9 August 1889: 3; 10 August 1889: 4, 5; Mitchell (n. 24), 212–13; Hartman (n. 24), 248.
29. *TT*, 13 February 1904: 11; Mitchell (n. 24), 213; Hartman (n. 24), 218, 253; Altick (n. 24), 258.
30. *LD* 124 (25 December 1937), 24–6; Douglas Frost, *FP* 26 (1967), 194.
31. *TL*, 1860 (ii): 592; *MTG*, 1873 (i): 274–5; *TT*, 8 March 1873: 11.
32. *TL*, 1840–1 (i): 479–82; 1844 (i): 638–9.
33. *TT*, 1 April 1847: 7; Alfred Taylor, *On Poisons, in Relation to Medical Jurisprudence and Medicine* (Philadelphia: Lea & Blanchard, 1848), 298.
34. J. Kratter, *WKW* 9 (1896), 1089–94; Taylor (n. 33), 297; Witthaus (n. 22), 567.
35. Witthaus (n. 22), 565; *TL*, 1840–1 (i): 258–62.
36. Victor Vaughan and James Dawson, *JAMA* 1 (1883), 115–16; *NR* 18 (1884), 562–8; Witthaus (n. 22), 574.
37. *TL*, 1838–9 (i): 246–8; 1838 (ii): 272.
38. John Snow, *TL*, 1838–9 (i): 264; Witthaus (n. 22), 566; Jean Gannal, *History of Embalming* (Philadelphia: Dobson, 1840), 210–25; *EMSJ* 64 (1845), 529–30; Edward Johnson et al., in Robert Mayer (ed.), *Embalming: History, Theory, and Practice* (New York: McGraw-Hill, 2000), 460.
39. Gannal (n. 38), 126; Robert Habenstein and William Lamers, *The History of American Funeral Directing*, 2nd edn. (Milwaukee: Radtke, 1962), 314–37.
40. Habenstein and Lamers (n. 39), 268–87; Johnson (n. 38), 464–70.

41. Habenstein and Lamers (n. 39), 321–8; Witthaus (n. 22), 565–7;
    Vaughan (n. 36), 116; Simon Mendelsohn, *Embalming Fluids* (New
    York: Chemical Publishing, 1940), 15.
42. Witthaus (n. 22), 130–1, 422, 567; Frederick Peterson and Walter
    Haines (eds.), *A Text-book of Legal Medicine and Toxicology* (Philadelphia:
    Saunders, 1904), 432–3.
43. Witthaus (n. 22), 570.

Chapter 11

1. Samuel Barton, *TL*, 1890 (ii): 119.
2. Robert Peck, in Sue Ann Prince (ed.), *Stuffing Birds, Pressing Plants,
   Shaping Knowledge: Natural History in North America, 1730–1860*
   (Philadelphia: American Philosophical Society, 2003), 11–25; Jean
   Gannal, *History of Embalming* (Philadelphia: Dobson, 1840), 168–9;
   NYT, 14 January 1885: 8.
3. George Rosen, *The History of Miners' Diseases* (New York: Schuman,
   1943), 8–38; Bernardino Ramazzini, *Diseases of Workers* (New York:
   Hafner, 1964), 16, 19.
4. Ramazzini (n. 3), 15; M. Harper, *BJIM* 45 (1988), 602–5; Agricola,
   De Re Metallica (New York: Dover, 1950), 215–16; James Scott, *Report
   of the Committee Appointed by the Westminster Medical Society, to Investigate
   the Subject of Adulterating Candles With Arsenic* (London: Painter, 1838),
   25; Rosen (n. 3), 61–2, 122–6.
5. Frank Booker, *The Industrial Archeology of the Tamar Valley* (Newton
   Abbot: David & Charles, 1971), 23–4, 143; S. Baring Gould, *JSCI*
   12 (1893), 692–3; Harper (n. 4), 603–5; Andrew Meharg, *Venomous
   Earth: How Arsenic Caused the World's Worst Mass Poisoning* (New York:
   Macmillan, 2005), 135–50.
6. J. T. Arlidge, *The Hygiene, Diseases and Mortality of Occupations*
   (London: Percival, 1892), 432–3; Thomas Oliver, *Diseases of
   Occupations* (New York: Dutton, 1909), 217–18; W. B. Kesteven,
   AMJ, 1856 (ii): 810–11; Gould (n. 5), 693.
7. *BMJ*, 1899 (i): 926; *MSR* 39 (1878): 385.
8. *TT*, 7 December 1874: 9.

9. *TT*, 8 February 1820: 3; *PJT* 9 (1849–50), 238; John Ayrton Paris, *Pharmacologia* (New York: Lockwood, 1822), 208; Kesteven (n. 6), 811; Alfred Taylor, *On Poisons in Relation to Medical Jurisprudence and Medicine*, 2nd edn. (Philadelphia: Blanchard & Lea, 1859), 382; N. T. Carrington quoted by Meharg (n. 5), 131.

10. Arlidge (n. 6), 435; William Guy, *PP*, 1863: XXV. 129–41; William Guy and David Ferrier, *Principles of Forensic Medicine*, 4th edn. (London: Renshaw, 1875), 478; William Guy, *AM* 1 (1860), 86–8; Taylor (n. 9), 388.

11. Guy, *PP*, 1863: XXV. 129–41; *TL*, 1845 (i): 139–40; Arthur Kerr, *BMJ*, 1875 (ii): 610; Golding Bird, *TL*, 1843–4: 98–101; W. Whalley, *MTG*, 1866 (ii): 222; Thomas Legge, in George Kober and William Hanson (eds.), *Diseases of Occupation and Vocational Hygiene* (Philadelphia: Blakiston, 1916), 4; Arlidge (n. 6), 437, 526.

12. Jabez Hogg, *SR* 10 (1879), 258; Hogg, *BMJ*, 1879 (i): 892; *BMJ*, 1862 (i): 474–5; Frank Draper, *CN* 26 (1872), 102–4.

13. W. D. Buchanan, *Toxicity of Arsenic Compounds* (Amsterdam: Elsevier, 1962), 38–40; Legge (n. 11), 9.

14. Donald Hunter, *The Diseases of Occupation*, 4th edn. (Boston: Little, Brown, 1969), 344–8; Buchanan (n. 13), 67–83; R. A. Witthaus, *Manual of Toxicology*, 2nd edn. (New York: Wood, 1911), 390; John Glaister, *Poisoning by Arseniuretted Hydrogen or Hydrogen Arsenide* (Edinburgh: Livingstone, 1908), 13, 100–204.

15. Arlidge (n. 6), 435–6.

16. P. W. J. Bartrip, *The Home Office and the Dangerous Trades: Regulating Occupational Disease in Victorian and Edwardian Britain* (Amsterdam: Rodopi, 2002), 2–11; *TL*, 1830–1 (ii): 450.

17. E. Symes Thompson, *MTG*, 1862 (i): 524.

18. *SR* 8 (1878), 223; *MTG*, 1858 (ii): 65.

19. Hunter (n. 14), 235–41; Bartrip (n. 16), 81–95; Christian Warren, *Brush with Death: A Social History of Lead Poisoning* (Baltimore: The Johns Hopkins University Press, 2000), 19–21.

20. Guy, *PP*, 1863: XXV. 138.

21. *Royal Commission on Employment of Children in Trades and Manufactures Not Regulated by Law. First Report* (London: Her Majesty's Stationery Office,

1863), 119–42; Bartrip (n. 16), 66–70, 148–54. Paper-staining was subsequently taken under the 1864 Factories Act Extension Act, but, as Bartrip has shown, government inspectors enforcing the law paid no attention to arsenic poisoning.

22. *Royal* (n. 21), 123, 127, 128, 130, 139.

23. Ibid. 123, 128, 142.

24. Ibid. 123–4, 133–4.

25. Ibid. 121–34, 140.

26. Quoted by Bartrip (n. 16), 155.

27. Thomas Oliver (ed.), *Dangerous Trades* (London: Murray, 1902); Bartrip (n. 16), 155–61; Kober (n. 11), 6.

28. John Pearse, *TL*, 1898 (ii): 107; *PJT* 11 (1851–2): 244–5; James Tunstall, *PJT* 11 (1851–2), 383.

29. Robert Crawford, *TL*, 1857 (ii): 127; *TL*, 1857 (ii): 181; *PJT* 11 (1851–2), 283–6; *PJT* 9 (1849–50), 302–3; Walter Watson, *TL*, 1857 (ii): 282.

30. Watson (n. 29); Crawford (n. 29); Taylor (n. 9), 384.

31. *PJT* 9 (1849–50), 302–3; Tunstall (n. 28); *PJT* 11 (1851–2), 283–6; ibid. 333–5; 18 (1858–9), 524–6.

32. *TL*, 1842 (i): 239.

33. *PJT* 9 (1849–50), 205–10; *TL*, 1842–3 (i): 838; 1842–3 (ii): 31–2; Alfred Taylor, *On Poisons, in Relation to Medical Jurisprudence and Medicine* (Philadelphia: Lea & Blanchard, 1848), 139; *Final Report of the Royal Commission Appointed to Inquire into Arsenical Poisoning from the Consumption of Beer and Other Articles of Food and Drink* (London: His Majesty's Stationery Office, 1903), 34; John Emsley, *Elements of Murder* (Oxford: Oxford University Press, 2005), 97.

34. Pearse (n. 28); *TL*, 1899 (ii): 1314.

35. Johann von Tschudi, *WMW* 1 (1851), 455; James Johnston, *The Chemistry of Common Life*, 2 vols., 8th edn. (New York: Appleton, 1856), ii. 169–70; Taylor (n. 9), 93; Charles Boner, *CJPLSA* 5 (1856), 91; W. B. Kesteven, *AMJ*, 1856 (ii): 810.

36. *TT*, 27 December 1855: 4; W. D. Husband, *AMJ* 3 (1855), 1020–1; *TT*, 31 July 1856: 11; Taylor (n. 9), 93; *PJT* 11 [3rd series] (1880–1), 681; *PJT* 20 [3rd series] (1889–90), 575; *PJT* 24 [3rd series] (1893–4), 640; Alexander Blyth and Meredith Blyth, *Poisons: Their Effects and Detection* (London: Griffin, 1920), 561; *MPC*, 1879 (ii):

488–9; J. Wheatcroft, *AMJ* 4 (1856), 17; *PJT* 11 (1851–2), 244–5; *TL*, 1899 (ii): 1314; Pearse (n. 28).

37. *TL*, 1901 (i): 988; *PJT* 14 [3rd series] (1883–4), 17; *PJT* 24 [3rd series] (1893–4), 578.

38. *TL*, 1901 (i): 988; 1849 (i): 71–2; Henry Fuller, *MTG* 19 (1848–9), 151; *PJT* 9 (1849–50): 207.

39. James Whorton, *Before Silent Spring: Pesticides and Public Health in Pre-DDT America* (Princeton: Princeton University Press, 1974); Booker (n. 5), 161.

40. Whorton (n. 39), 68–9; *BMJ*, 1892 (i): 741.

41. Whorton (n. 39), 133–7, 201–2, 248–9;

42. *First Report of the Royal Commission Appointed to Inquire into Arsenical Poisoning From the Consumption of Beer and Other Articles of Food and Drink* (London: Her Majesty's Stationery Office, 1901), 90; *TL*, 1909 (i): 286.

43. Edmund Davy, *PJT* 1 [2nd series] (1859–60), 187–90.

44. *PJT* 1 [2nd series] (1859–60), 287–8; Alfred Sibson, *PJT* 1 [2nd series] (1859–60), 286; E. S. Kensington, *PJT* 1 [2nd series] (1859–60), 287; *JSCI* 20 (1901), 190; Henry Scholefield, *PJT* 1 [2nd series] (1859–60), 464–5; *TL*, 1901 (i): 495.

45. *TL*, 1848 (i): 193; *TT*, 2 October 1860: 10; John Davy, *BMJ*, 1862 (ii): 425; *TL*, 1863 (ii): 53.

46. George Lefevre, *TL*, 1844 (i): 443.

47. Lefevre (n. 46), 442; Witthaus (n. 14), 422; *TL*, 1838 (ii): 625.

48. L. Geyer, *ADS* 43 (1898), 221–80; Martin Black, *PJ* 199 (1967), 593–7; R. A. Witthaus and Tracy Becker, *Medical Jurisprudence, Forensic Medicine and Toxicology*, 2nd edn. (New York: Wood, 1911), 421; *TT*, 6 January 1875: 3; 13 January 1875: 11.

Chapter 12

1. John Brown, *BMJ*, 1900 (ii): 1684; Brown, *TL*, 1900 (ii): 1728–9.

2. Peter Bartrip, *ENHR* 109 (1994), 893; T. N. Kelynack and William Kirkby, *Arsenical Poisoning in Beer Drinkers* (London: Ballière, Tindall & Cox, 1901), 1; Matthew Copping, ' "Honour Among Professionals": Medicine, Chemistry and Arsenic at the Fin de Siècle', doctoral

dissertation, University of Kent at Canterbury, 2003: 39–47; Ernest Reynolds, *BMJ*, 1900 (ii): 1492–3; T. N. Kelynack et al., *TL*, 1900 (ii): 1600–3; *MG*, 24 November 1900: 9; Henry Satterlee, *NEJM* 263 (1960), 676–84.

3. Ernest Reynolds, *TL*, 1901 (i): 166–70; *TT*, 28 December 1900, 4.

4. Reynolds (n. 3).

5. John Brown, *BMJ*, 1900 (ii): 1684; Kelynack and Kirkby (n. 2), 5.

6. Kelynack et al. (n. 2); *TL*, 1902 (i): 1221; *First Report of the Royal Commission Appointed to Inquire Into Arsenical Poisoning From the Consumption of Beer and Other Articles of Food and Drink* (London: Her Majesty's Stationery Office, 1901), 3; *TL*, 1901 (i): 644; Ernest Reynolds, *TL*, 1901 (ii): 385; James Niven, *BMJ*, 1900 (ii): 1724.

7. Reynolds (n. 3), 169–70; H. G. Brooke and Leslie Roberts, *BJD* 13 (1901), 121–48.

8. Niven (n. 6), 1725.

9. Kelynack and Kirkby (n. 2), 2, 9, 13; Reynolds (n. 3), 168–9; Robert Buchanan, *TL*, 1901 (i): 171; Kelynack et al. (n. 2), 1600; Nathan Raw et al., *BMJ*, 1901 (i): 11; R. D. Cran, *BMJ*, 1900 (ii): 1683; *TL*, 1901 (i): 980–1.

10. Buchanan (n. 9), 171; *TL*, 1901 (i): 171; Brooke (n. 7), 133; Kelynack et al. (n. 2), 1600; Leslie Roberts, *BMJ*, 1901 (ii): 863; Reynolds (n. 3), 168.

11. Niven (n. 6), 1724; Kelynack and Kirkby (n. 2), 2; Brooke (n. 7), 125; T. Lauder Brunton, *TL*, 1901 (i): 1259; Kelynack et al. (n. 2), 1600; *TL*, 1901 (i): 31.

12. Reynolds (n. 3), 168; *TL*, 1901 (i): 644; Reynolds (n. 2); F. W. Pavy, *BMJ*, 1901 (i): 396–8.

13. Reynolds (n. 3), 167, 169; Kelynack and Kirkby (n. 2), 9; Buchanan (n. 9), 171; Kelynack et al. (n. 2), 1600; *Final Report of the Royal Commission Appointed to Inquire into Arsenical Poisoning from the Consumption of Beer and Other Articles of Food and Drink* (London: His Majesty's Stationery Office, 1903), 6.

14. Cran (n. 9); Reynolds (n. 3), 169.

15. *Final* (n. 13), 4–5, 12; *BMJ*, 1901 (i): 415–16; *TL*, 1901 (i): 672–3, 904–5; 1901 (i): 1311.

16. *MG*, 23 November 1900: 10; *TT*, 28 November 1900: 9; *CTJ* 28 (1900), 421; *MG*, 26 November 1900: 10; 28 November 1900: 7; *TT*, 6 December 1900: 11; *PU* 120 (1901), 147; *MG*, 1 December 1900: 12.

17. Kelynack et al. (n. 2), 1602–3; Jim Phillips and Michael French, *RH* 9 (1998), 200.

18. *TT*, 26 March 1880: 9; R. H. Norman, *BMJ* 1900 (ii): 200–1; *TL*, 1900 (ii): 208.

19. *MG*, 27 November 1900: 12; Phillips (n. 17), 200.

20. *MG*, 26 November 1900: 10; *TL*, 1901 (i): 31–3; 1900 (ii): 1682; 1901 (i): 828-30; Michael French and Jim Phillips, *Cheated not Poisoned? Food Regulation in the United Kingdom, 1875–1938* (Manchester: Manchester University Press, 2000), 75.

21. *TT*, 28 December 1900: 4; 9 January 1901: 9; 16 January 1901: 5; 2 February 1901: 8; *TL*, 1901 (i): 644; *TT*, 21 January 1901: 8; 18 February 1901: 10.

22. *TT*, 17 January 1901: 8; 11 March 1901: 13.

23. *Final* (n. 13), 3–4, 22; *TT*, 11 March 1901: 13; 11 January 1901: 5; 22 January 1901: 7; 28 November 1900: 7.

24. *TT*, 8 February 1901: 11; 5 March 1901: 11; 21 March 1901: 7.

25. Reynolds (n. 3), 170; *PH* 13 (1900–1), 530; Raw (n. 9), 10; George Pernet, *BMJ*, 1901 (i): 560; John Glaister, *A Text-book of Medical Jurisprudence and Toxicology* (Edinburgh: Livingstone, 1931), 711; R. A. Witthaus and Tracy Becker, *Medical Jurisprudence, Forensic Medicine and Toxicology*, 2nd edn. (New York: Wood, 1911), 423.

26. Alexander Blyth, *A Manual of Practical Chemistry* (London: Griffin, 1879), 169; E. S. Reynolds, *BMJ*, 1901 (ii): 384–6; J. F. Hodgson, *TL*, 1902 (i): 399; E. Farquhar Buzzard, *TL*, 1901 (i): 1593–5; *Final* (n. 13), 7–11. The beriberi hypothesis is discussed by Copping (n. 2), 108–34.

27. John Brickwood, *TT*, 11 January 1901: 4; *Report of the Departmental Committee on Beer Materials* (London: Eyre & Spottiswoode, 1899), 3–4; *TT*, 28 November 1900: 9; 25 December 1900: 7; H. Stopes, *TT*, 8 January 1901: 11; *TT*, 14 February 1899: 10.

28. *TT*, 26 March 1896: 6; Sean Shesgreen, *Engravings by Hogarth* (New York: Dover, 1973), plate 75.

29. *TT*, 26 March 1896: 6, 9; 8 February 1896: 9.

30. Phillips (n. 17); *TT*, 21 January 1901: 8.

31. Graham Aldous, *TT*, 12 February 1901: 8; Cuthbert Quilter, *TL*, 1900 (ii): 1836; *TT*, 21 January 1901: 8; *Report* (n. 27), 5.

32. A. E. Berry, *TT*, 20 December 1900: 4; *TL*, 1900 (ii): 1764; Quilter (n. 31).

33. Copping (n. 2), 4–5.

34. *TT*, 12 January 1901: 6; 16 January 1901: 5; 17 January 1901: 8; *TL*, 1901 (i): 567; French (n. 20), 73.

35. *TL*, 1901 (i): 956; Brunton (n. 11), 1259–60; Cuthbert Quilter, *TT*, 15 June 1901: 12.

36. Charles Estcourt, *TT*, 19 December 1900: 12; Estcourt, *TT*, 24 December 1900: 10; L. Archbutt and P. G. Jackson, *JSCI* 20 (1901), 448–50.

37. *TT*, 7 February 1901: 12; John Brickwood, *TT*, 20 August 1901: 9; *TT*, 28 March 1901: 7; W. Harcourt, *TT*, 15 June 1901: 12; James Neech, *PH* 15 (1902–3), 138–42; *TL*, 1902 (i): 385, 466; Phillips (n. 17), 204–5; *Final* (n. 13), 9–10.

38. *Final* (n. 13), 26–30; *TT*, 30 August 1901: 8; *JSCI* 20 (1901), 208–9; S. H. Collins, *JSCI* 21 (1902), 221–2; William Thomson, *TL*, 1900 (ii): 1919–20; *JSCI* 20 (1901), 198.

39. *TT*, 28 November 1900: 7; John Brown, *TL*, 1900 (ii): 1837–8; James Keith, *TT*, 20 December 1900: 4.

40. *TT*, 11 January 1901: 5; *Final* (n. 13), 43–50; *JSCI* 20 (1901), 192; *TT*, 18 January 1901: 5.

41. Edward Willoughby, *Correspondence Respecting the Presence of Arsenic and Other Poisonous Pigments in Wall-papers and Textile Fabrics* (London: Harrison, 1883), 30; John Pearse, *TL*, 1898 (ii): 107; Henry Carr, *Our Domestic Poisons*, 2nd edn. (London: Clowes, 1884), 9–10; *TL*, 1899 (ii): 1314; Thomas Legge, in George Kober and William Hanson (eds.), *Diseases of Occupation and Vocational Hygiene* (Philadelphia: Blakiston, 1916), 4.

42. *TT*, 9 January 1901: 9; *Final* (n. 13), 50; H. Martin, *RR* 4 (1963), 26; James Whorton, *Before Silent Spring: Pesticides and Public Health in Pre-DDT America* (Princeton: Princeton University Press, 1974), 161–2; Andrew Meharg, *Venomous Earth: How Arsenic Caused the World's Worst Mass Poisoning* (New York: Macmillan, 2005), 11; French (n. 20), 78–80.

43. *JSCI* 20 (1901), 188.
44. Anna Carline, *SLS* 14 (2005), 215–38; *TNT*, 31 January 2007: A 4;18 April 2008: A3; David Caudhill, *CH* 27 (Spring, 2009), 20–5.
45. Dorothy Sayers, *Strong Poison* (New York: Garland, 1976), 336.
46. G. M. Fyfe and B. W. Anderson, *TL*, 1943 (ii): 614–15; David Wright, *MH* 27 (1983), 184–5; John Emsley, *Elements of Murder* (Oxford: Oxford University Press, 2005), 101–2; Kenzaburo Tsuchiya, *EHP* 19 (1977), 35–8; *TT*, 29 August 1955: 5; 30 August 1955: 6.
47. Patricia Miller, *CD* 7 (1991), 63–70; *TT*, 20 January 1932: 7; *TM* 68 (3 July 1956), 29; *NYT*, 17 July 1956: 25; Martin Gordon, *TL* 356 (2000), 170.
48. Virginia Sole-Smith, *GH* 244 (March 2007), 101–6; Paul Blanc, *How Everyday Products Make People Sick* (Berkeley: University of California Press, 2007), 240; Marianne Lavelle, *USNWR* 133 (16 September 2002), 58–9; Henry Peters et al., *JAMA* 251 (1984), 2393–6.
49. Meharg (n. 42), 1–7; Allan Smith et al., *BWHO* 78 (2000), 1093–103.
50. Meharg (n. 42), 17, 160, 170–81; Smith (n. 49), 1093.
51. Donald MacMillan, *Smoke Wars: Anaconda Copper, Montana Air Pollution, and the Courts, 1890–1924* (Helena, Mont.: Montana Historical Society Press, 2000), 32, 85–7.
52. Peter Dorman, *RRPE* 16 (1984), 151 64; *SPI*, 8 December 2004: A1.
53. Susan Gordon, *TNT*, 7 August 2004: B1; *TNT*, 2 August 2006: A1; Brian Everstine, *TNT*, 6 August 2008: B1; *TNT*, 21 June 2005: A1; Les Blumenthal, *TNT*, 24 August 2008: A1.

INDEX